1993

AIDS:
A Complete Guide to Psychosocial Intervention

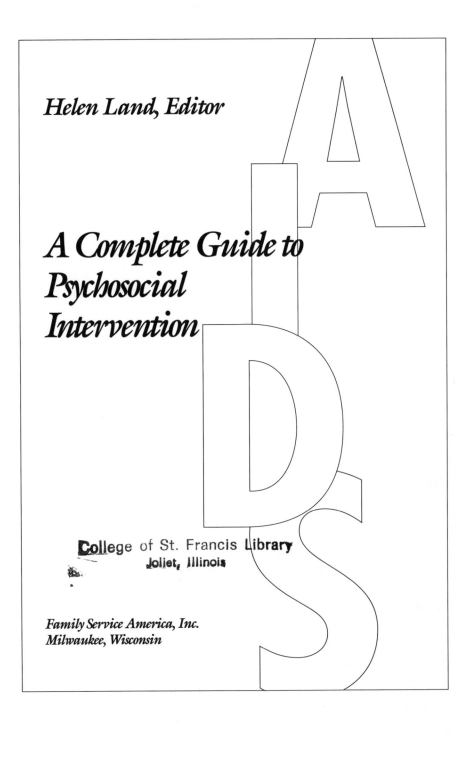

Helen Land, Editor

A Complete Guide to Psychosocial Intervention

Family Service America, Inc.
Milwaukee, Wisconsin

Library of Congress Cataloging-in-Publication Data

AIDS: a complete guide to psychosocial intervention / edited by Helen Land.
   p. cm.
  Includes bibliographical references.
  ISBN 0-87304-258-1
  1. AIDS (Disease)—Psychological aspects. 2. AIDS (Disease)—
Social aspects. 3. AIDS (Disease)—Patients—Services for.
I. Land, Helen Marianne.
RC607. A26A34522   1992
362.1'969792—dc20   92-18565

To Millie, who taught me the meaning of compassion,
and to those persons affected by AIDS with whom I have worked
and whose lives exemplify compassion.

ACKNOWLEDGMENTS

Many have been instrumental in the evolution and preparation of this book. I would like to thank George Harangody for first educating me about the AIDS crisis and its impact. I wish to express my deepest gratitude to friends, clients, students, and colleagues who have struggled with HIV; their lives have been exemplars of strength and courage. I thank AIDS Project Los Angeles for its service to the community and for allowing me to volunteer and learn. I thank all the contributors to this book, who helped me to expand my own knowledge of the field. My great appreciation is offered to the staff at Family Service America, Inc., especially Robert Nordstrom, whose conscientious efforts guided this book to completion, and to the Ittleson Foundation for its generous gift in aiding distribution of this book. Last, I wish to thank my friends and family for their support, particularly Robert Land and William Form for their insightful comments and consistent encouragement.

CONTENTS

Part 3
Special Topics in Clinical Work

FOREWORD

The second decade of the AIDS epidemic is under way. Individuals living with AIDS, their caregivers, and professionals in the field are caught in a vortex of life experiences and realities and their corresponding emotions. Early intervention with antiviral medications and new developments in treating opportunistic infections have allowed some individuals with access to sophisticated medical care to live longer with improved quality of life after diagnosis. The number of long-term survivors with AIDS is growing, taxing the scant resources available. Most long-term survivors are white, middle-class, gay men. Poor persons with AIDS—including most women with AIDS as well as most nonwhite people with AIDS—are still dying much more quickly than are middle-class people with the same condition.

Thus, the various populations affected by HIV/AIDS have reasons to feel cautiously hopeful but many more reasons to feel desperate, enraged, and overwhelmed. With more than one million Americans already infected, more becoming infected daily, and more than 100,000 Americans already dead, AIDS remains a political football rather than a public health crisis that warrants our complete and undivided attention and resources.

Most people living with AIDS or working in the field of AIDS are frustrated and angry. In this second decade of the crisis, no definitive leadership in the federal government has arisen to lead the charge against this epidemic. We have no centralized commitment to research on AIDS in the United States. Medical science is not any closer to a cure now than it was at the beginning of the crisis. Effective prevention efforts are still hampered by the influence of right-wing politicians who, it seems, would prefer to see more people become infected and die than teach adolescents how to become sexually responsible for protecting themselves and their sexual partners. Before we can initiate effective AIDS-prevention efforts at the national level, America must confront its schizophrenic attitudes toward sex, sexuality, and drug use. Such change is unlikely to occur under the current leadership.

On a daily basis, American teenagers watch television programs filled with sex and violence. Yet sex education throughout most of the country merely consists of lectures on reproduction and "plumbing" and advice to "wait until marriage," ignoring adolescents' need for adults who will talk honestly about passion, desire, sex, and love as well as restraint. Research shows that America's teenagers are engaging in sexual intercourse in growing numbers without protecting themselves against pregnancy or sexually transmitted diseases. Our message to youngsters is don't have sex until marriage, don't take drugs under any circumstances, and if you do, pay the price and die.

As a society, we have been unsuccessful in our attempts to stem the epidemic of drug addiction that is especially virulent in our inner cities. Yet, instead of funding drug-treatment centers and endorsing needle-exchange programs in an effort to stem the spread of AIDS, we suggest to individuals who inject illicit drugs that they are expendable, even deserving of death.

The lack of discussion about safer sex and safer drug-use techniques to stop AIDS parallels the failure of society and its institutions to discuss the relationships among racism, poverty, homelessness, unemployment, and drug addiction. As people with AIDS are blamed for having gotten themselves infected, the victims of urban neglect are blamed for their lack of investment in a society that has forsaken them. Although I do not condone urban violence, I understand the frustration, powerlessness, and hopelessness that have ignited rage and violence in our cities. By the same token, I continue to be amazed that organizations like the AIDS Coalition to Unleash Power (ACT UP) and People with AIDS have remained restrained in their protests about government inaction and indifference to this health crisis.

HIV/AIDS affects families. A growing number of grandmothers in our inner cities are now caring for two generations of their offspring who are ill and dying of AIDS. Entire friendship groups of urban gay men are infected with HIV, are concurrently sick, or have died.

The above merely touches upon the crises the nation, in general, and our service delivery systems, in particular, are facing. What do we do? First, we must become informed. The volume you are about to read is a masterpiece and a prime example of how members of the social work profession are on the front lines of service to the ever-growing number of individuals whose lives are affected by AIDS. This powerfully honest book bluntly presents the realities of the HIV/AIDS epidemic. It accurately and thoroughly describes the struggles and limits as well as successes encountered in working in the field of AIDS. It is essential reading for students and reflective professionals who wish, indeed need, to know and understand the pertinent issues affecting HIV/AIDS clients, caregivers, families, and professionals.

The authors of these chapters are pioneers in working with people with AIDS. They discuss how they talk with their clients, clients' families, and their colleagues about death and dying, sex and life, drug use and abstinence. They grapple with some of the most difficult client populations and issues of our time: homelessness, drug injection, prejudice, cultural differences, homophobia, and their own limitations as professionals and human beings. Their honesty is remarkable and, perhaps more important, extremely relevant to every professional who works in the field of AIDS as well as those who work with disadvantaged and oppressed members of our society.

This volume could very well become the seminal social work text for working with people affected by AIDS that takes the profession into the next century. The authors are skilled experts who embody all the best traditions of the social work profession. In reading and reflecting upon the chapters, each of us is challenged to examine his or her own work and professionalism to insure that it measures up to the highest standards of practice as described in this volume. If you are currently working in the field of AIDS, you will find much that validates as well as challenges you in this book. If you plan to enter the field, this book will inspire your efforts.

Michael Shernoff
New York, New York

CONTRIBUTORS

Marvin Belzer
Assistant Professor
Division of Adolescent Medicine
Department of Pediatrics
Childrens Hospital Los Angeles
Los Angeles, California

Rick Bidgood
Principal Consultant
JKRAssociates
San Francisco, California

Wendy Blank
Program Manager, Social Services
Los Angeles Gay and Lesbian
Community Services
HIV Healthcare Center
West Hollywood, California

Anthony T. DiVittis
Senior Health Care Program
Planner Analyst
Ambulatory Care/AIDS Program
Services
Woodhull Medical and Mental
Health Center
Brooklyn, New York

Wilbur A. Finch, Jr.
Associate Professor
School of Social Work
University of Southern California
Los Angeles, California

George Harangody
Social Worker
Home Health
AIDS Project Los Angeles
Los Angeles, California

Valerie Harragin
Social Worker
AIDS Programs
Department of Health Services—
Los Angeles County
Los Angeles, California

Paul D. Holtom
Assistant Professor
Chief of Infectious Diseases
University Hospital
University of Southern California
Los Angeles, California

Sally Jue
Mental Health Program Manager
AIDS Project Los Angeles
Los Angeles, California

Michele Cuvilly Klopner
Director, Haitian Mental Health Clinic
and the Cambridge Hospital
Cambridge, Massachusetts
Clinical Instructor in Psychiatry
Harvard Medical School
Boston, Massachusetts

Lee E. Klosinski
Hotline Coordinator
Department of Education and Training
AIDS Project Los Angeles
Los Angeles, California

Helen Land
Associate Professor
School of Social Work
University of Southern California
Los Angeles, California

Sandra Lew-Napoleone
Hospice Program Director
Kaiser Permanente Medical Center
Oakland, California

George Lewert
Social Work Supervisor
Department of Social Work Services
Presbyterian Hospital in the
City of New York
Columbia Presbyterian Medical Center
New York, New York

Gary A. Lloyd
Professor and Coordinator
Institute for Research and
Training in HIV/AIDS Counseling
School of Social Work
Tulane University
New Orleans, Louisiana

Richard G. MacKenzie
Director, Division of Adolescent
Medicine
Department of Pediatrics
Childrens Hospital Los Angeles
Los Angeles, California

Judy Macks
Partner, JKRAssociates
Organization Development Consultant
San Francisco, California

Joanne E. Mantell
Women and AIDS Resource Network
Brooklyn, New York

Luisa Medrano
Clinical Associate in Psychology
Department of Psychiatry
Massachusetts General Hospital
Harvard Medical School
Boston, Massachusetts

Julia N. Pennbridge
Coordinator of Clinical Research
Division of Adolescent Medicine
Department of Pediatrics
Childrens Hospital Los Angeles
Los Angeles, California

Robert Peterson
Registered Nurse
Home Health
AIDS Project Los Angeles
Los Angeles, California

Dina Rosen
Director of Client Services
All Saints AIDS Service Center
Pasadena, California

Arlene Schneir
Risk Reduction Program Coordinator
Division of Adolescent Medicine
Department of Pediatrics
Childrens Hospital Los Angeles
Los Angeles, California

Mark S. Senak
Deputy Director
AIDS Project Los Angeles
Los Angeles, California

Jack B. Stein
Director
Center for HIV/Substance
Abuse Training
Hi-Tech International, Inc.
Washington, D.C.

Catherine Sternberg
Medical Social Worker
Patient Family Counseling
St. Joseph Hospital
Denver, Colorado

Introduction

Meeting the AIDS Challenge: An Overview

Helen Land

As the AIDS epidemic enters its second decade, the challenges faced by service providers are formidable. The disease, once appearing only in a relatively small population of gay men, now has the potential to touch nearly every household in America. No American denies the threatening specter of AIDS. For many, however, it has become more than a calamity heard or read about in the media; for them, it is an intrusive and unwanted guest demanding change in every aspect of life.

AIDS terrifies most people. Some people compartmentalize the threat of AIDS by labeling persons with AIDS as being inherently different from themselves. Such stigmatization creates a psychological boundary that helps one feel protected from the disease. Others attempt to distance themselves from AIDS by "blaming the victim," asserting that persons who engage in high-risk behaviors are at fault for contracting the disease.

Although such stances are predictable, they are not justifiable. These postures are easily transformed into ideologies that validate abandonment or neglect of those who are most in need of care. Sadly, our history is replete with instances of isolating, ignoring, or underserving persons who need care because they are considered "different," are disenfranchised, or are otherwise divested of power (Janson, 1988). Persons with cancer have suffered in the back wards of hospitals; tuberculosis patients have been isolated from the public eye in sanatoriums. Similar disenfranchisement has been visited on the chronically mentally ill, as is witnessed by their incarceration without due process and then expulsion from institutions, which has forced many to live on the streets of our urban communities. Hence, our treatment of persons with AIDS is but one example of the callous way in which we treat vulnerable people in the United States.

In the face of widespread abandonment of the vulnerable, a commitment to and compassion for persons with AIDS represents a commitment to life. AIDS has stolen life from children and adolescents; women; gay, bisexual, and heterosexual

1

men; injection drug users; and people of color. At every point on the service continuum, these various groups need services and care. For HIV-infected persons, services need to be focused on early problem solving, including educating those who are HIV positive about how to stay healthy and asymptomatic. Treatment of those who have developed AIDS symptoms must center on containing the illness and on enhancing quality of life.

The battle against AIDS must be fought among other populations as well, extending beyond those who are HIV infected. Increasing efforts need to be directed at helping those who are seronegative to remain uninfected as well as to help them cope with the psychological distress of survivor guilt. Services must be provided to professionals and informal caregivers to help them meet their formidable challenges. Attention must also be focused on the healing and renewing of bereaved persons.

AIDS does not fit standard crisis models. It does not have a dramatic onset or a predictable course to its conclusion. Instead, its course is varied and diverse, both in terms of the populations affected and individuals' responses. AIDS is a crisis in which individuals anticipate the disease state; cope with the innumerable vicissitudes of the disease; undergo the physical, social, economic, psychological, and spiritual changes that the disease brings; and live with the devastating consequences of its aftermath. Providing services to counter the effects of such an atypical and prolonged crisis is a substantial challenge. Because AIDS diversely affects so many different populations, professionals in various settings need information and skills in order to provide adequate care.

To this end, this book presents and discusses the issues, goals, and nature of service provision across a continuum of care. Chapters include material on AIDS education and primary prevention as well as on programs and settings for HIV service provision, including outpatient and agency-based service models, inpatient hospital models, home health care, hospice service, and alternative service and grass-roots service settings. Case examples are used throughout the book to illustrate the didactic material.

For each of these service settings, issues that affect the ways in which services are delivered are examined. The discussions include descriptions of the populations served and analysis of the scope of the problem relative to those populations. Authors analyze the manner in which AIDS-related issues have changed over the years and discuss assessment, planning, and implementation of service models designed to meet the needs of diverse populations. The authors also discuss sociopolitical issues as well as how service settings' goals and locations affect delivery and quality of services.

The main tasks and roles of service providers within each setting are described, and information is provided on how the service role has evolved over the years and is defined at present. Direct service, administration, and supervision are analyzed. Both direct and indirect service models are presented, and the limitations of particular models, given the service setting and community, are discussed in detail. Authors outline specific treatment methods, including the issues involved in choice of method with respect to service goals and the needs of culturally diverse clients and the implementation and evaluation of these methods. Future service needs and changes in program design are suggested.

INTERVENTION ACROSS SERVICE SETTINGS

In this section, Klosinski addresses the topic of AIDS education and primary prevention, arguing that despite our considerable efforts to educate citizens about AIDS, HIV transmission has not been stemmed. This dilemma may exist because of the multiple factors operating at the personal and environmental levels that affect the behavior of individuals who engage in high-risk activities. Service providers need to be aware of these factors if they are to provide adequate HIV/AIDS education.

Earlier in the AIDS epidemic, the extent of HIV infection among the populace was not known. People avoided HIV testing because of fear of stigma as well as of possible loss of employment, insurance, or other resources. Medical intervention that delayed the course of HIV infection was not available; thus, for many people, the potential stress caused by knowledge of HIV-positive status outweighed the benefits of knowing their status (Buckingham, 1987; Reamer, 1988). Many people underwent testing only when life-extending drugs such as AZT and other prophylactics became available. With testing, the high rates of HIV infection were made public and the complex need for quality AIDS education became known. Klosinski discusses the means by which AIDS education is disseminated to diverse groups at risk of infection, showing how AIDS education is at the confluence of tensions existing among the needs of highly marginal groups, the interests of the medical profession, and American society's historical struggle to protect the rights of the individual in light of the common good.

The outpatient clinic or community agency is often the first line of service to clients concerned about HIV. In the chapter on outpatient service models, Jue traces the evolution of various HIV service agencies. Although program development often begins at the grass-roots level, programs and services may eventually find their home in a complex multiservice center. Because the demand for outpatient community services is steadily increasing and resources are often few, Jue proposes methods for setting priorities in program model development, providing diverse services, and meeting staff needs. She suggests that services must be tailored to meet the specific political, economic, cultural, and sociodemographic characteristics of the community.

Because community needs are diverse, program designs must be analyzed with regard to whether they truly meet those needs. To this end, Jue discusses empowerment and psychoeducational models as well as the use of long-term vs. short-term care. Because staffing needs may vary according to program priorities, Jue offers guidelines for using professional staff and volunteers. In addition, she provides problem-solving strategies for direct and indirect service and interagency collaboration.

HIV treatment in inpatient settings such as hospitals and residential hospices poses problems that require particular approaches to service design. Because a hospital stay often represents a medical crisis, hospital social service providers find themselves at the vortex of client care when providing information to the patient, family physician, nursing staff, and hospital system. Their multifaceted role requires flexibility in providing short-term counseling for patients and families, advocating for patient placements, and negotiating an often complex set of competing demands arising from physician directives, patient compliance, and family caregiving capabilities (Roberts, 1989). Sternberg discusses methods for managing patient–family stressors and for containing the complex conflicts that often occur in hospital systems. She discusses issues related to culturally defined health behavior among AIDS patients and their families in hospital settings, stressing the importance of patient advocacy in an environment where competing priorities of family, community, and the hospital system often adversely affect patient care.

Clients who are released from hospital settings often require home health care. Although the client's needs may be obvious, the considerable stress experienced by both the client and the family as a result of service providers' intrusion in the home setting is less obvious (Chinin, 1989). Service providers must define their roles clearly. As Harangody and Peterson discuss this issue, service providers achieve greater success when they target psychological problems that coexist with and result from the client's confrontation with AIDS. Harangody and Peterson describe common presenting problems of clients and offer guidelines for assessing client home health needs. Using short-term dynamic treatment and cognitive–behavioral approaches, they present practical steps for providing clinical treatment throughout the various phases of the disease process. Issues of countertransference and team management are discussed.

Both the hospice movement and its application to HIV-infected individuals are relatively new to this country. Hospice services are provided by a multidisciplinary team that emphasizes palliative and supportive care as opposed to aggressive treatment. The course of HIV, however, is often unpredictable, and services designed to help clients die well are uncertain at best (Moynihan, Christ, & Silver, 1988). Lew-Napoleone provides direction for treatment throughout the various phases of care—from assessment through termination—in both residential and home-bound programs. Interventions such as the life review and anticipatory bereavement care are discussed. In widening hospice care to multicultural populations, new services help preserve a sense of dignity and respect for each human life.

Many alternative service or grass-roots organizations evolved out of the inattention or unresponsiveness of funding sources or established services to underserved populations (Rothschild-Whitt, 1979). Over time, however, alternative service organizations' structure and program goals often change because of their dependence on larger established organizations or funding sources for financial stability. Finch discusses the evolution of alternative service organizations; key characteristics of program goals, structure, and process; as well as leadership and staffing patterns. He analyzes various end states as well as potential growth opportunities for single-focus and multifocus organizations. Because of the devastating effects of HIV on diverse populations, many alternative service organizations may be unable to respond to the crisis, thus increasing the pressure on traditional settings for meeting client needs.

SERVICE DELIVERY TO DIVERSE POPULATIONS

Part 2, on clinical issues in service delivery to diverse populations, includes material on various special populations affected by AIDS: gay and bisexual men, substance abusers, people of color, women, children, adolescents, the homeless, nonprofessional and professional caregivers, and the bereaved. Chapters focus on specific clinical issues in an effort to guide intervention strategies. Such issues include sudden changes in the expected developmental life course of individuals, ways that HIV has affected various populations, and how some populations share common concerns with other populations struggling with AIDS and HIV. Within an ecological framework, Part 2 examines the dynamics of common presenting problems from various theoretical and practice perspectives, including psychodynamic, interpersonal, systemic, cognitive, and behavioral. The authors provide an overview of treatment planning for both direct and indirect intervention strategies. With the help of case material, intervention is discussed from intake through termination and evaluation. The roles of service providers and their limitations, transference and countertransference issues, and population diversity and multicultural issues as they affect both service provider and client populations are discussed. Part 2 concludes with a discussion of the future of service provision with respect to populations being served.

Despite the changing demographics of those affected by the disease, gay men represent the largest population affected by HIV. Lloyd discusses the contextual and clinical issues in providing services to gay men infected with HIV. Lloyd's chapter focuses on the social and political impact of HIV on gay men as well as on how clinical interventions must reflect the complexity of the disease.

Clearly, HIV has had a devastating and far-reaching effect on gay men. Although the gay rights movement initially achieved positive results, including the removal of homosexuality from the *Diagnostic and Statistical Manual of Mental Disorders*, the connection between gay men and HIV has resulted in renewed homophobia in the United States (Tindall & Tillet, 1991). Gay men experience discrimination in nearly every aspect of life—from health care and employment to familial and community relationships (Ryan & Rowe, 1988). As a result, a significant number of bisexual men have remained closeted and continue to engage in high-risk behaviors, especially with female partners. As the number of AIDS deaths has risen, the gay community has undergone collective mourning and demoralization (Schindelman & Schoen, 1988). Through organizing collectively, as well as through political savvy, protective legislation has been initiated and new and innovative service organizations begun, thus creating new hope. Nevertheless, a comprehensive clinical armamentarium is needed to meet the needs of this population. Lloyd examines the multiple approaches that are currently being used to serve the various populations of gay and bisexual men coping with HIV.

To date, more than 30% of all reported cases of AIDS have been linked directly to injection drug use. To meet the needs of the growing population of injection drug users with AIDS, service providers must learn new ways to adapt their practice skills (Gerbert, Maguire, Bleeker, Coates, & McPhee, 1991). Stein provides an overview of the key issues in providing service to the traditionally underserved population of substance abusers who now face the additional stressor of HIV disease. Stein addresses the link between substance abuse and HIV, how social attitudes influence the delivery of service, key elements to understanding addiction, and recommended treatment goals and counseling strategies for serving clients who must cope with the double stigma of AIDS and injection drug use. Using an ecological, educative approach, Stein emphasizes the importance of engaging the client support system and other community resources while treating this vulnerable population.

People of color have been affected by HIV since the beginning of the epidemic, but only recently have these populations gained media attention in television and newspaper coverage of the AIDS crisis. People of color experience a greater rate of infection than do other at-risk groups (De La Vega, 1990). Hispanics, African Americans, and the various subcultures within these groups represent the largest groups of people of color infected by HIV. As a result of institutionalized racism and economic disenfranchisement, people of color with AIDS are particularly vulnerable. To work effectively with these populations, the service provider must examine the epidemiological, political, socioeconomic, cultural, and psychological needs of clients (Comas-Diaz, 1989; Diaz, 1991). Medrano and Klopner suggest in their chapter that the instrumental needs of these populations need to be stabilized before the therapeutic alliance can be secured. Clinicians need knowledge of cultural phenomena associated with health and illness in their clients. Services are more effective if they are adapted to the client's cultural mores.

The effects of AIDS on women have changed dramatically over the past several years. Currently, the rate of women with HIV disease is rising alarmingly (Noble, 1991). However, their traditional role as caregivers of the sick has not changed, thus leaving women with few physical and emotional supports. The majority of women with HIV/AIDS are poor, undereducated people of color. Until recently, the health care profession has neglected their special needs and issues (Chu, 1990). Resources that are currently available to men with HIV need to be broadened to include women. Educational materials need to focus on both homosexual and heterosexual women and their particular risk factors; women must be included in clinical research trials; AIDS-symptom criteria must include female-specific infections; and services must be designed to meet the special needs of women. Rosen and Blank address these pressing concerns and discuss the interventions for this high-risk HIV population.

Little is known about how a child's body responds to HIV infection. When women are infected with HIV, they may pass the virus on to their infant prenatally or congenitally. Children may also contract HIV as a result of sexual abuse by someone who is HIV positive. Children with HIV are a small but growing group that require special attention. Children need permanence and stability; however, the course of HIV/AIDS is often unpredictable, resulting in the need for repeated hospitalization or extended medical care away from family settings. In addition, when a parent is gravely ill or incapable of parenting, the HIV-infected child may require foster care (Boland, Allen, Long, & Tasker, 1988). Because children with AIDS often reside in families with few supports and resources, Lewert suggests that meeting the needs of children with AIDS involves meeting the family's needs. Many families fear stigma and rejection and thus may keep a child's HIV status a "family secret." Children fare better in an open and honest environment. Interventions designed to help families and children cope with HIV/AIDS are discussed and illustrated in this important chapter.

Adolescence is a period filled with experimentation and risk. Thus adolescents are especially at risk for contracting HIV disease as a result of sexual exploration and drug use (Gayle & D'Angelo, 1991). Moreover, other factors such as alcohol, marijuana, and cocaine use may impair judgment and increase the likelihood of high-risk behaviors. Adolescents of color residing in urban areas are disproportionately affected (Fullilove, 1989). In addition to specific HIV intervention, Pennbridge and colleagues urge practitioners to see adolescent clients as adolescents first and patients second; if adolescents' developmental needs are unattended, their medical needs will suffer as well.

Homelessness and AIDS are two grave problems in society today. Represented in this diverse group are persons who were homeless prior to contracting the virus and those who become homeless as a result of AIDS depleting their financial resources. Persons who have fallen through the holes of the so-called safety net into homelessness include people of color, children, drug addicts, immigrants without documents, and adolescents who become involved in survival sex. A major obstacle in treating this population is finding ways to engage them in order to provide education and medical care. Ironically, those who require the most intensive care may be least able to receive it. They may be unable to remember the location of service sites because AIDS has affected their cognitive capabilities. In addition, the connection between tuberculosis and AIDS is an increasing concern for the homeless, who are at risk for tuberculosis as a result of their impaired immune system and the high rate of contagion in shelters. Harragin discusses methods for using existing resources creatively and collaboratively to serve this highly vulnerable group.

Caregivers of persons with AIDS, including partners, family members, and friends, respond in various ways in their efforts to provide care to loved ones infected with HIV. Land explains how the relationship between the informal caregiver and the person with AIDS may predict caregiver responses. In addition, typical caregiver stressors and attendant coping styles are identified and chronicled throughout the course of the illness. Clinical intervention designed to ease the significant burden that caregivers face is discussed.

Professional caregivers struggle with a different kind of stress. Faced with the ongoing responsibility of caring for individuals who are terminally ill, inadequate community resources, a less than adequate health care system, and complex legal and ethical issues, professionals may feel helpless, hopeless, and angry. As a result, physical and emotional exhaustion may lead to burnout. Burnout is costly not only to the individual who suffers from the condition, but to the organization and the populations being served. Although an individual's capacity to cope with stress may explain some of the individual variability in response to burnout, the organizational milieu—job structure, role-related tasks, work distribution—often provides clues to why burnout occurs. Macks discusses AIDS-related burnout, proposing both individual and organizational strategies to tackle this disconcerting syndrome.

SPECIAL TOPICS

The last section of the book, on special topics in clinical work, focuses on matters such as bereavement, ethical and legal issues that need to be addressed when working with HIV/AIDS, medical phenomena and treatment procedures, and the role of research in service provision.

Professional and informal caregivers, as well as partners, family members, and friends of persons who have died of AIDS, struggle with bereavement. In fact, AIDS bereavement has been labeled "the second epidemic." Although grief-recovery models provide theory upon which to base interventions, coping with multiple AIDS losses presents unique challenges to the bereaved. Multiple losses, threat of harm to loved ones, and destruction of one's sense of community make AIDS bereavement similar to the emotional disturbance that follows an experience of trauma. Moreover, because of the stigma associated with AIDS, the bereaved may find disclosure of the loss and recovery more difficult (Schindelman & Schoen, 1988). Many bereaved persons feel cheated in their grief because their relationship to the deceased is unrecognized or invalidated by society (Anderson, Gurdin, & Thomas, 1989; Dick, 1989). Cultural or ethnic patterns may play an important role in the bereavement process. In his chapter, Bidgood discusses these issues and distinguishes the relationship between bereavement and trauma, outlining strategies that will help the recovery process.

AIDS has brought about monumental changes in how our medical systems administer treatment, creating legal and ethical crises in addition to the health crises. In his chapter on HIV and the law, Senak discusses how societal taboos involving sexuality, death, and nonprescription drug use have complicated the identification and treatment of persons with HIV. Advances in medical science, such as the development of the HIV-antibody test, have exerted pressures on our legal system. AIDS legislation often occurs within a context that pits the rights of the infected against the rights of those who are not infected (Gostin, 1987). Confidentiality, the right to insurance coverage, liability for health care providers, mandatory testing, and the criminalization of HIV transmission are major legal and ethical concerns. Clear guidelines on how to respond to these dilemmas are needed. Until the nation's underlying ethics and values are clarified, health care policy will exist in an unsettled state.

Medical issues in the treatment of HIV-related illness are equally complex. New diagnostic procedures as well as prophylactic, remedial, and palliative treatments are constantly being developed, tested, and administered. Patient compliance and the physical and psychological effects of such procedures on patients can create stress and strain in their own right, placing human service professionals at the vortex of medical conflicts. To serve client needs more comprehensively, practitioners must have knowledge of the disease process and procedures used to stem it. Holtom classifies and describes various causative agents that produce a host of medical disorders. He further discusses the common symptoms present with such disorders, the methods used to diagnosis them, and the types of therapy used to treat them.

In serving any population affected by HIV, evaluation of the effectiveness of services is key to developing effective programs. The urgency of the AIDS crisis requires an aggressive, nationwide research effort to document the efficacy of AIDS education, prevention, and service efforts. Furthermore, AIDS research can help community-based organizations and governmental agencies deploy scarce resources more effectively. However, conducting research on AIDS has proven to be a formidable task because of the wide scope and unpredictable nature of the disease. In addition, issues relating to human-subject studies and appropriate methodology complicate research efforts (Bharucha-Reid, Schork, & Schwartz, 1990). Mantell and DiVittis analyze obstacles to conducting AIDS-service research, discussing the politics of AIDS research, bioethical issues, methodological issues for both quantitative and qualitative research, selected measurement issues, and data-collection methods.

PURPOSE

This book is designed as a resource text for AIDS service providers and educators. As with any catastrophic illness, HIV/AIDS takes a devastating toll on both clients and service providers. But HIV/AIDS is more than a terminal disease; its presence affects the psychosocial disposition of the nation as a whole. To date, the majority of persons affected by AIDS have been those who traditionally have been disenfranchised and stigmatized by society. The task for service providers is to comprehend the interplay of the physical, social, and psychological factors affecting clients and society as a whole so that proactive services can be initiated. In this manner, we work to stem the devastating effects of AIDS and offer hope for the future.

REFERENCES

Anderson, G. R., Gurdin, P., & Thomas, A. (1989). Dual disenfranchisement: Foster parenting children with AIDS. In K. J. Doka (Ed.), *Disenfranchised grief: Recognizing hidden sorrow* (pp. 43–53). Lexington, MA: Lexington Books.

Bharucha-Reid, R. P., Schork, A., & Schwartz, S. A. (1990). Data linkage and subject anonymity for HIV testing. *AIDS and Public Policy Journal, 5,* 189–190.

Boland, M. G., Allen, T. J., Long, G. I., & Tasker, M. (1988). Children with HIV infection: Collaborative responsibilities of the child welfare worker and medical communities. *Social Work, 33,* 504–510.

Buckingham, S. L. (1987). The HIV antibody test: Psychosocial issues. *Social Casework, 68,*

387–393.

Chinin, E. (1989). Community care for the frail elderly: The case of the nonprofessional home-care worker. *Women Health, 14*(3), 93–104.

Chu, S. (1990). Impact of the human immunodeficiency virus epidemic on mortality in women of reproductive age, United States. *Journal of the American Medical Association, 254,* 225–229.

Comas-Diaz, L. (1989). Culturally relevant issues and treatment implications for Hispanics. In D. A. Koslow & E. P. Salett (Eds.), *Crossing cultures in mental health.* Washington, DC: SIETAR International.

De La Vega, E. (1990). Considerations for reaching the Latino population with sexuality and HIV/AIDS information and education. *SIECUS Report, 18*(3), 1–8.

Diaz, E. (1991). Public policy, women, and HIV disease. *SIECUS Report, 19*(2), 4–5.

Dick, L. C (1989). An investigation of the disenfranchised grief of two health care professionals caring for persons with AIDS. In K. J. Doka (Ed.), *Disenfranchised grief: Recognizing hidden sorrow* (pp. 55–65). Lexington: MA: Lexington Books.

Fullilove, R. (1989, July 3). Crack cocaine use and risk for AIDS among black adolescents. *CDC, AIDS Weekly,* p. 7.

Gayle, E. D., & D'Angelo, L. J. (1991). Epidemiology and acquired immunodeficiency virus infection in adolescents. *Pediatric Infectious Disease Journal, 10,* 322–328.

Gerbert, B., Maguire, B., Bleeker, T., Coates, T., & McPhee, S. (1991). Primary care physicians and AIDS. *Journal of the American Medical Association, 226,* 2837.

Gostin, L. O. (1987). The case against compulsory casefinding in controlling AIDS, screening and reporting. *American Journal of Law and Medicine, 13,* 7–53.

Janson, B. (1988). *The reluctant welfare state.* Belmont, CA: Wadsworth.

Moynihan, R., Christ, G., & Silver, L. G. (1988). AIDS and terminal illness. *Social Casework, 69,* 380–387.

Noble, G. (1991, April). Women and AIDS: The growing crisis, update. *CDC HIV/AIDS Prevention Newsletter,* pp. 1–2.

Reamer, F. G. (1988). AIDS and ethics: The agenda for social workers. *Social Work, 33,* 460–464.

Roberts, C. S. (1989, August). Conflicting professional values in social work and medicine. *Health and Social Work, 14,* 211–218.

Rothschild-Whitt, J. (1979). Conditions for democracy: Making participatory organizations work. In J. Case & R. C. R. Taylor (Eds.), *Co-ops, communes and collectives* (pp. 215–244). New York: Pantheon Books.

Ryan, C., & Rowe, M. J. (1988). AIDS: Legal and ethical issues. *Social Casework, 69,* 324–333.

Schindelman, E., & Schoen, K. (1988). Gay and grieving: Bringing grief out of the closet. In M. Shernoff & W. Scott (Eds.), *The sourcebook of lesbian and gay healthcare* (2nd ed.). Washington, DC: National Gay and Lesbian Healthcare Foundation.

Tindall, B., & Tillet, G. (1991). HIV-related discrimination. *AIDS, 4*(suppl. 1), 251–256.

PART 1

INTERVENTION ACROSS SERVICE SETTINGS

1

AIDS EDUCATION AND PRIMARY PREVENTION

LEE E. KLOSINSKI

The AIDS epidemic began on June 5, 1981, with the publication of a notice in the *Morbidity and Mortality Weekly Report* alerting physicians to the occurrence of rare opportunistic infections in several gay men who had been otherwise healthy (Centers for Disease Control, 1981). At that time no one realized that an unusual virus, which had already been transmitted around the world, was responsible for a set of diseases that eventually would be called acquired immune deficiency syndrome (AIDS). Affecting first gay and bisexual men, then injection drug users, their sexual partners, and their children, scientists concluded that the cause of this new malady was some blood-borne pathogen. By 1982, the first calls for more discreet sexual behavior and drug use were made. At the same time, community-based groups formed to assist those who were increasingly being diagnosed with previously unusual diseases and conditions. AIDS education had begun.

By 1984 the virus that causes AIDS was identified in laboratories in France and the United States. AIDS was recognized as a life-threatening stage of infection with the human immunodeficiency virus (HIV). Educators realized that infection with HIV was a far more pervasive problem affecting a much larger population than those who were actually diagnosed with full-blown AIDS. Efforts were directed toward information about HIV transmission. This basic information has not changed since the first years of the epidemic: HIV is transmitted only by blood, semen, vaginal secretions, and breast milk. Only unprotected anal, vaginal, or oral sex, blood-to-blood contact, and ingestion of breast milk transmits HIV. The basics of HIV transmission and prevention are readily accessible to the general public. Virtually every American has at least heard of AIDS, and the majority are familiar with how HIV is transmitted. Yet this has not stopped transmission of HIV (Centers for Disease Control, 1987, 1988).

HIV transmission occurs because a variety of factors operating at the personal and environmental level affect the behavior of individuals who engage in high-risk behaviors. HIV/AIDS education likewise has occurred within a context influenced by personal and environmental factors. By examining these personal and environmental factors, we elucidate the current state of HIV/AIDS education and are able to project future educational efforts. In the following sections, the development of educational strategies for gay and bisexual men, injection drug users, and others will be discussed. The chapter concludes by commenting on the critical issues facing HIV/AIDS education in the second decade of the epidemic.

ANTIBODY TESTING AND EARLY INTERVENTION

Information about the basic facts of HIV transmission is a critical component of HIV education. Another component of this education effort is providing the public with information about HIV antibody testing. When the HIV antibody test first appeared in 1985, HIV educators were reluctant to encourage testing. At that time, no proven medical intervention could delay the course of HIV infection. The stresses associated with knowing that one was infected seemed to outweigh any medical benefit. The social risks associated with a diagnosis of HIV infection or AIDS were substantial and included the loss of friends and family, employment, housing, and health insurance. Many people with HIV/AIDS feared physical violence. This fear was well-founded. Violence against gay men has occurred frequently. In Florida the family home of two brothers with AIDS was attacked with a fire bomb.

Attitudes toward testing began to change after the drug zidovudine (AZT) was approved in 1987 for those with full-blown AIDS. Because the drug proved effective for persons with AIDS, clinicians began prescribing it for persons in earlier stages of HIV disease. In 1989, AZT was approved for persons with moderate immune suppression, even if they did not yet have symptoms. Although AZT was and remains an expensive, toxic therapy, its efficacy is recognized by the medical establishment (National Institute of Allergy and Infectious Diseases, 1990). The drug is available, however, only to persons who have been diagnosed as being HIV positive and who have private health insurance to pay for this extremely costly medication.

In the late 1980s, advances were made in primary prophylaxis against *Pneumocystis carinii* pneumonia, the major cause of death among people with AIDS. The availability of early intervention to delay the progression of HIV disease and to relieve symptoms as well as prophylaxis against the leading cause of death among people with AIDS caused a rapid, dramatic shift in attitudes toward testing.

Several factors at the societal level contributed to the growing support for antibody testing. One factor was the publicizing of Rock Hudson's AIDS diagnosis, an event that underlined the reality of AIDS for the American public. Suddenly, everyone knew of someone with AIDS. Legislation in most large urban jurisdictions and several states offered those with HIV infection explicit protection from discrimination. The federal government made funds available to purchase AZT for individuals who could not afford it. Several court decisions, beginning with the Supreme Court decision in 1987 on *School Board of Nassau County v. Arline*, made it clear that those with contagious diseases like AIDS must be afforded the same protection that other persons with physical handicaps receive (Gostin, 1990).

By late 1989, almost all HIV educators encouraged anonymous antibody testing for persons at risk for HIV infection. As more individuals tested positive for HIV infection or were diagnosed with AIDS, the immensity and complexity of the HIV epidemic became clearer. The personal challenges of living with HIV disease, as well as the demands that the epidemic placed upon the public health system and the bureaucracy that regulates it, resulted in the creation of diverse grass-roots organizations dedicated to supporting persons with HIV disease and advocating for funding for treatment, research, and education. Such advocacy ranged from traditional lobbying to scripted acts of civil disobedience. Although the means differed, the objectives were the same: to put pressure on elected officials who were unresponsive to the urgency of the needs of people with HIV.

While some in the HIV community took to the streets or visited offices of elected officials, the established community organizations serving the needs of people with HIV formalized and expanded their educational efforts. The movement was directed toward enabling clients to be proactive about their health and welfare. Educational programs were established to help individuals become knowledgeable about antiviral therapies; prophylaxis against opportunistic infections; access to clinical trials of new drugs; and the general principals of health, nutrition, insurance, and public benefits.

As the epidemic begins its second decade, major efforts are under way to carry information about prevention and testing to the general public. Outreach efforts have been made to the heterosexual population, especially adolescents. Sexually active adolescents and college students are at high risk for sexually transmitted diseases and unplanned pregnancies because they often do not use condoms during intercourse. Hence, they are also at high risk for HIV. Also, adolescence is a time when experimentation with alcohol and drugs is common. Even adolescents who might otherwise be committed to abstinence or safer sex may engage in high-risk behaviors while under the influence of a chemical substance (Oskamp et al., 1988).

Another area of growing concern involves women and HIV. Women with HIV infection tend to be diagnosed at a later stage of infection and live shorter lives than do men with HIV. The manifestations of HIV among women include chronic yeast infections, chronic pelvic inflammatory disease, vaginitis, and cervical dysplasia. These symptoms are often overlooked by gynecologists, many of whom were trained before the advent of the epidemic or assume that HIV does not affect female patients. Hence, professionals practicing in general medicine need to update their knowledge (Minkoff & Dehovitz, 1991).

This brief history of HIV/AIDS education demonstrates some of the unique aspects of the HIV epidemic. Tension exists among the personal needs of people infected with HIV, advances in science and technology, and the broader cultural and societal context. On the personal level, the challenge of living with HIV can produce acute anxiety, compromised health, an uncertain future, stigmatization by society, the threat of abandonment by friends and family, and the loss of basic rights to privacy. Modern medicine can assist people with HIV infection, but medical interventions are available only to people who are tested and diagnosed as HIV infected. In addition, society has been reluctant to respond to an epidemic that seems to affect primarily highly marginalized people.

As the tension among these factors plays itself out over time, HIV/AIDS educators are faced with the challenge of primary prevention of HIV infection. This task involves addressing the personal and environmental factors that contribute to high-risk activities. By examining the experience with gay and bisexual men and injection drug users, it is possible to understand what some of these factors are and to glean some general principals for HIV/AIDS education.

GAY AND BISEXUAL MEN

AIDS was first identified among gay and bisexual men. This population has received more concentrated educational efforts than has any other group. The initial success of this campaign is well-known: gay and bisexual men quickly either abandoned anal intercourse or began practicing it with a condom. This change in behavior, supported by dramatic drops in the number of new cases of rectal gonorrhea and hepatitis B, represented a rapid, dramatic modification of sexual behavior and subcultural ethos (Handsfield, Krekeler, & Nicola, 1989; Judson, 1983; Handsfield, Krekeler, & Nicola, 1985; Peterson, Sondergaard, & Wantzin, 1988).

What accounted for the rapid transmission of HIV in this population, and how is the rapid change in personal sexual behavior to be explained? The transmission of HIV is easily understood as a result of environmental and personal phenomena. The modern gay/lesbian liberation movement began in the summer of 1969 among drag queens and people of color at an obscure bar in New York City, where patrons fought back against a routine police raid. After the Stonewall Riots, gay men began to come out of the "closet" and identify themselves as gay. A variety of educational, recreational, and social groups were organized by and for gay men and lesbians. At the societal level, gay liberation did many things: it allowed gay men and lesbians to surface as a visible group in the larger population, it motivated them to organize themselves, and it allowed them to lobby for the passage of laws to protect sexual minorities from discrimination.

On a personal level, most gay men did not openly identify themselves as such until after high school or college. This meant that many gay men experienced sexual adolescence 10 years after their heterosexual peers. Bath houses or sex clubs provided casual, recreational sex for many people. Before AIDS, the greatest risk associated with such activity was sexually transmitted infection. Promiscuous sexual activity among gay men paralleled the sexual revolution that was occurring in society as a whole during the 1960s and early 1970s. This casual approach to unprotected sex, however, changed dramatically with the advent of AIDS (Shilts, 1987).

Several factors accounted for changes in sexual behavior and activities. Multimedia campaigns aimed at the gay and bisexual community broadcast the risks and safety of various sexual practices. In addition, less risky sexual practices were promoted.

Another factor that contributed to changes in sexual behavior among gay and bisexual men was the maturation of the gay/lesbian liberation movement. Across the country, especially in large urban areas, the AIDS epidemic provided a focus for social and political energy. Efforts of gays to organize social services and to secure funding for educational materials through political lobbying helped to organize the gay community, which traditionally had lacked a political and social center. Because governmental funding was slow in coming, a great deal of creative energy went into fund raising and organizing. At the same time, the movement became involved in battling political attempts to secure mandatory HIV testing, the issue of reporting HIV-infected individuals to state health departments, and even more extreme efforts to quarantine those with AIDs. Thus, the AIDS epidemic served to organize the gay and lesbian community in ways that the sexual liberation movement could not. It helped to create a new ethos in the gay community, whereby safer sex became part of the community's discourse and behavior (Bolton & Joseph, 1988).

The many gay men who were developing HIV-related symptoms or who were being diagnosed with AIDS also significantly modified gay and bisexual behavior. No one could deny the reality of HIV disease, and the resulting suffering, grief, and caregiving challenges were the greatest influence on forcing changes in sexual behavior. As a result of all of these factors, the incidence of new infections dropped dramatically by the mid-1980s (Hessol, O'Malley, & Lifson, 1989).

The issues of education and primary prevention among gay and bisexual men have changed in the second decade of the epidemic. Educational efforts still focus on disseminating basic information about transmission of HIV, particularly to the next generation at risk. Today, however, most educational efforts focus on issues concerning HIV testing. Studies suggest that a small but significant proportion of gay and bisexual men have not yet been tested for HIV (Kanouse, Berry, Gorman, Yano, & Carson, 1989). For those who test positive for HIV infection, medical interventions can slow the progression of the disease. For those who test negative, efforts can be made to sustain the behaviors that prevent transmission.

Alarmingly, recidivism among gay and bisexual men is occurring. Sex clubs allegedly devoted to safer sex have opened in urban centers. The ongoing debate about the relative safety of oral sex suggests that some gay men are willing to engage in a practice that under certain conditions clearly leads to HIV infection. The incidence of rectal gonorrhea among gay and bisexual men is also on the rise. Anecdotal reports from some therapists suggest that survivor guilt among some HIV-negative gay and bisexual men may cause them to practice unsafe sexual behaviors (Handsfield, Krekeler, & Nicola, 1989; Ekstrand, Stall, Coates, & McKusick, 1989).

The implications of these developments for primary prevention are not clear. It appears that the gay community needs to develop mechanisms by which members' anger and grief associated with HIV and AIDS can be addressed. At the individual level, the negotiation skills necessary for sustaining behavioral changes need to be taught. Before exploring these issues in greater depth, it may be helpful to examine other populations that are affected by HIV.

INJECTION DRUG USERS

The drug-using population remains the most complex, misunderstood, and politically charged population at risk for HIV infection (Klosinski, Longshore, Gorman, Yano, & Sekler, 1989). The use of drugs can create various behaviors that place individuals at risk for HIV. Sharing drug-injection equipment for purposes of intravenous, intramuscular, or subcutaneous injection can transmit HIV. This risk also applies to persons who use unsterile needles for body piercing or tattoos. The sexual partners of persons who share unsterile drug-injection equipment are also at risk. Moreover, some women trade sexual favors for drugs and are thus at risk of infecting their children through perinatal transmission. Finally, even if a person is committed to safer-sex practices, judgment can be impaired while under the influence of alcohol and other drugs.

The following discussion focuses on persons who share drug-injection equipment, a population that is often misunderstood because of the stereotypes associated with it. Sharing drug paraphernalia is a social phenomenon that affects all socioeconomic groups. Moreover, not all people who use injection drugs are irresponsible, antisocial, or users on a daily basis.

The challenge of reaching injection drug users (IDUs) is compounded by several personal and environmental factors. Many such people are at the lower end of the social and economic spectrum and their drug use intensifies their alienation from society. The risk of HIV infection may seem remote compared with more immediate concerns such as obtaining income, food, housing, and drugs. Other factors that motivate drug use beyond simple experimentation include pain, depression, anger, and addiction. Because of these factors, HIV/AIDS education is difficult to provide to this population (Klosinski, Longshore, Gorman, Yano, & Sekler, 1989). Some IDUs have little or no education and are alienated from or distrustful of authorities. They tend to organize their lives around short-term rather than long-term goals. Drug addiction can be accompanied by various psychosocial and medical problems that produce a stress cycle; IDUs may seek to relieve this stress through increased drug use. This is especially true for users who are aware of their HIV infection or AIDS diagnosis. Unfortunately, drug use puts them at a greater health risk and in a more precarious social position, thereby causing more stress.

Finally, the phenomenon of drug addiction itself intensifies the risk of HIV. Mere possession of a drug and anticipation of its use may stimulate or intensify the symptoms associated with drug withdrawal. This can cause an IDU to use whatever injection equipment is available to get a fix (Des Jarlais & Hopkins, 1985; Connors, 1989). Many of the symptoms of drug withdrawal mirror the symptoms of HIV infection. Drug users may mistake the latter for the former and increase their drug use as a means of relieving what are in reality HIV symptoms.

Other factors that influence high-risk behavior among IDUs are rooted in their environment, including lack of opportunities, peer pressure, and neighborhood culture. The use of drug-injection equipment is a learned skill passed down from one generation of users to another. It is a social phenomenon that promotes sharing of equipment. The practice is such a fundamental aspect of the subculture that many users do not consider the use of injection equipment by friends or sexual partners as sharing, but as an activity that defines friendship. In addition, many states allow the possession of syringes only by prescription, which creates a scarcity and thus promotes sharing of needles or renting of needles in shooting galleries (Watters, 1989; Kleinman & Mockler, 1988; Des Jarlais & Friedman, 1987; Murphy, 1987; National Academy of Sciences, 1989).

Politicians have been reluctant to support programs for distribution of bleach and condoms to addicts or needle-exchange programs. Their resistance is based on the belief that such programs condone or encourage drug use, although available evidence suggests that this is not the case. Rather, such efforts appear to encourage addicts to seek treatment or to clean their works (Des Jarlais, Friedman, & Stoneburner, 1988; Jackson & Rotkiewicz, 1987; Selwyn, 1987).

Because some IDUs lack education, economic resources, and good health and because the drug subculture is predatory in nature, IDUs lack the social organization that characterizes the gay/lesbian community. Their lack of social organization makes it more difficult to disseminate information and to change the subculture's ethos.

Finally, as with many other populations, the use of condoms is not normative behavior among IDUs (Celentano, Vlahov, Anthony, & Bernal, 1989; Peterson & Bakeman, 1989). More men than women use drugs, and many women may not be aware that their partners use drugs or that they are bisexual. Among poor drug users, women may be economically dependent on their husbands and involved in relationships in which traditional sexual roles are strongly reinforced. Women may not have the social position or negotiation skills to insist upon condom use (Cohen, Hauer, & Wofsy, 1989; Cochran & Mays, 1988; Conviser & Rutledge, 1989; Peterson & Bakeman, 1989; Selwyn, Carter, Schoenbaum, Robertson, Klein, & Rogers, 1989; Solomon & DeJong, 1989). Women need education about the risks associated with unprotected sex. Family planning and prenatal clinics are ideal settings in which such discussion can be initiated and supplies provided.

Faced with these personal and environmental factors, how can HIV education proceed? The optimum setting for HIV education is a drug-treatment program. By controlling drug dependency, the major risk of HIV transmission is eliminated and other risk-reduction techniques can be taught. Energies directed to obtaining the next fix can be redirected to long-range personal health and risk-reduction goals. Drug users can be tested for HIV infection, taught risk-reduction techniques, and directed toward early intervention programs when appropriate. Contrary to the popular stereotype that drug users are recalcitrant, IDUs who are aware of their serostatus frequently desire admittance to drug rehabilitation programs or begin to take precautions by cleaning their drug paraphernalia. Unfortunately, few publicly supported treatment programs are available for IDUs without financial resources. The greatest challenge of HIV education is reaching out to users not in treatment programs (Klosinski, Longshore, Gorman, Yano, & Sekler, 1989).

HIV education to IDUs occurs in various contexts: family-planning clinics, emergency rooms, hospitals, jails. Aggressive, direct community outreach to IDUs has also been successful. Outreach workers are especially effective in communicating with users who are alienated from conventional sources of information or who are interested in reducing their risk for HIV but not in stopping their drug habit. The outreach workers with the most credibility are former users with firsthand experience with the IDU community.

Regardless of the context, successful HIV education for IDUs includes at least three components. First, information should be provided in blunt language about what can be done to reduce the risk of HIV transmission through drug use and sexual activity. Second, practical skills about how to sterilize needles and use condoms should be demonstrated. Once the skills are demonstrated, they must be practiced. Practice reinforces the techniques, promotes incremental learning of the skills, and provides the IDU with feedback and positive reinforcement. Third, supplies such as bleach, condoms, and sterile needles should be exchanged for used equipment. This is especially important for users who cannot afford these supplies. Also, the availability of bleach and condoms promotes their use. Anecdotal reports suggest that when HIV-education programs include these three components, IDUs do begin to adopt new behaviors. Indeed, supermarket owners from urban areas with many IDUs report that they are finding an increasing number of bleach bottles with needle holes in them.

EDUCATION IN THE WORKPLACE

It is currently estimated that approximately one million Americans have HIV infection (Centers for Disease Control, 1990). People diagnosed with AIDS are living longer, and more people speak openly about their diagnosis or request time off from work for medical appointments or sick leave. At the same time, however, fear, rejection, discrimination, and acts of violence against HIV-infected individuals are still occurring. Thus, an ongoing need exists for socialization of this population into the broader population, particularly in the workplace.

The workplace was one of the first places where the American public encountered HIV education. Many business leaders quickly recognized the implications of the HIV epidemic for the workplace. Several factors motivated early educational efforts for employees. Businesses recognized that HIV was creating fear and disruption in the work setting, losses in productivity, more expensive health care programs, and possible litigation. Companies recognized that education was the best means of prevention and the best guarantee that employees would respond compassionately and rationally to fellow employees with HIV infection. Thus companies began to develop their own programs or looked to national organizations such as the American Red Cross or local AIDS service providers to provide education. Early workplace programs focused on key concepts such as why AIDS is not contagious in the workplace, how HIV is spread, what behaviors put one at risk, how risk behaviors can be reduced, and why the stigma associated with HIV/AIDS can lead to irrational, unfair, or illegal behavior.

Today, new challenges face HIV education in the workplace. A significant challenge is educating management about laws that protect HIV-infected employees. Such employees, like other employees with communicable diseases, are considered handicapped and thus are entitled to reasonable accommodations extended to other handicapped individuals, including flexible hours, changes in the work environment to allow physical access, or even working at home. Other workplace issues include ensuring continuation of benefits, preparing the work group for the return of a person with AIDS to the workplace, ongoing educational efforts, and dealing with employees who refuse to work with people with HIV/AIDS.

CONCLUSION

Successful HIV/AIDS education includes three components: (1) discussion in blunt language of the necessary steps for reducing transmission of HIV through sexual practices and drug use, (2) demonstration and supervised practice of skills in condom use and sterilizing injection equipment, (3) distribution of supplies such as bleach, condoms, and sterile needles.

HIV/AIDS education works most effectively for populations who are receptive to its message. Unfortunately, most of these receptive populations are groups who are directly affected by HIV infection either because they themselves or their family members, friends, or co-workers are infected. Early intervention with antiviral drugs and prophylaxis against opportunistic infections means that people with HIV infection and AIDS are living longer, healthier lives. The HIV-infected population is becoming more visible; as HIV becomes more prevalent in the workplace, the need and desire for education will spread to the general public.

HIV education alone will not stop the AIDS epidemic. Knowing the facts about how HIV is transmitted does not change the personal and environmental factors that contribute to transmission. Personal factors are rooted deep in the human psyche: sexual identity, habitual behaviors, religious beliefs and moral judgments, and addiction. The environmental factors are equally complex. They include society's attitudes toward marginalized groups such as gay men and injection drug users, the inadequacy of women's health care, the fear and stigma attached to persons with chronic life-threatening illness, the reticence of society to speak frankly and openly about sexual practices and drug use, the unwillingness of elected officials to provided basic risk-reduction supplies such as condoms and bleach, and societal factors that lead to drug use.

HIV/AIDS prevention and education face tremendous challenges in the second decade of the epidemic. Our experience with gay and bisexual men and injection drug users proves that those who engage in high-risk activities can change their behavior. The hope for the future is that those less directly affected by HIV/AIDS will be as conscientious and responsible about adopting risk-reducing practices.

REFERENCES

Bolton, M. H., & Joseph, J. G. (1988). AIDS and behavioral change to reduce risk. *American Journal of Public Health, 78*, 394–410.

Celentano, D., Vlahov, D., Anthony, J. C., & Bernal, M. (1989, June 12–15). *Is condom use an independent risk for HIV in IV drug users?* Paper presented at the Fifth International Conference on AIDS, Montreal, Quebec, Canada.

Centers for Disease Control. (1981). *Morbidity and Mortality Weekly Report, 30*(22), 204.

Centers for Disease Control. (1987). *Surgeon General's Report on Acquired Immune Deficiency Syndrome.* Rockville, MD: U.S. Public Health Service.

Centers for Disease Control. (1988). *Understanding AIDS.* Rockville, MD: U.S. Public Health Service.

Centers for Disease Control. (1990). HIV prevalence estimates and AIDS case projections for the United States; report based upon a workshop. *Morbidity and Mortality Report, 39*(7), 110–119.

Cochran, S. D., & Mays, V. M. (1988). Women and AIDS-related concerns. *American Psychologist, 44*, 529–535.

Cohen, J. B., Hauer, L. B., & Wofsy, C. B. (1989). Women and IV drugs: Parenteral and heterosexual transmission of human immunodeficiency virus. *Journal of Drug Issues, 19*, 39–56.

Connors, M. (1989, June 12–15). *The role of IV drug withdrawal symptoms and symptom anticipation in AIDS risk reduction.* Paper presented at the Fifth International Conference on AIDS, Montreal, Quebec, Canada.

Conviser, R., & Rutledge, J. H. (1989). Can public policies limit the spread of HIV among IV drug users? *Journal of Drug Issues, 19*, 113–128.

Des Jarlais, D. C., & Hopkins, W. (1985). Free needles for intravenous drug users at risk for AIDS: Current developments in New York City. *New England Journal of Medicine, 23*, 1476–1477.

Des Jarlais, D. C., & Friedman, S. R. (1987). *AIDS and the sharing of equipment for illicit drug injection: A review of current data.* Paper prepared for the National Institute on Drug Abuse, Washington, DC.

Des Jarlais, D. C., Friedman, S. R., & Stoneburner, R. L. (1988). HIV infection and intravenous drug use: Critical issues in transmission dynamics, infection outcomes, and prevention. *Review of Infectious Diseases, 10*, 151–158.

Ekstrand, M. L., Stall, R. D., Coates, T. J., & McKusick, L. (1989, June 4–9). *Risky sex relapse, the next challenge for AIDS prevention programs: The AIDS Behavioral Research Project (Abstract).* Fifth International Conference on AIDS, Montreal, Quebec, Canada.

Gostin, L. O. (1990). The AIDS litigation project. A national review of court and human rights commission decisions, part II: Discrimination. *Journal of the American Medical Association, 263*, 2086–2093.

Handsfield, H. H., Krekeler, B., & Nicola, R. M. (1985). Decreasing incidence of gonorrhea in homosexually active men—minimal effect on risk of AIDS. *Western Journal of Medicine, 143*, 469–470.

Handsfield, H. H., Krekeler, B., & Nicola, R. M. (1989). Trends in gonorrhea in homosexually active men—King County, Washington, 1989. *Journal of the American Medical Association, 262*, 2985–2986.

Hessol, N. A., O'Malley, P., & Lifson, D. (1989, June 4–9). *Incidence and prevalence of HIV infection among homosexual and bisexual men, 1978–1988* (Abstract). Fifth International Conference on AIDS, Montreal, Quebec, Canada.

Jackson, J., & Rotkiewicz, L. (1987, June 5–8). *A coupon program: AIDS education and drug treatment.* Paper presented at the Third International Conference on AIDS, Washington, DC.

Judson, F. N. (1983). Fear of AIDS and gonorrhea rates in homosexual men. *Lancet, 2*, 159–160.

Kanouse, D. E., Berry, S. H., Gorman, E. M., Yano, E. M., & Carson, S. (1991). *Response to the AIDS epidemic: A study of homosexual and bisexual men in Los Angeles County.* Santa Monica, CA: Rand.

Kleinman, M. A. R., & Mockler, R. W. (1988). *AIDS and heroin: Strategies for control*. Washington, DC: The Urban Institute.

Klosinski, L. E., Longshore, D., Gorman, M., Yano, E., & Sekler, J. (1989). *Ideas for AIDS reduction among intravenous drug users*. Office of AIDS, California State Department of Health Service, Sacramento, CA.

Minkoff, H., & Dehovitz, J. A. (1991). HIV infection in women. *AIDS Clinical Care, 3*, 33–35.

Murphy, S. (1987). Intravenous drug use and AIDS: Notes on the social economy of needle sharing. *Contemporary Drug Problems, 14*, 373–395.

National Academy of Sciences. (1989). *AIDS: Sexual behavior and intravenous drug use*. Washington, DC: National Academy Press.

National Institute of Allergy and Infectious Diseases. (1990). AZT therapy for early HIV infection. *Clinical Courier, 8*(5), 1–8.

Oskamp, S., Hoffman, V., Donaldson, S., Winter, D., Kane, K., Bird-Westerfield, D., Parra, R., Paulson, A., & Wegbreit, R. (1988). AIDS knowledge, attitudes, and sexual behavior of California students. *California Sociologist, 11*, 91–116.

Peterson, C. S., & Bakeman, J. (1989). AIDS and IV drug use among ethnic minorities. *Journal of Drug Issues, 19*, 27–37.

Peterson, C. S., Sondergaard, J., & Wantzin, G. L. (1988). AIDS related changes in pattern of sexually transmitted disease (STD) in an STD clinic in Copenhagen. *Genitourinary Medicine, 64*, 270–272.

Selwyn, P. A. (1987). Sterile needles and the epidemic of acquired immunodeficiency syndrome: Issues for drug abuse treatment and public health. *Advances in Alcohol and Substance Abuse, 7*, 99–105.

Selwyn, P. A., Carter, R. J., Schoenbaum, E. E., Robertson, V. J., Klein, R. S., & Rogers, M. F. (1989). Knowledge of HIV antibody status and decisions to continue or terminate pregnancy among intravenous drug users. *Journal of the American Medical Association, 261*, 3567–3671.

Shilts, R. (1987). *And the band played on*. New York: St. Martin's Press.

Solomon, M. Z., & DeJong, W. (1989). Preventing AIDS and other STDs through condom promotion: A patient education intervention. *American Journal of Public Health, 79*, 453–458.

Watters, J. K. (1989). Observations on the importance of social context in HIV transmission among intravenous drug users. *Journal of Drug Issues, 19*, 9–26.

2

HIV OUTPATIENT SERVICES

SALLY JUE

As of October 1991, the Centers for Disease Control (CDC) reported 195,718 cases of AIDS in the United States (Centers for Disease Control, 1991b). On June 17, 1991, the *Morbidity and Mortality Weekly Report* predicted that "AIDS will be the second leading cause of death among men 24 to 44 years of age, and one of five leading causes of death among women aged 15–44 in the U.S. by the end of 1991" (Centers for Disease Control, 1991a, p. 25). At several points during the course of infection, these individuals and their loved ones will need various social services to help them cope with the effects of the illness. But before discussing current service needs, it may be helpful to examine the historical development of HIV social services.

In the early years of the HIV epidemic, most AIDS clients were educated, white, middle-class, gay men. In seeking services from traditional providers, they initially experienced AIDS phobia, homophobia, and discrimination. These experiences caused infected persons to become reluctant to seek services until a crisis occurred. Some clients began to internalize society's "blame-the-victim" mentality, which only augmented their depression and lowered their self-esteem. Because existing services failed to meet their needs, the gay community created its own service organizations. According to the Report of the Presidential Commission on HIV (1988), "community based organizations have led the response to the HIV epidemic in this country" (p. 110). Most of the care-delivery models used today were developed by gay community organizations in the early 1980s. It is also important to note that services were created primarily by and for white, middle-class, gay men.

During their infancy, AIDS service organizations were volunteer agencies with minimal staff and funding. Volunteers provided nearly all direct and indirect services. Agencies had an informal, nonhierarchical, familial structure, with staff performing various functions ranging from direct services to clerical work and fund raising. Fighting AIDs became a personal commitment rather than a job and was perceived as crucial to the survival of the gay community.

146,646

Due to the relatively short survival period after diagnosis (12–16 months), many clients viewed their diagnosis as an immediate death sentence. AIDS services focused on crisis intervention, helping clients and their loved ones confront mortality issues and helping them cope with the psychosocial impact of the disease. Legitimate fears of rejection and discrimination and the lack of information about AIDS, opportunistic infections, treatments, and transmission exacerbated feelings of anxiety, depression, and powerlessness.

Volunteer training focused heavily on AIDS transmission, safer sex, death and dying, how to provide emotional support, and bereavement issues. Staff and volunteers operated on the premise that an average client's relationship with the agency would last six months to a year at best, so all programs and treatment plans took on a short-term, present-oriented, problem-solving focus. Agencies did not initiate long-range planning because of the crisis mode under which they operated, the lack of information about AIDS, and the hope that a cure for the disease would be found in a few years.

During the mid-1980s, medical and scientific advances led to major changes in AIDS social services. The discovery of the HIV virus and the development of the HIV antibody test expanded knowledge of the disease continuum and created a new type of client—the HIV-positive asymptomatic individual. When medical advances made possible early treatment to delay the onset of HIV symptoms, early medical intervention programs were initiated and information, referral, advocacy, and emotional-support services for asymptomatic clients were developed.

The development of the antiviral drug zidovudine (AZT) as well as earlier diagnosis and more effective treatments for opportunistic infections also had a dramatic impact on AIDS service providers. The client's survival time was more than doubled, and enhancing the quality of that person's life became a more pertinent issue. These developments led to a slower client attrition rate and to utilization of agency services over a longer period. Along with the increases in the number of newly diagnosed cases, these factors generated larger agency case loads.

Clients began to establish more in-depth relationships with staff and volunteers, made more long-term plans, and did not feel such an immediate need to complete tasks and accomplish personal goals. Issues such as living with HIV dementia, whether to return to work, financial planning, long-term care, and guilt about outliving other clients began to emerge. Thus services began to respond to new needs generated by changes in the course of HIV infection. In addition to helping end-stage clients take care of unfinished business before dying, services now also helped healthier clients learn to live with AIDS and to plan ahead.

Another factor that has seriously affected AIDS outpatient agencies is the relentless increase in the number of HIV-infected people seeking assistance. Along with the slower client attrition rate due to greater client longevity, agency staff must now cope with rapidly increasing case loads at a time when most agencies do not have the resources to continue expanding staff and volunteers. For example, in 1985 AIDS Project Los Angeles (APLA) had 120 clients. By 1991, the active client case load was nearly 3,000. When APLA started its case-management program in 1986, case managers had an average case load of 75 clients. By 1991, most managers had case loads of 150 to 200. Such numbers preclude a hands-on approach to service delivery for all clients. However, continuous staff expansion is unfeasible due to costs and the large, unwieldy organizational structure such expansion inevitably creates.

By the late 1980s, the demographics of HIV infection began to change. White gay men no longer represented the vast majority of AIDS cases. The Centers for Disease Control reported significant increases in AIDS among women of child-bearing age, many of whom had young children, and among heterosexual substance abusers and people of color, especially African Americans and Hispanics. An increasing number of HIV-infected clients were also homeless or had psychiatric problems. Many clients had multiple and interacting problems such as mental illness, substance abuse, and homelessness, and in some cases several members in one family were HIV symptomatic. These newer client populations come from groups that historically have experienced discrimination and difficulty accessing social services. Their needs are usually numerous, varied, and increasingly complex. Many of these clients live in communities with few resources and little HIV information and expertise. Thus they lack the community support that many gay clients receive.

The change in client demographics poses several dilemmas for service providers. Should gay-oriented organizations retool their programs to accommodate heterosexual clients and, if they do so, to what extent? And how do gay agencies deal with heterophobia? If gay-oriented organizations take on heterosexual clients, will they still be gay agencies or will they become AIDS agencies serving anyone who is HIV infected? If they are AIDS organizations, what is the role of historically dominant populations such as gay staff and volunteers within the agency?

Agencies in smaller, more conservative communities have an advantage in being seen as an AIDS service agency in that such a designation implies that the organization serves all people with AIDS and is not supported by a particular constituency. These distinctions are important when an organization tries to raise money, form alliances and partnerships, conduct outreach programs, and deliver services (Carbine & Lee, 1988). Because no one agency can do it all, AIDS service organizations need to decide what populations they are willing and able to serve and with what types of services.

Some non-AIDS organizations may be better equipped to serve a particular population of HIV-infected persons. A number of agencies in minority communities, substance-abuse treatment and prevention programs, and agencies specializing in service to women or to the homeless have added an HIV component to their existing services because many of their traditional clients are HIV infected and funding became available for these agencies to expand their services. These agencies need to decide how much of a priority HIV services are within their programs and how best to work with AIDS service providers to help educate staff and to coordinate client care.

In 1987, the National AIDS Network sponsored a national conference to develop strategies for how to respond to the AIDS epidemic in the '90s. According to the conference report, participants agreed that no single service-delivery model was appropriate for every community because "services and programs must be tailored to the unique political, economic, cultural and sociodemographic characteristics of the community" (Carbine & Lee, 1988, p. 1). Macks (1987) states that "an effective approach in any community will link hospital based services with public health, mental health and substance abuse systems, private practitioners, community based groups, AIDS agencies, volunteers and representatives of the populations that are most heavily affected by AIDS" (p. 35). Service models also need to be able to change as conditions dictate. Thus "flexibility must be part of all strategic planning, program development, resource mobilization and partnership building initiatives" (Carbine & Lee, 1988, p. 5).

SERVICE MODELS

AIDS service organizations rely heavily on volunteers to provide the majority of direct and indirect services. Professional volunteers provide mental health, legal, insurance, dental, pastoral, and nutritional services, and lay volunteers provide emotional support, socialization, transportation, assistance with household chores, food delivery, hospital visits, and information and referral. Volunteers also assist with clerical work, fund raising, and advocacy. The use of volunteers is not only cost effective, but their presence and commitment enhance agency and client morale.

Most agencies have a volunteer coordinator or department responsible for recruitment, orientation to the agency, maintenance of volunteer records, and volunteer recognition. Volunteer programs are usually supervised by a staff person who is responsible for screening, training, assignment, and ongoing supervision. Personal satisfaction from volunteer activities; easy access to staff for consultation and support; and the quality of a volunteer's relationships with staff, clients, and other volunteers affect volunteer retention. Volunteers need not only support and recognition but also clear expectations and guidelines for their job functions, assistance in establishing well-defined boundaries in their relationships with clients, and easy access to staff should a crisis occur.

Problems occur when volunteers are unclear about their role in the agency, when they do not follow agency policies and procedures, and when staff do not discipline or fire volunteers for inappropriate behavior or poor performance. A volunteer program structure that has good screening, training, supervision, and support components will enhance volunteer retention and decrease burnout. Poor volunteer management leads to high volunteer attrition, thus jeopardizing services and having a negative effect on staff and client morale. Such problems can lead to difficulties in replacing volunteers, especially in smaller cities and rural areas where the volunteer supply may be low.

HIV-infected clients are an invaluable and often underutilized source of volunteers. They can provide a variety of direct and indirect services, bring a unique perspective to program development, and be in a position to reach their peers more effectively. Volunteer work can enhance client self-esteem, help provide structure in the client's daily life, and, unlike a job, give the client more control over the number of hours he or she is able to give. HIV-infected client volunteers wanting to work in programs that require more intense personal contact with other clients need to be carefully screened and monitored to ensure that countertransference issues do not interfere with work. Contingency plans also need to be made should the client volunteer develop serious health problems during the course of volunteer work.

EMPOWERMENT MODELS

Partnership or client-empowerment models are especially helpful to people with AIDS, particularly because clients are living longer and healthier lives and are capable of doing more for themselves. A partnership model "promotes alliances between those providing services and those receiving them" (Carbine & Lee, 1988, p. 16). Rather than telling clients what's best for them, service providers give clients information, present options, assist with skill building, and then allow clients to decide what they want to do. Such strategies help clients escape from the victim mind-set and its ensuing feelings of helplessness by giving them a sense of power and control over their lives.

Agencies with a diverse clientele require a service model that can accommodate more self-sufficient, lower-need clients as well as those who have greater needs and are less able to manage their lives without assistance. At APLA, for example, when a new client registers with the agency, the intake department assesses the client's needs, then determines if the client should be assigned a case manager. Clients with fewer resources or more complex needs may be permanently assigned to a specialist or generalist case manager. Specialists have expertise in a specific area such as non–English-speaking clients, the homeless, or the chronically mentally ill. They also have consistent cooperative relationships with agencies that work with those populations. Clients can be assigned temporarily to a case manager until their current needs are met.

Clients not assigned to case management are given the information they need at the time. Then, via client-education forums, the client-information line, legal/public benefits, and insurance counselors, they are able to access the necessary skills and information to meet their needs independently. Phone volunteers provide ongoing client contact to ensure that clients do not fall through cracks in the system. This is especially important for clients who are isolated, do not have a strong support system, or are uncomfortable in seeking assistance. If, at any time, the client's family, friends, or volunteers feel the client's needs have changed, the intake department will reassess that client and, if it is deemed appropriate, will assign a case manager.

ADVOCACY

Many of the larger AIDS service providers are becoming more involved in influencing public policy. Advocating for individuals can be very time consuming and does not address problems and inequities inherent in existing public social service systems. Public policy staff and volunteers work to change local, state, and national systems in ways that benefit numerous clients. For example, the recent passage of the Americans with Disabilities Act protects all physically challenged individuals from discrimination, including people with HIV infection. AIDS service providers participated in lobbying for passage of this legislation.

Because no single agency can provide all the necessary services, a successful service model must include collaborative relationships with other service providers. Such efforts are essential to the delivery of coordinated care to all clients. Building coalitions can help AIDS service providers influence policy and community programs, define HIV as a community rather than an interest-group problem, and help raise funds and influence how funds are allocated (Carbine & Lee, 1988).

EVALUATION

To maintain a successful service model, agencies must implement evaluation and quality-assurance mechanisms to determine which programs and service-delivery strategies are working and to monitor staff and volunteer efforts. Evaluation need not be overly complex and time consuming. It can be as simple as regularly reviewing client files, calling randomly selected clients on a regular basis to see how satisfied they are with services, and monitoring complaints and service-utilization rates.

Within the basic structure of a volunteer-based, client-empowerment model, agencies can employ various treatment modalities. Choices must take into consideration available resources, accessibility to clients, client needs, and cultural differences. Because it would be impractical to discuss modalities for all the needs that clients present, this chapter limits discussion to strategies for information and referral, case management, food, shelter, transportation, emotional support, and advocacy programs.

AIDS service providers utilize several methods to provide information and referral to clients along the entire spectrum of HIV infection. Several communities operate publicly funded HIV hotlines staffed primarily by trained volunteers. These hotlines provide HIV transmission and treatment information as well as referrals to a wide variety of community services available to clients, friends, and families. Hotline volunteers undergo intensive training and are closely supervised by agency staff. Some communities also have HIV hotlines staffed by volunteers who speak Spanish or other foreign languages or they may have a transmission device for the deaf or hearing impaired. The APLA has tape recorded HIV information in several Asian Pacific languages and dialects in conjunction with bilingual/bicultural HIV-sensitive community agencies that persons can call for more detailed information or services. The advantage of hotlines, especially those with toll-free numbers, is that they are easy to access and the caller can remain anonymous. Confidentiality is important because of the stigma attached to HIV and the discomfort most people experience when discussing sexual behaviors.

PSYCHOEDUCATION

Educational forums such as those developed by APLA or time-limited, structured psychoeducational groups such as those used by the University of California–San Francisco's AIDS Health Project provide information and skill building to

clients in a safe, supportive setting. The APLA has monthly forums on public benefits, insurance issues, safer sex, nutrition, legal issues, stress and symptom management, and clinical drug-treatment trials. These forums, presented by staff and volunteers, educate clients in a more time-efficient manner and empower them to make
informed decisions, then act upon them. Clients who require more assistance are
referred to other staff or to agencies that can assist them. This system frees staff
from having to go over basic information with clients individually and therefore
allows them to spend more time with clients whose situations are more complicated
or who lack the resources to function independently.

San Francisco's AIDS Health Project uses an eight-week psychoeducational
group model that deals with basic HIV information, safer sex, and stress management with a problem-solving approach. This structured group provides information,
emotional support, and skill-building activities. A short-term approach not only is
cost effective but also allows time for practicing new skills and group bonding,
while precluding the development of dependence on the facilitator or other group
members (Acevedo, 1989).

OUTREACH

Street outreach programs have been very effective in engaging and educating
hard-to-reach populations such as the homeless, runaway youth, substance abusers,
and people who trade sex for drugs or money. Many of these clients do not trust
institutions and often do not seek assistance unless they feel providers are trustworthy and nonjudgmental. The fact that staff or volunteers make a consistent effort to
reach out to clients who traditionally have felt alienated from care providers con-
veys a credible message of care and concern and facilitates the building of trust.
Outreach workers who at one time were part of the targeted population are especially helpful because they understand the needs of the population. Moreover, they have
greater credibility and function as positive role models.

CASE MANAGEMENT

Case management is an integral part of nearly all outpatient services. By 1988,
the U.S. Public Health Service and the Robert Wood Johnson Foundation had funded 22 AIDS service-delivery demonstration projects (Report of the Presidential
Commission, 1988). All projects were required to have a case-management component to ensure continuity of care. The primary functions of case management
include the following: assessment, planning and coordination of services, monitoring services, and following the client's medical and psychosocial condition (Muk-
and, Starkson, & Melvin, 1991). Many case managers will also provide advocacy
for the client and his or her support system.

Although few disagree on the necessity of the above functions, professionals
have not reached consensus as to how these functions should be implemented. For
example, at one agency, linking a client with a needed resource such as the Social
Security office can include anything from giving the client the name and telephone

number of a contact person to making an appointment for the client, transporting the client to the Social Security office, and assisting with the paperwork. Case managers whose case loads are light may be able and inclined to provide more hands-on assistance. Such services are not likely to be possible in agencies with heavy case loads.

In some large urban areas, such as New York and Los Angeles, not all clients are assigned to a case manager or they are assigned on a temporary basis to take care of immediate needs only. In communities where several agencies provide case management but not all agencies provide it in the same way, services may be duplicated unnecessarily and clients who are receiving services from several agencies may become confused. In these situations, case managers need to explain clearly to their clients how case management is defined and implemented in each agency and who is eligible for those services. Agencies also need to decide who will be responsible for managing the cases of clients who use services from more than one agency.

NECESSITIES OF LIFE

Basic necessities such as food and affordable housing or shelter are essential client services. Most clients are on fixed incomes and have difficulty making ends meet, especially if they are also paying for a portion of their medical care. In the early years of its existence, APLA purchased food vouchers to distribute to low-income clients. The vouchers could be used to purchase food as well as necessities such as soap and toilet paper. As the number of clients increased, the agency could no longer afford to purchase food vouchers. Thus, the Necessities of Life Program (NOLP), a mini-grocery store/food pantry, was created. The NOLP is subsidized by donations, small grants, and purchases through wholesale distributors or food pantry coalitions. Volunteers coordinate weekend food drives to obtain donated items. They also stock shelves as well as pack groceries that clients order in response to lists distributed weekly and monthly. A ride-share board is available for clients who do not have transportation. As APLA's clients have diversified, so have NOLP items. Some ethnic food products and personal items for women are now available. Clients who are too ill to cook are referred to agencies that provide free or low-cost home-delivered meals.

Affordable transitional and permanent housing are important services because so many HIV-infected homeless people are too ill to continue living on the streets and many AIDS clients lose their current housing when they begin receiving public benefits. Education and developing collaborative relationships with local homeless- and shelter-service providers help to generate more resources for clients. Some agencies have started their own HIV shelters or transitional-living programs. Others have bulletin boards and newsletters whereby clients can advertise for housing or roommates. Being Alive, an AIDS organization in Los Angeles, offers a roommate referral service, and Shanti, in San Francisco, provides low-cost permanent housing in small-group living situations. The APLA started its own government-subsidized housing program.

When clients can no longer afford to maintain their own vehicles or become too ill to drive or use public transportation, they need to find someone who can regularly provide such services. A variety of community resources may be available to assist these clients. Most public transportation systems offer discounts to the physically challenged, and some community agencies sell low-cost taxi and medi-van coupons or coordinate ride-share programs. The APLA has started its own volunteer transportation program, wherein volunteers transport clients to medical appointments and occasionally to support groups. Agencies with large case loads cannot always guarantee volunteer drivers for all client requests, so it is best to offer a variety of options. Smaller agencies may choose to finance their own van and driver, but repair, insurance, and maintenance costs can make this option impractical.

EMOTIONAL SUPPORT SERVICES

Emotional support and counseling services are often needed by clients and their loved ones during all phases of the illness. Most people are devastated by the disease and its ensuing psychosocial problems. In May 1991, APLA polled 500 clients, nearly half of whom were women and people of color. Survey results showed that emotional support was one of the most important services the agency provided. Most HIV service providers offer a combination of lay and professional staff and volunteer programs.

Support groups for clients, families, and partners remain one of the most cost-effective treatment interventions. Groups offset isolation and offer additional support by providing clients with the opportunity to discuss issues with others experiencing similar problems. When groups focus on information sharing, emotional support, problem solving, and enhancement of coping skills, they empower clients to manage their lives. Useful group modalities include cognitive behavioral therapy and self-help (Macks, 1989). Groups may be ongoing or time limited, drop-in or closed membership, or focused on specific client populations such as women or persons with impaired vision due to retinitis.

Due to the diversity of its clients, APLA offers a variety of support groups. Drop-in groups are useful for people who need immediate support or who feel unable to make a regular, ongoing commitment. Most APLA clients prefer ongoing, closed support groups that focus on emotional support, problem solving, information sharing, and enhancement of coping skills. Professional mental health staff and volunteers facilitate these groups and thus require less training and supervision than group facilitators who have no experience in the mental health field. Some advantages to using mental health professionals include their expertise in assessment, group process, and management of countertransference as well as their ability to provide clinical interventions should the need arise.

For closed groups the intake process is essential for screening out inappropriate clients or those who are unable to benefit from the group experience. The intake process also alleviates client anxiety about the group, allows clients to make informed decisions about their participation in a group, and cuts down on group attrition.

Using a longer-term group model allows clients to establish relationships with one another and to resolve more complex issues. In order to expand member support

33

outside the group meetings, participants are encouraged to socialize with one another between meetings and to pool their transportation resources. When clients become too ill to leave home or when they have lengthy hospital stays, other group members, with the ill client's permission, often decide to hold the group meeting at that member's home or hospital room. Such efforts send a message to all members that the same support will be available to them if they become too ill to go out on their own. Thus homebound clients do not feel abandoned by the group and consequently have to experience yet another loss.

The primary disadvantage to ongoing closed groups is that some clients experience difficulties if they outlive several other members of the group. The multiple losses and the emotional energy required to reinvest in new members takes its toll. These clients may decide eventually to drop out of the group. Should this occur, it is important for group members to have the opportunity to say good-bye and to provide departing clients with other support options.

Counseling services, particularly crisis intervention, are an integral part of emotional support services. Medical and psychosocial crises often lead to anxiety, depression, suicidal ideation, or, for some clients, alcohol and drug abuse. Most agencies find it impractical to offer long-term counseling. Clients requesting more intensive therapy are referred to private practitioners or community mental health centers. Most AIDS service providers have a list of affordable, HIV-sensitive, and knowledgeable mental health practitioners who can be easily accessed by clients. Innovative programs such as Los Angeles' Pacific Counseling Center and San Francisco's AIDS Health Project have recruited therapists to see one client at no charge. These programs screen and match clients with a therapist, then monitor the outcome. Northern Lights, also in Los Angeles, runs a similar program for clients who are homebound. Their volunteer therapists provide counseling services in the client's home. Many agencies also have licensed mental health staff or volunteers supervise mental health interns who provide group and individual treatment. Intern programs are not only cost effective, but they can also help offset staff burnout and create future volunteers or referral sources.

VOLUNTEER SUPPORT SERVICES

For clients who do not require counseling but are feeling isolated or for clients who are unwilling to burden a support system they feel is already overwhelmed by AIDS, HIV service providers have created a variety of nonprofessional volunteer support programs. "Buddy" programs exist in HIV service agencies across the country. A buddy volunteer is a trained layperson assigned to a client to provide emotional support, social contact, and assistance with practical needs such as grocery shopping or sorting through medical bills. Buddies usually have weekly contact with their clients, either in the client's home, by telephone, or an outing. As clients live longer, buddy relationships can last several months to a few years. Because buddies are lay volunteers and their client contacts occur outside the agency, most programs do not assign buddies to clients who have a documented history of violent behavior, ongoing substance abuse, or an unstable psychiatric condition. Agency staff supervise the buddies and provide clinical backup when clients experience severe HIV dementia, suicidal ideation, or when buddies have difficulty with countertransference issues.

Telephone volunteer programs are helpful to homebound clients and to those in rural areas far from services. The APLA phone volunteers come to the agency weekly to call their clients, who are contacted twice a month or more frequently if the client needs more contact. Telephone volunteers not only provide emotional support, but also alert agency staff to changes in the clients' status that may require staff intervention.

In order to provide support and socialization to hospitalized AIDS clients, APLA developed a hospital visitation program. The APLA obtained permission to station trained volunteers at hospitals on a regular basis. Each hospital assigned a staff person, usually a nurse or social worker, to be the volunteer's hospital contact and to orient the volunteer to the hospital, staff, and procedures for treating AIDS patients. Volunteers also "float" to unassigned hospitals if a patient calls the agency and requests a visit. For many patients, the volunteer is their first contact with APLA. Volunteer reports on agency clients also help keep staff informed of their clients' progress and possible service needs upon discharge.

Partners of people with AIDS also require emotional support. In addition to partner, couples, and bereavement groups and counseling services, APLA has a buddy program for partners called Significant Others for Each Other (SOFEO). These volunteers are people who have lost a partner to AIDS at least a year prior to the time they become volunteers. They provide emotional peer support to other partners who are in their first year of bereavement or who are caring for someone who is ill. The primary appeal of the program is being able to talk to someone who has already gone through a similar experience. For family members, comparable peer-support programs such as Mothers of AIDS Patients and Families Who Care are available.

ADVOCACY SERVICES

Advocacy programs that assist clients with legal, insurance, and public-benefits issues are also important services. For clients who are more self-sufficient, educational workshops can provide basic information. Staff and volunteer specialists can then provide individual services to clients with specific or more complex needs and to advocate on an individual basis for them if they are having difficulties obtaining services from other agencies.

At APLA, staff and volunteers working directly with clients document trends and recurrent social, legal, and health-care-system problems. Armed with this information, APLA's public policy department can then advocate for legislation, policy, or funding that will help change systems in ways that benefit clients. In addition to policy analysis, lobbying, and coalition building, APLA has also developed the Citizen's Network. This program consists of a large group of volunteers who, when notified by public policy staff, write and call elected officials at all levels of government to urge them to vote for or against proposed legislation affecting HIV clients. Such efforts also help generate more funds for service delivery, make more services available, or provide easier access to services, thus enabling staff, clients, and volunteers to feel more empowered.

ORGANIZATIONAL ISSUES

Working as an HIV service provider, especially in an AIDS service agency, presents unique personal, professional, and organizational challenges. Unlike most work settings, volunteers and co-workers are often affected by the same illness as the clients. Many staff and volunteers are dealing with HIV in their personal life, either as a result of their own infection and illness or that of a partner, family member, or friends. Many workers feel that they can't get away from the illness, that it encroaches into all areas of their life. Thus, service providers often experience an issue paralleling that of their clients—how to live with HIV infection.

Service providers must cope continuously with loss and grief, often without even having the opportunity to say good-bye to clients or to close their relationships with staff and volunteers who become too ill to continue working. Simultaneously, they must reinvest in relationships with new clients, staff, and volunteers before they are able to finish grieving over personal losses. Thus, staff are very vulnerable to burnout. Staff may become less empathic and more aloof in an effort to distance themselves from painful feelings. They may also become irritable, angry, and judgmental, especially with clients who are manipulative, demanding, and seemingly ungrateful, or they may overidentify with clients and develop co-dependent relationships.

Staff may also displace their anger and frustration onto the agency, attempting to compensate for their feelings of powerlessness by inappropriately trying to dictate agency policy or by making unrealistic demands on agency resources. Staff need to be supported and given opportunities to express their feelings constructively. If they are not given such opportunities, morale drops, the quality of work declines, and people eventually leave the agency with bad feelings.

Agency administrators need to create programs, policies, and procedures to help staff cope with these painful issues. Management style should focus on team building and staff empowerment. Discussions during staff meetings and individual supervision, support groups facilitated by an outside professional during work hours, and employee assistance programs can help make staff members aware of their feelings and provide safe outlets for expressing their emotions.

Staff also need to feel heard, supported, and empowered by agency administrators. They need to have their efforts acknowledged, to know that they are making a difference, and to feel that they have some control over their work lives. This can be accomplished by assisting staff with stress and time management, providing in-service education, funding staff to attend conferences, requiring that staff take their vacations, avoiding overtime, and making job expectations clear. Involving staff in program design, planning, and the development of policies and procedures that affect their work also provide staff with a greater sense of control and ownership of their work.

Having several employees with AIDS can create managerial dilemmas when these employees become too ill to perform their jobs. Work is often a source of self-esteem and a measure of one's health. It may be difficult for an employee who is ill to acknowledge that his or her job performance may be deteriorating along with his or her health. Managers need to approach this situation with sensitivity and care. It is best to be honest with an employee when reviewing job performance and to help the employee review possible options, such as part-time work or a change in job duties. Co-workers can become resentful if they have to take on an unmanageable share of someone else's work, yet feel guilty about saying anything because that co-worker is ill. Budgeting for temporary staff or building a volunteer backup system are other possible solutions.

Another issue that affects HIV service providers, especially in gay or smaller communities, is the blurring of boundaries between one's personal life and work. Staff have reported running into their clients at the gym, the grocery store, or at bars and social events. Such encounters appear to be more awkward for staff than for clients. Staff say they feel inhibited and uncomfortable. They do not feel free to behave in any way that they perceive weakens their professional image. Some staff have discovered that they have personal or business relationships with friends of their clients, so they worry about accidentally breaching confidentiality or having a conflict of interest. Such situations are bound to occur, but it is helpful if the supervisor is sensitive to the issues and provides opportunities for staff to discuss them and obtain feedback and support.

Just as mainstream organizations have had to become more sensitive to gay and HIV issues, HIV service providers are now finding that they must also diversify their own staff, volunteers, and board members in order better to serve their more varied clientele and to remain competitive for funding. This transition has not been easy, because it requires AIDS service providers to become more culturally sensitive to groups with whom they have not developed close relationships in the past. Most HIV services were started *by* white gay men *for* white gay men. Though AIDS is not a gay disease, gay persons have understandably felt a certain ownership of HIV services. In traditionally gay agencies, it may be difficult to hire staff who come with varying perspectives as well as to work with clients with diverse values, needs, and communication styles. Sharing power and control with these newer groups has created tension, resistance, and a sense of loss for senior staff and volunteers, who may talk about "the good old days." However, successful resolution of these differences can be a powerful and positive experience for staff who learn to respect differences and find ways to work together.

CONCLUSION

Despite the increasing number of AIDS cases and the impact on every segment of society, the United States has not yet developed a national plan for managing the HIV epidemic and fighting further spread of HIV infection. As public funding for health and social services decreases, AIDS service organizations are forced to try to fill the gaps, often without having the resources to do so. As an agency's clientele becomes more diverse, so must its board, staff, volunteers, funding sources, and service models. No single segment of society can or should bear the major responsibility for the service needs of HIV-infected persons and their loved ones.

The U.S. Public Health Service (1986) issued the Coolfont Report, a plan for preventing and controlling AIDS. Their recommendations for health care also apply to social services. The report concluded that the response to AIDS must "reflect the pluralistic character of the American health care system and must involve the coordinated participation of the public, private and voluntary sectors" (p. 348). Only with the cooperation and mobilization of diverse social groups, systems, and institutions can our society provide consistent, quality care for everyone who is affected by HIV/AIDS. Without leadership from the federal government, it is unlikely that coordinated efforts of this magnitude will occur.

REFERENCES

Acevedo, J. (1989). A group model for AIDS prevention and support. In J. W. Dilley, C. Pies, & M. Helquist (Eds.), *Face to face: A guide to AIDS counseling*. San Francisco: AIDS Health Project, University of California, San Francisco.

Carbine, M. E., & Lee, P. (1988, January). *AIDS into the 90s: Strategies for an integrated response to the AIDS epidemic*. Washington DC: National AIDS Network.

Centers for Disease Control. (1991a, June 17). *AIDS weekly report*. Atlanta, GA: Author.

Centers for Disease Control. (1991b, October). *HIV/AIDS surveillance report*. Atlanta, GA: Author.

Macks, J. (1987). Meeting the psychosocial needs of people with AIDS. In C. Leukefeld & M. Fimbres (Eds.), *Responding to AIDS: Psychosocial initiatives*. Silver Spring, MD: National Association of Social Workers.

Macks, J. (1989). The psychosocial needs of people with AIDS. In J. W. Dilly, C. Pies, & M. Helquist (Eds.), *Face to face: A guide to AIDS counseling*. San Francisco: AIDS Health Project, University of California, San Francisco.

Mukand, J., Starkson, E., & Melvin, J. (1991). Public policy issues for the rehabilitation of patients with HIV-related disability. In J. Mukand (Ed.), *Rehabilitation for patients with HIV disease*. New York: McGraw-Hill.

Report of the Presidential Commission on the Human Immunodeficiency Virus Epidemic. (1988, June 24). Washington, DC: U.S. Government Printing Office.

U.S. Public Health Service. (1986, July–August). Coolfont report: A PHS plan for prevention and control of AIDS and the AIDS virus. *Public Health Reports, 101*, 341–348.

3

AIDS IN HOSPITAL AND ACUTE-CARE SETTINGS: THE SOCIAL WORK PERSPECTIVE

CATHERINE STERNBERG

Hospitals were the first systems to be affected by the AIDS epidemic, which had an overwhelming impact on physicians, nurses, hospital staff in general, and social workers. With AIDS and HIV, hospitals had more medical questions than answers. Personnel and community resources were inadequate, and the epidemic generated a tremendous amount of negative emotion and fear, not only from outside the hospital setting but also from within. During the early years of the AIDS health crisis, hospitalization for patients with AIDS was generally long term, in part because of the lack of community resources available for aftercare. As a result of the great number of cases diagnosed in areas such as New York City and San Francisco, with the backing of local and state government, eventually home-care and alternative-living programs were developed and support networks established to handle the emotional impact of this disease. Mid-size cities, however, were much slower to develop programs and even now struggle with lack of resources. For example, Denver has approximately 10,000–12,000 new HIV-positive cases and 350 new AIDS cases diagnosed yearly. However, the city has only three alternative intermediate living facilities with approximately 30 beds and three skilled nursing homes that will provide care for patients with AIDS. The local AIDS organizations, which provide various services for people diagnosed with HIV or AIDS, have had their budgets reduced or eliminated as a result of funding cutbacks by state and local governments, even though the number of persons newly diagnosed has risen.

Many hospitals, such as St. Joseph Hospital in Denver, do not have a specific unit for patients diagnosed with HIV or AIDS. The decision not to have such units is often made to eliminate the stigma attached to a particular disease and to ensure confidentiality of diagnosis. In addition, AIDS patients require extensive care; by not designating a unit or a staff to provide exclusive care for them, AIDS patient care is distributed more evenly among staff and less burnout occurs.

At St. Joseph Hospital an AIDS task force was developed early to deal specifically with problems created by the epidemic. The task force suggested policies to the hospital administration concerning patient care, patient and staff rights, laboratory procedures and precautions, and so forth. Although the task force could not mandate policy, it was able to initiate substantial changes with regard to these issues. The task force was a multidisciplinary team, similar to the teams utilized for caring for AIDS patients within the hospital. Teams include physicians, including specialists in infectious disease, pulmonology, oncology, internal medicine, and psychiatry; nursing staff; physical, occupational, and respiratory therapists; pastoral care counselors; home health care coordinators; and social workers.

Although St. Joseph Hospital attempted to respond quickly to the needs of persons with AIDS, patient needs were not met consistently throughout the hospital departments or units. For example, attitudes regarding homosexuality and the potential influence of those attitudes on patient care and the fear of contagion by hospital staff were not adequately addressed by hospital policies. Despite hospital infection-control guidelines, many staff members were distrustful of the information that was provided.

THE PROFESSIONAL'S ROLE

Referrals of HIV-positive and AIDS patients to social workers can be made in various ways and through various sources. Weekly team-care meetings are held in order to identify problem areas that may affect patient care during hospitalization or with discharge planning. The nursing staff, because of their close relationship with patients, can sometimes pick up information that is useful to other professionals. Team-care meetings provide a good forum for discussing potential problems before a crisis develops. Diagnosis of AIDS is now viewed as a risk factor that warrants an initial evaluation and assessment by a social worker. Patients are typically identified through physician referrals, interdisciplinary rounds, or through the utilization review process. Patients and families are given information about social work services upon admission; they often self-refer.

In some hospitals, policies dictate that only physicians can initiate referrals to other members of the team. However, such policies inhibit social work intervention in that physicians often have little time to spend with patients. Moreover, doctors' focus during time spent with patients is generally related to medical aspects of the disease, an inadequate approach given the diverse physical, social, and emotional problems experienced by persons with AIDS.

The hospital social worker is often the first nonmedical staff person to see the AIDS patient, especially if the person has not sought services in the community. The first hospitalization is a very difficult experience for a person diagnosed with AIDS. Often, hospitalization represents the first confirmation of the diagnosis. At this time, patients must deal with the physical impact of the disease as well as with emotional reactions, changes in their role performance, and changes in their relationships with others (Furstenberg & Olson, 1984). Many AIDS patients have suspected the diagnosis for some time but have been afraid to see a physician to confirm their suspicions. Many people of color felt AIDS was a disease that affected whites and gays and thus did not relate directly to them.

Denial of the diagnosis and its implications is common initially. For some people, denial continues throughout the treatment phase of the disease. Young people who are diagnosed as HIV positive or with AIDS are forced to confront a terminal disease at a stage in their lives when they may feel "invincible." Patients experience anger and depression. Multiple hospitalizations are common as a result of acute episodic illnesses, thus exacerbating feelings of loss and powerlessness. The role of hospital social workers is to normalize and validate such feelings.

Feeling a lack of control and a sense of powerlessness over one's life is caused by various aspects of the disease and its treatment. Hospitals, however, can exacerbate such feelings among patients. Patients may feel that they are being constantly bombarded by staff at all hours of day and night for the monitoring of vital signs, taking samples and specimens for laboratory tests, examinations by numerous medical personnel, and interventions by respiratory therapists, dieticians, and social workers. If patients refuse interventions they can be labeled "noncompliant" by staff.

Sometimes patients are rendered powerless by a lack of information. Although many physicians and other medical staff take the time to explain the purpose of tests, medications, or treatment, some do not. Many diagnostic and treatment procedures elicit fear because patients do not know what to anticipate. Furstenberg and Olson (1984) state,

> Social workers may have to act to help patients exercise as much control over their diagnostic workup and treatment as they want. Direct and straightforward communication with patients to encourage and support their efforts to communicate with physicians and other health care staff may be required (p. 52).

Social workers can help health care staff understand how patients may feel violated by procedures that they do not understand; workers thus can assist medical staff in working more fully with patients. Social workers can facilitate discussions during patient–staff conferences and can help the patient prepare for such conferences through role-playing activities. Patients may be reticent about bringing up care issues or concerns with their physicians or with nursing staff out of fear that their care will be compromised. Social workers can alleviate such fears by bridging the gap in communication between the patient and staff.

Information can help patients reacquire a sense of control over their life in general and medial treatments in particular. For example,

> a young black male refused to allow staff to insert a central intravenous (IV) line that would make it easier for the staff to draw blood and more comfortable for the patient to receive IV medications and transfusions. The staff were unaware of the patient's fear of the procedure and his perception of loss of body image. The social worker was able to help the patient understand what to expect and reassure him that such feelings and responses were normal.

As do other chronic, progressive diseases, AIDS brings life changes that require patients to make alterations in many areas of their lives. Often, the need for

41

these changes becomes evident when symptoms are most acute and the individual requires hospitalization. At such times, patients may need a wide range of services, such as financial assistance, legal services, housing, home health care, long-term care, hospice care, child care, and transportation. Social workers' knowledge of community resources as well as of the psychosocial implications of AIDS places them in an ideal position to link patients with resources. Sometimes, however, social workers need to go beyond established programs and find creative solutions to unique problems that may arise for individuals in this population group.

People with AIDS often face severe financial crises as a result of job loss due to multiple hospitalizations and progressive debilitation. For many patients this occurs at a point in their life when their career and financial status have just begun to solidify. Due to their impaired ability to work and to depleted funds, patients may suddenly need to apply for state and federal disability funds. Regardless, it is essential that patients obtain financial assistance as quickly as possible to avoid lapses in insurance premiums and disruptions in other critical areas of their lives. Health insurance coverage becomes a critical issue as patients face the expenses of medications, hospitalization, and outpatient services.

Public fear about contagion may make it difficult for AIDS patients to obtain housing. For persons who are in a stable housing situation, financial stresses can make it difficult to meet their rent or mortgage payments. Also, the physical layout of the residence (e.g., stairs, bedroom and bath on upper level) can make it impossible for persons with AIDS to remain in their home.

Alternative housing options are inadequate, forcing some patients to remain in unsafe or difficult living situations. Patients are currently being discharged from hospitals more quickly than ever before. As a result, they require more follow-up care at home, sometimes as a transition to independent care. Most persons with AIDS have home-care needs when they leave the hospital. For example, they may need IV medications that require instruction and monitoring by a home health care professional. Depending on the patient's support system, the extent of home care needs may vary from intermittent weekly visits to 24-hour care. Agencies such as visiting nurse organizations have formed special teams that work specifically with AIDS patients. However, such services may provide insufficient home care due to inadequate insurance reimbursements and the personal financial limits of patients. Family, friends, and volunteer agencies are often asked to pick up the burdens of home-care needs. Social workers can coordinate services and care needs by helping patients and families develop a care plan, thereby enhancing physical and psychological well-being.

Helping patients attend to legal concerns is another area in which hospital social workers can provide service. Living wills, power of attorney, wills, and child custody after the death of a parent are important legal issues for persons hospitalized with AIDS-related illnesses. Social workers can encourage and assist patients to attend to legal matters early. By outlining the legal options available for the patient, workers encourage patients to address important issues before it is too late. Legal assistance is especially important for gay patients who wish their partners to retain power of attorney, in that the gay relationship is not protected by law. Legal documentation can protect patients from their family intervening in their affairs if such is their wish (Macks, 1989). In some instances, a lover or a close friend has received no inheritance because a will was not completed even though that person may have been the patient's only caregiver prior to death.

In many hospitals, the social worker's primary goal (as defined by the hospital) is discharge planning. Hospitals emphasize early discharge while trying to provide necessary physical and emotional supports to patients in order to obviate unnecessary readmissions. Because of the time constraints imposed on social workers by the hospital system, discharge planning is often viewed as planned short-term intervention. Patients and families should be told as soon as it is medically appropriate that they need to look at care alternatives, to solve problems, and to determine mutually agreed-upon goals.

During the early years of the AIDS epidemic, appropriate resources and services for people with AIDS were often unavailable. Untimely provision of financial assistance, housing, skilled nursing home care, and hospice services caused substantial delays in patient planning. Because AIDS patients require extensive care and services from various agencies, even now it is difficult to connect patients to services that will meet all their needs. Mantell, Shulman, Belmont, and Spivak (1989) state that problems related to agencies outside the hospital system, such as bureaucratic delays in approval of Medicaid benefits, and programs for home care followup, such as home care allowance and home- and community-based services through the department of social services, present barriers to appropriate and timely posthospital planning. In addition, lack of appropriate intermediate care facilities and the unwillingness of skilled nursing facilities to provide beds for people with AIDS continue to be obstacles to discharge of these patients.

With other community agencies, social workers need to advocate for patients by identifying gaps in services and by mobilizing resources in an effort to establish programs for this population group. Social workers must assume the role of community advocate as well as that of the skilled clinician who addresses psychosocial issues.

The strength of the patient's support system plays a critical role in the timeliness of patient discharge. Patients with strong, intact support systems often return home with few problems. Patients with minimal or weak support systems, however, have fewer alternatives for post-hospital care. Some cultural groups place a higher value on family interdependence than they do on self-reliance and autonomy (De La Cancela, 1989). For example, if the person with AIDS is Hispanic, a culture that values family bonds highly, family members can play an important role in developing care plans. Such bonds often override negative feelings and beliefs regarding homosexuality and AIDS.

Today, many patients with AIDS are either caring for or being cared for by someone who has also been diagnosed as HIV positive. In such cases, the caregiver with AIDS may at some point lose the physical stamina necessary to provide adequate care, even though the caregiver may remain emotionally supportive of the other. Conversely, in families that are physically able to handle the day-to-day care, members may be afraid of contracting the disease or have unresolved emotional conflicts that prohibit them from providing care.

A person caring for someone with AIDS experiences the same burdens and strains that confront caregivers of other chronically ill people. To provide care, they may need to restructure their personal and social lives, which in turn may adversely affect their employment and cause financial hardship. Reorganizing one's life can lead to emotional and physical exhaustion (Raveis & Siegel, 1991). For example, one mother who ran a hairdressing business out of her home eventually refused to care for her son because she was afraid that her clients would be infected or that she would lose them due to their fear of contagion. In another situation, three gay men, all diagnosed with AIDS, found it increasingly difficult to manage one another's care, especially as each became more symptomatic. And a family who outwardly expressed support and a desire to be totally involved with their son who had AIDS refused to allow him to interact with the young children in the family because of their fear of contagion. The social worker must be able to tolerate shifting scenarios or ambiguities in finding the best solution to diverse problems.

INTERVENTION MODALITIES

GROUP INTERVENTION

Because both patients and families experience a sense of isolation and aloneness as well as intense feelings or emotions related to HIV or AIDS diagnosis, support groups work well with this population. Participation in groups provides patients and families with an outlet to express their feelings and to share experiences with others who are experiencing similar problems. Kelly and Sykes (1989) state,

> Families sometimes need help not only in dealing with AIDS but also with their feelings about homosexuality and drug abuse. A support group can provide an opportunity for the members to ventilate their feelings about these situations and learn how others dealt with similar ones (p. 241).

Groups can also help patients establish a measure of control over their lives and help others who are coping less well. Various community groups, as well as hospitals, provide support groups not only for patients with AIDS but for families, partners, and friends. Social workers can use the group setting as both a means and context for achieving individual and group objectives for the purpose of growth and change.

In some instances, however, groups may not be as successful within the hospital setting as they are in community settings. Hospitals may be seen as good, safe places to go when one is sick or symptomatic, but when a person with AIDS is doing well, the hospital may be a reminder of times when the disease is active. Often, patients tend to move toward groups that are not affiliated with the hospital, if such options exist. However, the hospital setting can be used to link families with other families in a peer-counseling relationship, that is, a parent-to-parent group. Some families may not wish to become involved in a group yet have a strong need to relate to someone who understands their problems and emotions on a one-to-one basis.

FAMILY INTERVENTION

Working with the families of AIDS patients may be as important as is working directly with the patient. The problems and issues that arise as a result of an AIDS diagnosis create intense stress among family members. Families as well as patients are confronted with a homophobic society and consequent fear of social rejection. A gay or bisexual son may not have revealed his homosexuality to family or friends out of fear of rejection or condemnation. Thus, parents may be faced with the diagnosis of AIDS and disclosure of their son's homosexual life-style simultaneously.

Under the best of circumstances, family conflicts are normal; however, an illness as emotionally laden as AIDS can exacerbate latent conflicts and stress. Reactions to an AIDS diagnosis and/or revelation of homosexuality vary enormously from family to family, but generally stem from families' belief system or religious orientation. Some families report having had previous knowledge or suspicions of the son's homosexuality while choosing not to discuss it because they did not want to open issues that they were not ready to confront. Other families may feel that AIDS is God's punishment to homosexuals and that the patient brought the problem on himself. Still other families feel guilt and self-blame for being inadequate parents and for causing their son's homosexuality and ultimately his diagnosis of AIDS.

Families need encouragement and support to express the hurt, anger, and fear they are experiencing as a result of the diagnosis. Fathers often have the most difficulty resolving their feelings about their son, whereas mothers typically revert to some degree to their care-taking role. Social workers need to help families identify their conflicting emotions and help them make sense of and establish some control over their overwhelming situation.

Many families who are seen at large metropolitan hospitals live in small rural communities that may be less tolerant of alternative life-styles. Parents from these communities may have less exposure to information regarding HIV and AIDS and consequently may have misconceptions regarding transmission and contagion. Social workers need to reeducate families about the disease and help them feel more comfortable about providing care for the patient.

Families also need support and assistance in dealing with friends and neighbors. Often, families are forced to cope with the emotional reactions of others at a time when they have not resolved issues for themselves. Moreover, intervention needs to be culturally sensitive. For example,

> In minority cultures, especially Latino, discussion of homosexual activity or communication between men and women or parents and children regarding sex is supposedly not the norm. Other cultural factors that supposedly inhibit AIDS awareness include fatalism, Catholicism, machismo and familism (De La Cancela, 1989, p. 143).

Social workers need to provide culture-specific interventions to obtain optimal results.

If patients have been separated from their families as a result of conflicts or geographical factors, spouses, partners, or friends may assume a more primary role in the patient's life. The social worker needs to learn which "family" patients most closely align themselves with so that the patients' interests remain the focus of the intervention (Kelly & Sykes, 1989). Early in the AIDS epidemic, hospital social workers needed to advocate for patients within the hospital setting to expand the definition of family to include partners and friends as well as family. Today, hospital staff are more aware of this issue. However, power struggles sometimes develop between the patient's family and his lover or friends. Social workers may need to mediate between these groups, help the patient anticipate possible problems, and deal with conflicts as they occur during the patient's hospitalization.

Such problems can continue after discharge, complicating aftercare planning for the patient. The following case illustrates problems that can arise when persons who are significant to the patient assume adversarial roles.

> Grant, a 37-year-old gay male, was diagnosed with AIDS two years earlier. He had multiple hospitalizations due to *Pneumocystis carinii* pneumonia, Kaposi sarcoma, cytomegalovirus retinitis, and, toward the end of his life, AIDS dementia. Grant had been living with his lover, who eventually was also diagnosed as HIV positive. Upon diagnosis, Grant initially reacted with denial and noncompliance with treatment. Grant chose not to reveal his diagnosis to his family. However, as the Kaposi sarcoma advanced, Grant found it increasingly difficult to deny the diagnosis and sought solace from his friends and lover.
>
> Grant's family became more aware of Grant's situation, but also chose not to deal openly with the issues. Philosophically, they felt his life-style was immoral and had difficulty separating their beliefs from the love they still held for their son. With the assistance of a social worker and physician, the diagnosis was dealt with openly. Although Grant's family remained involved and supportive, they forced Grant to disassociate himself from the gay community. Thus Grant found himself in the position of having to choose between his "families."
>
> The care issues were complex: family members worked full time and Grant's lover and friends were the only support people around to provide the ever-increasing home care. Given the emotional intensity of feelings between the two factions, the social worker's role became that of getting the involved parties to identify Grant's needs and resolve how these needs were going to be met and working with family regarding their feelings about Grant's friends and lover. Although good relations were never achieved, a schedule was set up in terms of who would provide care at what time so that everyone contributed to the patient's care. These conflicts placed a lot of strain on Grant. It was felt that earlier intervention with the patient and family might have resolved issues more successfully.

CONSULTATION AND EDUCATION

The social worker must educate not only patients and their families about AIDS but hospital staff as well. Hospitals are microcosms of society and, more specifically, of the communities in which they are located. They mirror the values, prejudices, and fears of the area. As Furstenberg and Olson (1984) state, "Health professionals, like others within the community, bring to their workplace strong feelings, attitudes and beliefs about health and illness" (p. 56). AIDS raises issues of contagion and elicits conflicting feelings regarding disease transmission, homosexuality, and drug use. The attitudes of hospital staff have a direct influence on patient care. Thus physicians and other hospital staff need to explore their feelings and fears regarding these issues. Social workers, too, must be cognizant of their feelings and biases regarding homosexuality, drug use, parents of children with AIDS, and other issues if they are to work effectively with HIV-positive patients.

During the early years of the epidemic, hospitals required staff to put on gowns, masks, and gloves prior to entering an AIDS patient's room. Nurses were sometimes observed handing medication to visitors in the room to give to the patient in order to avoid direct contact with the patient. Much has changed over the past decade. With better information about the disease and its transmission, health care professionals have become less guarded in their interactions with patients. For example, as mentioned previously, at St. Joseph Hospital in Denver, an AIDS task force was established to deal with the questions and problems that arose regarding the care of HIV-positive patients. Universal precautions were established for providing care to all patients with infectious diseases regardless of their diagnosis. Moreover, social workers have helped staff communicate with patients more fully with regard to hospital precautions and procedures so that misconceptions and resentments do not occur.

Patients continue, however, to raise concerns about their relationships with physicians and other staff members. At such times, social workers can assist the medical staff in raising their level of awareness about patient needs and concerns as well as sort through their feelings and fears regarding AIDS. Social workers and physicians sometimes have very different perspectives on working with patients. Physicians tend to be concerned primarily with saving lives, whereas social workers focus on improving the quality of life of an individual. Because AIDS is currently an incurable disease that primarily affects young people, physicians may feel that the disease threatens their professional competence and may unconsciously express anger toward patients or withdraw from them. As Roberts (1989) states, "A physician can experience a sense of defeat when he or she fails to save a life. Although physicians are indoctrinated on the whys and wherefores of saving lives, they are given little support or help in dealing with their feelings when they fail" (p. 213). Social workers can help physicians acknowledge their frustrations and sense of helplessness by allowing them to ventilate their feelings in a supportive environment. The social worker can model therapeutic skills that the physician can use with patients. Sometimes, however, the social worker may need to take a more direct approach, possibly facilitating a conference with the patient, "family," and physician to allow everyone concerned to express his or her feelings.

In teaching hospitals, each year brings new interns and residents to the staff. Often their focus is solely on the medical problems of a patient, and they pay little attention to the psychosocial issues that may affect the total treatment of a patient.

Social workers can help these physicians make the necessary connections in order to see the patient as a whole.

Medications used in the treatment of AIDS to prolong life can, at times, cause side effects, some severe enough that patients choose to discontinue the medication or treatment. Some patients choose an aftercare plan at discharge that the physician does not feel is appropriate given the patient's medical condition. Physicians and other medical staff find it difficult to allow patients to participate in making decisions regarding their treatment because health care workers' professional goal is to extend an individual's life, not necessarily the quality of that life. Social workers need to advocate for the patients' right to participate fully in decisions affecting their life by educating hospital staff and helping patients devise treatment goals.

Patients may not comply with treatment plans, especially if they have not been involved in designing the plan. Roberts (1989) states, "Patients who do not comply and risk their life in the process may well have deep, underlying questions, or ambivalence regarding whether they want to live or die" (p. 214). Many patients express a strong desire to live while simultaneously feeling that they do not want to live under the conditions imposed by the disease. One young patient felt strongly about being with his wife and children for as long as possible, but as his pain increased, he questioned his ability to endure under such conditions. Social workers can help bridge the gap between patients' and physicians' values as well as enhance the working relationship between themselves and physicians by understanding the differences in their respective professional orientations. Although social workers and physicians may hold different views regarding professional goals, most physicians are grateful to social workers for attending to their patient's psychosocial needs, an area in which they feel that they do not have the time or expertise to be effective.

COMMUNITY OUTREACH

Hospitals have been forced to cope with the impact of AIDS on their programs and departments. As a result of new medical care and drug protocols, more people with HIV will survive longer. Consequently, the demands on our health care systems and resources will increase and programs will need to be expanded. The multidimensional problems that affect this population demonstrate the need for coordinating all areas of care with community resources. Social workers must identify service gaps within the various systems and advocate for expanding existing programs and developing new ones. The availability of outpatient services are very important in terms of quality and cost-effective care. The costs for caring for a person with AIDS in inpatient hospital settings is approximately twice that of treating other patients in the same setting. More than 30% of AIDS-related hospital costs is not reimbursed; thus, caring for patients with AIDS is not profitable to hospitals. In communities where extensive outpatient services meet the psychosocial and basic housing requirements of persons with AIDS, long hospital stays have been reduced. The availability of residential programs as alternatives to hospitals and broader home-care services are cost effective and more emotionally satisfying for people with AIDS.

Social workers have provided services to patients and their families since the onset of the AIDS epidemic. Even before that time, social workers were working with patients within the health care setting by counseling individuals regarding the physical, emotional, and social consequences of their particular disease. With the AIDS epidemic, social work skills dealing with patient advocacy, program development, and community outreach become even more important. Workers must provide leadership in getting communities to expand resources for this client group.

CONCLUSION

Social workers must not only educate the community at large regarding the AIDS crisis and the need for resources, but must also continue efforts to educate the hospital administration and staff about the role social workers can play in working with this population. Hospital administrators, physicians, and staff generally have a narrow perspective with regard to the roles social workers can play in the overall care plan for AIDS patients. In hospitals, emphasis is placed on discharge planning. However, such plans cannot be developed if the multiple needs of patients are not met. In many hospitals, social work staff is insufficient to provide adequate coverage of each patient care area. With the growing demands placed on workers by the influx of AIDS patients, the problem is exacerbated.

The social worker's role within the hospital setting focuses on the psychosocial aspects of AIDS and involves seeking attempts to minimize the negative impact of AIDS on the patient by linking the patient with available resources. The phenomenon of AIDS, perhaps more than any other disease, demonstrates that our health care system cannot treat only the physiological or medical aspects of disease, but must understand that every health condition affects the physical, psychological, social, economic, and political lives of individuals (Furstenberg & Olson, 1984).

REFERENCES

De La Cancela, V. (1989). Minority AIDS prevention: Moving beyond cultural perspectives towards sociopolitical empowerment. *AIDS Education and Prevention, 1*(2), 141–153.

Furstenberg, A. L., & Olson, M. M. (1984) Social work and AIDS. *Social Work in Health Care, 9*(4), 45–61.

Kelly, J., & Sykes, P. (1989). Helping the helpers: A support group for family members of persons with AIDS. *Social Work, 34*, 239–242.

Macks, J. (1989). Meeting the psychosocial needs of people with AIDS. In J. W. Dilley, C. Pies, & M. Helquist (Eds.), *Face to face: A guide to AIDS counseling* (pp. 2–13). San Francisco: AIDS Health Project, University of California, San Francisco.

Mantell, J. E., Shulman, L. C., Belmont, M. F., & Spivak, H. B. (1989, February). Social workers respond to the AIDS epidemic in an acute care hospital. *Health and Social Work, 14*, 41–50.

Raveis, V. H., & Siegel, K. (1991, February). The impact of care giving on informal or familial care givers. *AIDS Patient Care*, pp. 39–43.

Roberts, C. S. (1989, August). Conflicting professional values in social work and medicine. *Health and Social Work, 14*, 211–218.

4

A MODEL FOR AIDS HOME CARE

GEORGE HARANGODY AND ROBERT PETERSON

Home care as a medical treatment modality has existed since the beginning of the 20th century. Its focus of intervention was based on the medical model, and its goal was to provide alternative care in the most cost-effective way possible. But the complexity of problems confronting people with AIDS as well as the psychological terror it engenders has challenged the home health care profession, causing professionals to develop specific standards for managing AIDS cases. This chapter discusses the development and implementation of a model of home health care for persons afflicted with AIDS. Discussion focuses on the interactions among ecological, medical, and psychological factors that make AIDS clients particularly vulnerable as well as the services that best meet their needs.

AIDS affects every aspect of a client's life. In the words of one AIDS patient,

> I never dreamed that at 32 I would be dealing with my own mortality by a disease that there is no cure for. My health has declined dramatically over the last six months, as I contract infection after infection. My day seems to have lost focus on the life I used to live and has become obsessed with what time my infusion begins, what pills do I take at this moment, what stranger will be entering my home today to tell me how I have to eat when I have no appetite and how I should not smoke in my own home when this is the last enjoyment that I have left in life. AIDS has impacted every facet of my life. Nothing has been left untouched. I can't do the things I did before—like jogging, going to the gym, shop, visit friends, plan a trip, drive out of town, work. I just don't have the energy or stamina—I am too fatigued. People have forgot who I used to be—I am a person with feelings. I am always asked how I feel today, but the questions refer to my physical condition. I must not forget who I used to be. I must keep connected to that part of me that used to laugh and cry and get angry. I must remember how to live again.

This case example demonstrates that mental health cannot be separated from medical intervention. In addition to dealing with minimal community resources, the person with AIDS must also confront his or her altered relationships with friends, family, and co-workers (Christ & Wiener, 1985).

51

From the onset of the AIDS pandemic, it took the state of California six years to recognize the vital need for a home health program. In April 1986, the California State Department of Health Services awarded a contract to AIDS Project Los Angeles (APLA) to analyze the costs of home health, attendant, or hospice care for persons with AIDS or AIDS-related complex (ARC). The program, *AIDS Home Health, Attendant or Hospice Care Pilot Study,* assigned social workers without graduate level degrees as primary case managers to coordinate services among available community resources. Care included homemaker, attendant, skilled nursing, psychosocial counseling, and hospice placements. Before pilot study funds were made available, both private and public benefits programs (Medi-Cal, Medicare, private insurance) were used to fund the program.

However, the multiple and complex needs of AIDS patients soon required that registered nurses and social workers with expertise in the field of AIDS provide case-management services. Multidisciplinary teams were established to provide regular assessment of the medical, nursing, psychological, and social needs of the client. Team members also provide advocacy, referral and/or brokering of services, and coordination of care (Littman & Siemsen, 1989).

During the first year of the pilot study, it was soon realized that resources that were assumed available for AIDS clients were few or did not exist. Hospices and skilled nursing facilities accustomed to dealing with Alzheimer's disease and cancer populations were not equipped to deal with AIDS. Several factors contributed to this problem: inadequate education, fear of contagion, and homophobic fear of the infected populations. It also became apparent that registered nurses were needed as case managers because they had the medical expertise to manage the disease process. Clinical social workers focused on the mental health and psychosocial components of home care.

Housing became a major issue as clients lived longer but were increasingly debilitated for longer periods. Public benefits programs had difficulty covering the high rental costs in Los Angeles County, leaving little or no funds for utilities payments and food. These problems were evaluated, and pilot funds were set aside for housing subsidies. The APLA-run Necessities of Life Program currently provides for basic nutritional needs, alleviating some of the problems. However, because some clients still required food subsidy, such funding was established. Despite these efforts, government threats to reduce spending for home health have had a negative effect on AIDS home health care programs.

POPULATIONS

Several populations are served by the home health care program—each of which has unique needs and issues. Before clients are admitted into the home health care program, they must demonstrate a need for home health services and medical case management. Clients often enter the program after insurance policies are exhausted and they are at home, recently discharged from the hospital, and unable to care for themselves or maintain their home environment.

FIGURE 1. KARNOFSKY PERFORMANCE STATUS SCALE.

STAGE I (Diagnosis)	100	Normal, no complaints, no evidence of disease.
	90	Able to carry on normal activity, minor signs or symptoms of the disease.
	80	Normal activity with effort, some signs or symptoms of disease.
STAGE II (Early chronic)	70	Cares for self. Unable to carry on normal activity or to do active work.
	60	Requires occasional assistance, but is able to care for most of care needs.
STAGE III (Late chronic)	50	Requires considerable assistance and frequent medical care.
	40	Disabled, requires special care and assistance.
STAGE IV (Critical)	30	Severely disabled, hospitalization is indicated although death not imminent.
	20	Hospitalization necessary, very sick, active supportive treatment necessary.
	10	Moribund, fatal processes progressing rapidly.
	0	Dead.

"The clinical evaluation of chemotherapeutic agents in cancer," D. A. Karnofsky (1949). In *Evaluation of chemotherapeutic agents.* © Columbia University Press, New York. Adapted with permission of the publishers.

Clients enter the home health program at various points along the HIV disease continuum. Some are newly diagnosed and symptomatic, whereas others are in the terminal stages of the disease. In order to fulfill the purpose of the pilot study (comparing home care costs vs. hospital costs over the course of the disease), clients at various levels of independence were accepted into the program. The Karnofsky Performance Status Scale, which measures clients' level of independence, is used in the initial assessment. This assessment is then updated monthly. Clients eligible for the study consisted of those who were defined as falling in the chronic functional level rating (70 or lower) (see Figure 1).

Gay white males in their late 20s and early 30s form the largest group affected by HIV/AIDS. Because of the stigma surrounding this population, home health care professionals and staff must be aware of their own potential prejudices (Lukes & Land, 1989). A gay client who may have experienced a lifetime of isolation and oppression as a result of society's homophobia should not be forced to deal with homophobic health care workers.

The second largest HIV-infected population is injection drug users and their sexual partners. In large cities, these persons are located disproportionately in black and Latino communities. Survival sex and prostitution contribute to the spread of HIV infection. In minority communities, the majority of injection drug users are heterosexuals (Tiblier, Walker, & Rolland, 1989). Again, it is imperative that the home health care team understand the dynamics of drug addiction and how multiple stressors increase vulnerability. The home health team must also be aware of their own countertransference issues and focus on helping the drug user enter a drug-treatment program rather than on projecting their value judgments on clients.

A growing number of women and children also require home health care. Women who have sexual contact with bisexual men or injection drug users or who use injection drugs themselves are at high risk for contracting HIV. Often, women do not know that they are infected until after their child is diagnosed with AIDS. The disease process may be accelerated by pregnancy and the mother may die before her child. Minority women living in poverty form the largest group of women with AIDS (Tiblier et al., 1989). Many of these women have not been documented as having HIV and thus do not qualify for public benefits. These women face insuperable odds in their fight to live with AIDS while caring for their children, some of whom also have HIV. Home health team professionals need to be sensitive to the psychosocial dynamics operative in such circumstances and to recognize and validate the incredible energy it takes for the mother to care for her child while fighting for her life. The number of children with AIDS is increasing, particularly in black and Hispanic communities. It is essential that one of the members of the home health team be bilingual and that all team members be sensitive to the cultural background of the patient. When providing services for a child, case managers must evaluate the child within the context of the family system. Services need to be provided to both the child and mother. If the mother collapses in a state of exhaustion or develops another opportunistic infection, no one may be available to care for the child. Because of the stigma of AIDS, extended-family members may be unaware of the diagnosis, thus increasing the level of stress for the mother.

Persons who have contracted HIV through blood transfusion are likely to be heterosexual. As with other groups, they experience the social stigma and isolation associated with HIV. Home health care team members must work with the families of HIV-infected individuals in an effort to increase the infected person's support network. Because few support groups exist for this population, home health care workers can play a vital role in serving these clients' needs. Often members of this population are served by community resources and do not receive home health care services. Because stress can cause life-threatening bleeding, social workers need to help clients and family members keep tension under control (Tiblier et al., 1989).

TASKS AND ROLES OF THE SERVICE PROVIDER

The APLA pilot project interdisciplinary team, consisting of a registered nurse (RN) case manager, licensed clinical social worker (LCSW), primary physician, and home health agency RN, begin treatment by generating a problem list with the client and his or her significant other. It is important that clients be involved in this process so that they maintain some level of control over their life. Initially, the RN case manager assesses the client's physical and medical status. The assessment includes the client's ability to care for self, progression of the disease, compliance with medication regimen, ability to secure resources, and safety. The initial assessment is lengthy and may take several visits to complete if the client's concentration span and energy are compromised.

The LCSW completes a psychosocial assessment. After the initial assessments have been completed, the nurse and the social worker develop a service plan to meet the client's needs. If clients are functioning well and in the early stages of the disease process, case-management efforts focus on securing public benefits, insurance, and housing. Issues concerning mental health and coping with a terminal illness are addressed.

When the client enters the end stages of the disease, the case manager must provide extensive services needed by the client while finding resources to pay for such services. For example, APLA is funded to provide each client with only 2.75 hours of attendant care each week, which is not nearly enough for clients who need 24-hour care during certain periods of the disease process. Because of the limited service hours, it is critical that clients be enrolled in home care early in the disease process in order to stabilize their situation and make additional hours available for clients in the end stages of the disease. Early intervention helps preclude problems that may occur later.

The following case example illustrates the multiple needs of home health care clients.

> A family that included a male injection drug user, female injection drug user, and their one-year-old daughter was enrolled in home health care services. The family's needs were enormous. Because the father and the child had extreme health care needs, the mother was overwhelmed and neglecting her own care. The family had numerous concrete and psychosocial needs: safe, clean, affordable housing; nutritious food for the toddler and the parents; and education regarding general health and child care.
>
> The outcome of this case was disappointing and sad. The father died relatively quickly. The mother reverted to her old coping mechanisms and resumed drug use, engaging in prostitution to obtain drugs. The child was removed from the home and placed with the mother's sister.

Although services for this family included instrumental support for ecological hardships as well as direct clinical intervention (i.e., working through issues of separation and grief), the stressors relating to AIDS were very potent and often created a set of new problems. These problems for the most part were not medical but reflected the psychosocial issues of HIV disease. The social work intervention in this case should have had a major impact on the outcome. But no one can predict how anyone will respond to the repeated loss of family and friends.

SERVICE MODELS

Determining what services and levels of care clients require is the primary responsibility of RN case managers. Their task is to coordinate quality services while ensuring that budgetary guidelines are maintained. This task can be very frustrating indeed.

The following paragraphs briefly describe the various levels of care as stated in the Case Management and Home/Community-based Care (CHC) Pilot Project (Home Health Study) report (Department of Health Services, 1986).

Homemaker services include household services necessary for maintaining clients in the home setting in order to prevent institutionalization. Such services are provided when long- or short-term illness and disability require supportive, therapeutic, or compensatory services to maintain independent living.

Attendant care is nonmedical personal care provided by a home health aide or nurse attendant.

Skilled nursing care is professional nursing care provided by an RN or a licensed vocational nurse. Skilled nursing interventions include the following:

♦ Treatment, diagnostic, and preventive procedures requiring substantial specialized nursing knowledge and skill

♦ Preventive and rehabilitative nursing procedures to ensure the clients' safety

♦ Observation of signs and symptoms in the clients' condition and needs and informing the RN case manager of any changes

♦ Supervision and training of other nursing, paraprofessional, and service personnel

♦ Counseling and instructing the client and family about nursing and related needs

♦ Documentation of progress

Both the home care worker (who is an employee of a community agency) and the client need to understand the expectations and limitations of the job assignment. When RN case managers oversee homemaker, attendant care, or skilled nursing services, it is advised that they do not generalize services under the umbrella term of nursing care. Most people have clear expectations of what an RN does in the home. Roles need to be clearly defined to prevent role conflict and to prevent clients from feeling that they are losing their sense of autonomy and privacy (Chichin, 1988).

Donovan (1986) indicates that half of all home care workers are foreign born and almost all are female. These findings are not surprising in that this type of work attracts persons who are poor and poorly educated, with few job opportunities. These home care workers receive an hourly wage that is approximately $2.75 more than minimum wage. However, they are confronted with enormous responsibilities. They are often the first to recognize changes in the client's medical and psychological condition (Jenkins, 1984) and in emergency situations are the only persons available to assist clients. They may also provide emotional support and are sometimes forced to resolve problems or deal with situations for which they have been inadequately trained (Auman & Conry, 1985). Some home care workers are unwilling to care for clients who are suffering with HIV disease out of fear of contagion. For example, a woman described the first day of her eight-week training course to obtain a certified nursing attendant license. When the class was informed that a certain percentage of class hours would be focused on the care of AIDS patients, more than one-half the class left, saying that they didn't want any contact with "those people."

Tardiness, absenteeism, rough care, abusive treatment, and failure to complete assigned tasks on the part of home care workers often result in clients feeling vulnerable yet reluctant to identify such problems because they believe that reporting problems will sabotage the care they are receiving. Moreover, inadequate or abusive care is often minimized or excused by care providers. Sometimes a client's behavior may be considered manipulative and angry by care team members when such behavior is in fact a legitimate response to inadequate care. Team meetings may degenerate into criticizing the client to avoid examining failures in service provision. Case managers must take the lead in such situations by remaining objective and advocating for the client.

CLINICAL PROBLEMS AND INTERVENTIONS

ASSESSMENT PHASE

Shortly after the medical assessment is obtained, the social worker should conduct a psychosocial assessment. The client should be told that the reason for the assessment is to help determine the level of psychosocial support that he or she needs. At the same time, the social worker should establish that a significant portion of the session will focus on mental health issues of the client and how the client is coping with multiple stressors in his or her life. Clients need to understand that in many instances some level of depression or perhaps cognitive impairment is normal, given the psychological trauma they are experiencing. Clients need to understand that it is OK to talk about problems beyond the medical and social issues that they are confronting.

In an institutional setting, social workers have more freedom to enter a patient's room and obtain the information they need to develop an intervention plan. However, when social workers or nurses enter a client's home, they are on the client's turf, and their presence may be considered an intrusion. Clients have been let down by many people and institutions—government, insurance companies, drug companies, society, religious institutions, health care. Thus the home health care team must establish trust and rapport with the client before attempting to assume a significant position in the client's life.

Upon entering a client's home, the social worker should attempt to join with the client by initially talking about *anything except AIDS*. Wells (1982) labels these efforts the *reconnaissance phase*. A very simple but powerful psychotherapeutic intervention is "bringing the world" to a client who is shut in and isolated because of the social stigma attached to AIDS. Spending 10 minutes talking about "life before AIDS" helps establish a rapport and trust, while simultaneously eliciting assessment information from the client. For example,

> When a social worker entered the home of a male client (R), the client appeared agitated, hostile, and suspicious. R stated that he did not have much time to spare because he had a number of

errands to run. (In fact, the client was not ambulatory and was self-isolating as a result of the overwhelming number of friends who had died of AIDS in the past year.) When the worker passed the television, an alarm sounded from a portable security system that plugged into a near-by outlet. The worker was fascinated by the inexpensive yet effective security system that R had rigged throughout his house. The client began explaining how the system worked, where one could purchase it, and how he had made the system more sophisticated. Thus, for a brief moment, the client felt empowered, productive, and helpful. R began showing the worker items he had collected from his travels before he got sick. He felt that it was safe to talk and eventually provided all the necessary information for the psychosocial assessment. He talked about the loss-es he was experiencing in his life as a result of his entire support network dying as well as about the slow death he was experiencing in his own body.

As a result of this initial assessment, the team obtained a clearer understanding of the kinds of interventions that would establish emotional equilibrium in R's life. In a single 90-minute ses-sion, R was able to ventilate his catastrophic experience. Because he was not ambulatory and suf-fered from extreme fatigue, he could not be referred into the community for psychotherapy. Short-term crisis intervention is generally performed over a period of 8–12 sessions (in this case example, 8 sessions). During that period, a referral was made to APLA's "buddy" program, which arranged for a companion to come to his home twice a week to help decrease his sense of social isolation. During psychotherapy, R was able to connect with the multiple losses in his life and begin the grieving process. As his sense of trust increased, he began talking about issues relating to his own death and dying. The last four sessions focused on termination of the thera-peutic relationship.

At the beginning of the interview, the social worker should let the client know that if any questions are uncomfortable for the client, he or she does not have to answer. This statement communicates to the client that he or she is in control and that the social worker's mission is not to pry into the client's personal affairs but to help the home health care team obtain a better picture of how the client is coping with multiple stressors and, most important, identify how the team can help. Areas covered in the psychosocial assessment include, for example, personal data, insur-ance coverage, health service options, source of income, occupation, or when the client last worked.

In exploring issues relating to mental health, the worker should begin by asking the client to describe his or her reaction to the discovery that he or she was HIV posi-tive. Clients generally remember this event in detail. By verbalizing their reaction, clients often begin grieving over the catastrophic losses they have experienced since diagnosis. It is important that the interviewer not rush the client. At this point the clini-cian has the opportunity to join with the client through empathy and active listening. If the dialogue moves in a relaxed and unpressured manner, the client is more likely to disclose information. Ideally, clients will offer information about past psychiatric his-tory, the extent of the family's emotional and financial support, and so forth.

During the psychosocial history, the worker should evaluate the client's men-tal status, including appearance; behavior and attitude; mood and affect; and thought process and content. Suicidal ideation is common and often reflects clients' efforts to exercise some control over the disease process. Thus, the social worker should allow the client to verbalize these feelings, providing an opening for intervention. Other times, the worker might ask, "You've been under so much pressure. Have you experienced any concentration problems?" In addition, normalizing client responses to memory loss or impaired concentration helps reduce anxiety. Symptoms of depression may be manifested during the interview. Crisis intervention begins by identifying problem areas, finding resources to meet clients' concrete needs, then initiating work on issues such as loss of autonomy, dependence, changing mental competence, and denial of illness.

Those working in the field of AIDS should note that at diagnosis or during the initial psychosocial interview many health care providers fail to recognize the client's immediate and long-term needs for psychological support. If these mental health needs of the client are identified, a referral may have to be made to yet another individual or agency. Consequently, coordination of services becomes increasing complex. Psychosocial intervention by qualified mental health professionals working closely with the home health team and attending physician should begin immediately. Other issues that are evaluated during psychosocial assessment include how medical treatment will be paid for, how clients will support themselves if they are unable to work, and how clients will disclose their diagnosis (and perhaps life-style) to family and friends (Christ & Wiener, 1985).

During the psychosocial assessment, the social worker should assess for dementia. If forgetfulness and concentration problems appear to exist, the clinician must attempt to differentiate between the effects of depression and early signs of AIDS dementia (Buckingham & Van Gorp, 1988).

MIDDLE PHASE

After rapport is established, day-to-day conflicts must be addressed. For example,

B, a female client, was progressively becoming more ill and was resistant to the placement of a feeding tube to prevent wasting syndrome. She was determined to fight AIDS and resume the active life she had once lived. Since her diagnosis three years earlier, she had developed friendships with many people who were also struggling with AIDS. All of those who had medical intervention, such as a feeding tube, had died. B experienced overwhelming fatigue and was unable to eat. To her, the feeding tube symbolized death.

B and the social worker initiated short-term psychodynamic therapy over a period of 12 sessions. Therapy focused on B's depression by helping her begin to exercise some control over AIDS, verbalize her fears, and understand the implications of engaging in or avoiding medical interventions. After three sessions, the social worker and B established a deeper trust and were able to address B's paralyzing fears of her own death. They discussed the benefits of extending her life through medical intervention as well as the repercussions of stopping medical intervention and dying naturally. By including the nurse in the sessions, B's fears about the feeding tube were diminished. By the fifth session, B had spoken with her physician and agreed to go ahead with the feeding tube.

B began to gain weight and her fatigue decreased somewhat, which helped lift her depression by making her feel self-empowered. As the sessions continued, B talked about her fears and eventually disclosed the shame and guilt she felt over the fact that her virus had been sexually transmitted. Through cognitive restructuring (i.e., by labeling HIV as a virus rather than as a reflection of her sexual morality), B began to understand HIV disease and cope with the associated chaos in her daily life. Sometimes she could not find the language to interpret or make sense of the multiple stressors she was experiencing. But the worker's presence allowed B to grieve over the numerous changes and losses in her life while giving her the strength to continue to live with AIDS. At the end of each session, B would become very angry that the 60-minute session was over and would cry. She stated that during this one hour in the week, she was able to feel alive again. But then she knew she had to return to her bedroom and lose touch with the world. (Because of her psychological and physical fragility, B was reluctant to having another service provider, such as a "buddy," visit her.)

Although B's family was very supportive in terms of home care, family members did not speak about the disease. Their religious faith did not permit them to discuss issues remotely connected to sexuality. They connected AIDS with punishment. B's mother was referred to Mothers of AIDS Patients, a community support group. Her brother was uncomfortable with support groups but was willing to see a psychotherapist for individual treatment.

TERMINAL PHASE

Social workers must avoid rigidity during the course of treatment and intervention. A clinician might develop a "brilliant" treatment plan and set an agenda for sessions, but AIDS is unpredictable and workers must meet clients where they are in the process of living with the disease. Opportunistic infections might interrupt psychotherapeutic treatment, or the client might get sick and die suddenly and unexpectedly. Clients may sabotage their treatment by avoiding or canceling appointments.

In B's case, the last four treatment sessions centered on the impending loss of the therapeutic relationship. The worker attempted to explain the limitations in mental health resources; however, when someone is slowly dying, it is difficult to rationalize budget cuts or public policy issues.

B was able to confront her death and dying issues and to confront her family about their condescending attitude. She completed her will and designated her brother as the agent for durable power of attorney. During the last session, B cried and expressed her gratitude for the worker's bringing life to her again. Three months later, B was admitted into the hospital for CMV retinitis. She began to lose her eyesight and was frightened. The social worker visited B several times while B was in the hospital. But the worker's heavy case load made it difficult to resume ongoing treatment. One month later, B died of lung complications. Her life was in order and she was at peace with the state of her life.

DEMENTIA AND IMPLICATIONS FOR CLINICAL PRACTICE

Approximately 3 out of 10 people who have AIDS develop dementia. It is estimated that 30% of people with AIDS and 5% of those with ARC symptoms (diarrhea, fatigue, fever, weight loss, generalized lymphadenopathy, and thrush) eventually develop clinically significant dementia. AIDS dementia requires special attention (McArthur, 1990).

Cummings and Benson offer a useful neurobehavioral definition of dementia:

Operationally, dementia can be defined as an acquired persistent impairment of intellectual function with compromise in at least three of the following spheres of mental activity: language, memory, visuospatial skills, emotions or personality, and cognition (abstraction, calculation, judgment, etc.) (Buckingham & Van Gorp, 1988, p. 372).

Diagnosis is divided into those maladies that affect the outer covering of the brain, such as in Alzheimer's disease (cortical dementia), and those that affect the deep subcortical structures, such as in Huntington's disease (subcortical dementia). A third, mixed category has been proposed whereby both the cortical and subcortical structures are affected, as might be seen in mixed dementias. By understanding which part of the brain is affected by the virus, the social worker can better identify patterns resulting in mental abnormalities. In turn, by recognizing the characteristic pattern of cognitive disturbance associated with AIDS, clinicians can strategically plan interventions based upon the types of changes associated with the disease (Buckingham & Van Gorp, 1988). Sadly, such detailed information, culled from a complete neurological workup, is often unavailable because of the client's limited contact with the health care system.

A marked loss of functioning ability occurs with subcortical dementia. Clients manifest slowed motoric and thought processes, have difficulty concentrating, and demonstrate impaired language functioning and capacity to learn. Such symptoms occur in other dementias, such as Alzheimer's disease. Clients may manifest visuospatial deficits that make it difficult for them to negotiate new environments. In addition, they may experience difficulty performing complex tasks that require them to divide their attention between two tasks or to shift between mental sets. This dementia pattern is distinct from behaviors resulting from a cortical dementia, in which slowing is not evident (Buckingham & Van Gorp, 1988).

Generally, the client is the first to notice memory impairment, poor concentration, and slowed thought processes. When this occurs, clients may become paralyzed with fear that they are losing control over their mental capacities, which connect them to life. Clinicians should assess any subtle differences in cognitive abilities, behavioral changes, and motor functioning. For example,

> When a social worker telephoned T, he seemed confused and had trouble finding a paper to write down a date. He eventually found a writing pad. When the social worker asked T to repeat the date and time, there was a long pause before T responded in a flat, low tone of voice. He had forgotten to write down the time. Upon arriving at T's house, the worker found T sitting on the curb in his bathrobe. It was apparent that he was unable to maintain personal hygiene. T had forgotten about the scheduled visit. When the worker explained why he was there, T was able to recall the scheduled meeting, saying, "I haven't looked at my calendar book." When assessment began, T struggled for words to answer the questions. He began crying, saying that he could not remember things anymore and tried to verbalize how lonely he felt. T's support network had died from AIDS and his family lived on the East Coast.
>
> During their conversation, the social worker noticed that the gas burner on the stove had been left on. When the worker asked T about the burner, T became agitated and frustrated about forgetting to turn it off. T allowed the worker to contact his family by telephone. T's mother was most helpful and concerned about his care. Fortunately, his family was financially able to help pay for attendant nursing care; otherwise, it would have been dangerous for T to continue living at home.

Typical questions that workers should consider when assessing dementia include the following: Is the client's speech slurred or does he or she have difficulty finding words to express him- or herself? Can a client complete a routine task or follow a three-step command? (Testing a client with a three-step command helps to establish a diagnosis of AIDS dementia and avoids the error of misdiagnosing dementia in cases of depression.) Such procedures should be embedded in the interview process; interrogative styles should be avoided. Is the client less verbal than usual? Does the client have a history of drug or alcohol use? (Acute intoxication may produce apathy, delirium, hallucinations, and agitation as well as decrease cognitive and motor functions. Chronic drug and alcohol abuse can cause some of the symptoms described above. Persons who previously relied on drugs and alcohol to cope with stress may manifest inappropriate and even primitive behaviors when they are drug free [McArthur, 1990].)

Dementia has four stages. The initial stage involves slowed ocular or extremity movements, although gait and physical strength appear normal and the client is able to work and perform activities of daily living. Mild deterioration in performance of demanding work and in living skills may be evident, and impaired intelligence or motor ability may be present. In stage two, the client shows moderate impairment. The client is able to perform basic self-care tasks but is unable to work or handle the more demanding aspects of daily living. Although the client may be ambulatory, he or she may require an assistive device such as a walker. In stage three, the client manifests severe impairment in intellectual capacity. The client is unable to follow current events or maintain his or her personal life. The client cannot sustain complex conversation and may move very slowly and clumsily. During stage four, the end stage, the client is in a vegetative state. Intellectual and social comprehension and speech are rudimentary. Urinary and fecal incontinence occurs.

Many home health care agencies that provide attendant care or licensed nursing care consider clients who manifest symptoms of HIV dementia as "troublesome to the staff." In such cases, it is important that trained mental health staff be available.

TREATMENT PLAN

Professionals who care for clients with AIDS-related dementia need special training so that they do not attribute clients' forgetfulness or noncompliance to willful stubbornness or manipulation (Buckingham & Van Gorp, 1988). For example, in the case of T, simple and practical aids helped him negotiate his environment and thus cope with his deteriorating cognitive functions. Environmental aids were placed throughout his apartment. He was encouraged to carry a small appointment book with him and to refer to it throughout the day for reminders of when he should take his medication. Notes were taped on the walls in every room of the house to remind him of things he needed to do—for example, turn off the gas burner. Because T had difficulty remembering telephone conversations, a tape recorder was used to record all of his conversations. Replaying a conversation helped decrease his loneliness as well as remember important things in his daily life. A neighbor in the building, who also had AIDS, visited him periodically, which again helped decrease his (and her) sense of isolation.

Because T had intermittent periods of cognitive impairment, the social worker made good use of the days when T was able to engage in psychotherapy. During the sessions, intervention focused on helping T understand his feelings of frustration and anger with regard to losing his cognitive abilities. Anticipatory planning helped T determine the course of his life when he would no longer able to make decisions.

In addition, the social worker alerted the primary physician to the episodic changes that were occurring with T. He underwent a battery of neurological tests in an effort to determine the severity of his condition. The primary physician prescribed zidovudine (AZT), which helped to slow the progression of the disease.

COUNTERTRANSFERENCE ISSUES

All professionals who work in the field of AIDS experience, at some point, emotional overload associated with the death and dying of their clients. They tend to minimize the work and energy it takes to care for persons with AIDS. Team members need to explore the numerous stresses of their work.

It is important that the multidisciplinary team establish collectively a treatment philosophy that embraces their emotional investment and personal commitment to persons with AIDS. When hiring professionals for home health care positions, the entire team should participate in the screening process so that new members fit the philosophy of other team members. It is also important that team members challenge one another regarding the level of care provided to clients.

The hiring process should evaluate an applicant's understanding of the multiple, complex behaviors of clients with AIDS. Persons who are dying become increasingly needy and often regress in psychological functioning. Consequently, clients sometimes act out their anger and rage in unproductive ways. The home health care provider must be able to understand and interpret such behavior while setting limits and finding constructive ways for clients to express their frustrations. Team members must be aware of possible neurological impairment that may contribute to the inappropriate behavior. When the home health care team focuses primarily on clients' negative behaviors, members lose sight of the fear, pain, and losses clients are experiencing.

Sometimes professionals cope with the stresses of treating AIDS clients by distancing themselves from the client. They may become very "clinical" and thus fail to develop trusting relationships with clients. Or professionals may dehumanize clients by labeling them "druggies" or believing that particular clients are "getting what they deserve." Professionals may victimize clients by projecting their anger onto the client. If negative statements are tolerated by other team members, quality of care and professionalism are likely to deteriorate.

Structured weekly team meetings help members process their own feelings of sadness, frustration, and pain. Such meetings also offer opportunities to share touching and rewarding experiences in members' work with clients. Often, meetings are most successful when facilitated by a mental health professional outside the agency.

OUTLOOK FOR THE FUTURE

The cost effectiveness of home care services as well as client satisfaction with them clearly make home care more desirable than hospitalization or institutionalization. Hospital and hospices will continue to experience bed shortages for AIDS patients. Moreover, with most third-party payors and public programs refusing to reimburse for basic services, the need for community-based care will become even more extreme. Home care is an obvious alternative.

Using RNs and social workers as primary case managers in a multidisciplinary team approach is an effective approach to home health care treatment of AIDS clients. Because the disease process is chronic and slowly debilitating, psychosocial issues of the client are as important as are the medical issues. Despite inadequate funding, it is imperative that professionals advocate for quality care and services for persons with AIDS. Professionalism, integrity, and cultural sensitivity are critical in work with this population.

REFERENCES

Auman, J., & Conry, R., (1985). An evaluation of the role, theory and practice of the occupation of homemaker. *Home Health Service Quarterly, 5*(3–4), 135–158.

Buckingham, S., & Van Gorp, W. G. (1988). AIDS dementia complex: Implications for practice. *Social Casework, 69,* 371–375.

Chichin, E. (1988). Community care for the frail elderly: The case of non-professional home care workers. *Women and Health, 14*(3–4), 93–104.

Christ, G., & Wiener, L. (1985). Psychosocial issues in AIDS. In G. Christ & L. Wiener (Eds.), *AIDS: Etiology, diagnosis, treatment, and prevention* (pp. 275–279). Philadelphia: J. B. Lippincott.

Department of Health Services. (1986). *The case management and home/community-based (CHC) pilot project (home health study).* Sacramento, CA: Author.

Donovan, R. (1986). *The health and social needs of home care workers: Preliminary report.* New York: Hunter College School of Social Work.

Jenkins, E. H. (1984). Homemakers: The core of home health care. *Geriatric Nursing, 5*(1), 28–30.

Karnofsky, D. A. (1949). The clinical evaluation of chemotherapeutic agents in cancer. In *Evaluation of chemotherapeutic agents.* New York: Columbia University Press.

Littman, E., & Siemsen, J., (1989, November). AIDS case management, a model for smaller communities? *Caring, 8,* 26–31.

Lukes, C., & Land, H. (1989). Bi-culturality and homosexuality. *Social Work, 35,* 155–162.

McArthur, J. (1990). AIDS dementia: Your assessment makes all the difference. *RN, 53*(3), 36–42.

Tiblier, K. B., Walker, G., & Rolland, J. S. (1989). Therapeutic issues when working with families of persons with AIDS. *Marriage and Family Review, 13*(1–2), 81–128.

Wells, R. (1982). *Planned short-term treatment.* New York: Free Press.

5

HOSPICE SERVICE AND AIDS

SANDRA LEW-NAPOLEONE

Human immunodeficiency virus presents an ongoing challenge to those who are infected, their friends and families, and the systems providing care for this population. Established care options are constantly being evaluated and new ones created. Patients more than ever before are assuming an active role in traditional, experimental, and alternative treatment procedures. The choice of care options runs from aggressively fighting the disease to allowing the disease to run its course with minimal intervention. For patients who choose the latter, hospice care is a dignified, respectful treatment option.

Hospice care is a relatively new concept in the United States, especially for the HIV-infected person. The word "hospice" is derived from the medieval word for a place of shelter for travelers on a difficult journey. During the early 1900s, hospices for the terminally ill were established in London. In the United States, hospices opened in the mid-1970s with the pioneering efforts of New Haven Hospice, Inc., Hospice of Marin in California, and St. Luke's Hospice in New York City (Stoddard, 1978). In 1983, Medicare adopted a hospice benefit for the terminally ill, a monumental step in sanctioning an alternative-care option in this country.

Hospice care differs from traditional health care in that its focus is not curative or treatment oriented but rather palliative and supportive. Hospice care manages symptoms and pain, not the disease. Care is usually provided by a team of professionals that includes a physician, nurse, social worker, home health aide, pastoral worker, volunteers, and a bereavement care worker. Early hospices in the United States were run by volunteer staff. In fact, even today many hospices are run by health care professionals who volunteer their time and services. With Medicare's assumption of payment for hospice care, however, the trend in hospice staffing has moved toward having some paid employees and a pool of volunteers who provide concrete and emotional support. Some hospices have opted to become certified by

Medicare in order to bill Medicare for services rendered. As a result, the administration, monitoring, documentation, and evaluation of services are more closely scrutinized.

Hospice care can be provided in various settings ranging from inpatient hospital units in skilled nursing facilities to a patient's home. The range of medical needs of patients, their level of comfort and safety in managing these needs, and the wishes of patients and family help determine the setting where care can best be provided. Settings can also alternate from an inpatient facility to the patient's home as needs change. Throughout the course of a patient's terminal illness, the level of care may vary. These care levels, as established by Medicare, include 24-hour care at home or at the hospital during periods of crisis, a short inpatient hospitalization to provide respite to caregivers, hospitalization when the patient's symptom and pain management require more skilled care, and finally routine care in the home. Hospice care views the patient and family as a single unit of care; family can be defined as blood relatives or a network of friends and neighbors. But patients without families or support systems are not usually turned away. However, these patients are often the most needy; the role of team members, especially that of the social worker, is to assist with developing a network of community support to supplement the hospice team.

HISTORICAL REVIEW OF AIDS AND HOSPICE CARE

One of the first hospices to see an HIV patient, or what was referred to then as a gay-related immune deficiency (GRID) patient (Napoleone, 1988), was the Visiting Nurses and Hospice in San Francisco, in 1981. Because medical technology was unprepared to treat this new disease, the average life span from diagnosis to death was relatively short. In many cases, a person with AIDS qualified for a hospice program shortly after diagnosis. The disease often progressed quickly, with essentially no treatment for the opportunistic infections that invaded the suppressed immune system. As the AIDS crisis escalated, the numbers of infected individuals exceeded researchers' predictions, especially in major metropolitan areas such as San Francisco, Los Angeles, New York, and Miami (Napoleone, 1988). Health care systems thus began to take the necessary steps to plan and respond effectively and economically to this disease. Hospice programs expanded and educated staff about infection precautions regarding the delivery of services in the home, the unique psychosocial concerns of patients and families, and the new drug therapies being developed to combat the multitude of opportunistic infections.

Hospices critically examined their philosophy of providing symptom management and pain control vs. aggressive treatments. What might be viewed as an aggressive treatment procedure might also be seen as managing opportunistic infection symptoms to enhance the quality of a patient's life. One example of this controversy is the debate whether to provide ganciclovir (DHPG), a common intravenous (IV) drug used in cases of cytomegalovirus retinitis in order to prevent blindness (Byne, 1988). With few effective drugs available to combat a multitude of infections, new drug protocols constantly being developed, and drug companies racing for patents and the opportunity to make millions of dollars, hospices were forced to evaluate whether they could afford to take on AIDS patients and to pay for all the medications and treatments under the per-diem hospice rate offered by Medicare and Medicaid (U.S. Department of Health and Human Services, 1983). Hospices needed to develop admission criteria for HIV patients.

At what point is hospice care appropriate for an AIDS patient? For example, is a patient with a six-month prognosis who is receiving aggressive treatment and, as a result, shows a dramatic turn in health status a candidate for hospice treatment? At what point should treatment be discontinued? With the onslaught of AIDS, the profile of a typical hospice patient changed from a 70- to 90-year-old end-stage cancer, heart, or lung patient to include a 30- to 40-year-old HIV patient in the prime of life. How could hospice facilities impart their traditional palliative care when these patients needed and desired aggressive state-of-the-art treatment until the end? Moreover, when does HIV infection reach an end stage? Answers to these questions continue to be explored.

In November 1985, the National Hospice Organization (NHO) adopted a policy statement that publicly supported the growing demand for AIDS-related serves.

> The National Hospice Organization (NHO) believes that the care of persons with AIDS is as important as the cure of the AIDS disease. Member hospices of the NHO have been, since the discovery of AIDS in this country, providers of palliative care to persons with AIDS. NHO affirms the pioneering work of our members in making hospice care accessible to persons with AIDS and responsible to their needs. Those hospices which have pioneered palliative care for persons with AIDS symbolize what hospices ought to do in fulfilling the standards and principles of the NHO. NHO encourages all hospices to serve persons with AIDS. . . . The significant issues posed by persons with AIDS to hospice care must not result in avoidance, denial, or desertion by those to whom these persons have turned for help. The special needs of persons with AIDS call for the best in us as hospice and as hospice people (Kilburn, 1988).

HOSPICE CARE AND SPECIAL POPULATIONS

Despite these questions and concerns, hospices are committed to providing services to HIV-infected individuals and their families. Traditionally, hospice care has been an option pursued by white, middle-class persons. This population has access to medical care, knowledge of health care options, and the education to be knowledgeable consumers of health care. The HIV hospice population initially mirrored this population group. However, the unique psychosocial problems that affect the HIV patient as well as the changing demographics of AIDS infection increasingly force hospice workers and organizations to confront issues related to cultural minorities, racism, social oppression, homophobia, AIDS phobia, IV drug use, and the stigma of sexually transmitted disease. Minority populations, who often have strong cultural and spiritual practices with regard to death and dying, have forced hospice organizations to broaden their scope of services.

Reluctance to serve the culturally different or socially oppressed is an obstacle that can indeed be overcome. Hospice workers need to confront their subconscious feelings about cultural minorities as well as their feelings regarding who is "truly deserving" of such care. Workers must explore their comfort level in working with the culturally different and be receptive and open to various customs, traditions, and cultural taboos. In many minority communities, members will reject assistance from providers outside the community and in many instances will accept help only from the family. Often such reactions are the result of minority peoples' view of outsiders as "oppressors." This stance is very prevalent in some Asian communities (Aoki, 1989). Some cultures view seeking assistance outside the family as equivalent to insulting the family, failure, weakness, and lack of dedication, devotion, and strength.

Bilingual, bicultural staff need to be recruited to meet the needs of minority hospice patients. Cultural differences must be recognized and respected as they pertain to illness, death, and dying. As Meyers (1990) states, "Failure to market to minority peers . . . impoverishes existing hospices as they deny themselves the insights and enrichments that these peers would bring to the team. Minority peers could provide unique insights around the special needs and concerns of minority patients and families, thereby making hospice more appealing to minorities" (p. 19).

The drug user with HIV is another special-needs patient with whom hospices have not traditionally dealt. Drug users often do not seek or accept assistance from what they perceive as the establishment. Their survival may have depended on manipulation, lying, and stealing in order to maintain their habit, which presents tremendous challenges to hospice workers whose goal is to provide physical comfort and emotional support. Drug-use behavior may carry over into drugs used for palliative care, raising issues of drug misuse, keeping drugs away from other IV drug users in the home, and the safety of the patient. Hospice workers must be prepared to confront initial resistance, distrust, and suspicion regarding services. Working collaboratively with community services that are knowledgeable about this population may be necessary in order adequately to meet the needs of these patients and families. In-service training must be provided in order to equip staff with the tools and knowledge needed for working with addiction issues, HIV in women and children, and the effects of life-long discrimination, poverty, and oppression.

HOME HOSPICE TEAM

The typical profile of an HIV-infected individual in San Francisco and other large metropolitan cities is a Caucasian, gay, middle-class, educated man. Financial resources and health insurance are generally available to ensure adequate medical follow-up. His support system often includes a significant other and/or friends who provide additional assistance and emotional support. The biological family may or may not be available or supportive. These patients take an active role in their medical treatment, often challenging their physicians with questions about the latest drug trials or alternative therapies.

By the time that hospice care is introduced, the patient and family may have been fighting an emotional and physical battle for several years. Finances and insurance coverage may be exhausted. Often, significant others and caregivers have also contracted HIV. Biological families may be more involved with caregiving or may be called in as the last resort. After having experienced tremendous losses, patients must now face the ultimate loss—their own life.

The hospice worker is not a welcome guest in every patient's home. The health care team operates in unfamiliar territory with each new case. Team members begin treatment equipped only with the preliminary information provided by the discharge planner or physician on the initial referral form. The hospice team contacts the patient's physician for authorization, assessment of appropriateness, and to verify terminal illness with a prognosis of six months or less. The patient may not have a clear understanding of the referral to hospice services or of hospice care. When the hospice worker first meets the patient and family, he or she may be greeted with emotions ranging from gratitude and relief to hostility and resentment. Whereas a general examination and routine tests may have felt natural in a physician's office, patients may feel differently about such procedures when they are performed in the home. Workers must take cues from the patient and proceed gently and cautiously, respecting the patient's boundaries. Workers need to ask numerous questions and must disseminate extensive information about the program. Although the initial visit may be long and tedious, it is critical for establishing a trusting and supportive relationship with the patient.

HOSPICE SOCIAL WORK AND PSYCHOSOCIAL ISSUES

ASSESSMENT PHASE

For patients and families, social work intervention in the hospice tends to be more nebulous in comparison with the task-oriented approach of the nurse. Often, patients have a stereotypical notion of the social worker as a "welfare" worker. Titles such as counselor or therapist tend to connote psychological deficits. If the nurse properly prepares the patient and family, most patients willingly accept an initial assessment visit. Offering concrete services and referrals in addition to explaining the role of the social worker help put patients at ease and facilitate the gathering of information for a psychosocial assessment.

The psychosocial assessment typically includes the following: patient demographics, emergency contact, financial information, funeral plans, patient's mental status, coping abilities, support systems, other significant losses, religious affiliation and beliefs, and the need for a volunteer referral. The beginning phase of treatment or discussion of concrete services may include exploring the need for a will, durable power of attorney, and funeral arrangements. Generally speaking, many of these items have been taken care of or are in the planning stages. These subjects are not as difficult to discuss with an elderly hospice patient as they are with younger patients. Because gay relationships are not legally recognized in the United States, legal issues with regard to wills and power of attorney for a significant other are especially important.

The therapeutic or counseling role of the social worker is generally well accepted by the HIV patient. Patients generally feel the need for psychological support toward the end stage of illness. Previous relationships with mental health professionals may have been terminated due to the patient's deterioration and homebound status. The therapeutic relationship established between the patient and social worker may be heightened and accelerated when time plays a critical role in the process.

The social worker begins where the patient is, utilizing a client-centered, supportive-therapy model. The patient may be in any one of Kübler-Ross's (1969) stages of dying: denial, anger, bargaining, depression, acceptance, or experiencing a combination of several stages. In general, however, social workers need to help patients come to terms with early death. Clichés such as "you've lived a long and full life" cannot be used with a 30- to 40-year-old HIV patient. The plight of the HIV patient is analogous to a soldier returning from war. Reality of death and dying has been experienced, and friends and comrades have been lost. Counseling can assist patients to develop a new perspective, indeed wisdom, with regard to their life.

MIDDLE PHASE

Life review. Life review is a useful and therapeutically necessary tool during the middle phase of treatment in helping the patient reach a level of acceptance with regard to his or her situation. Life review is a "spontaneous process, a retrospective survey of one's life experience" (Hospice by the Bay, 1987). Such reminiscence often generates reflection and insight into the patient's actions, behaviors, and feelings, allowing the patient to critique his or her life. Life review can increase feelings of self-esteem and self-awareness and decrease feelings of loss and isolation. Throughout the life-review process, a patient may anticipate and grieve about approaching death. By examining past experiences and relationships and working to integrate these memories into their perceptions of life, patients are able to maintain some control and power over their remaining life (Hospice by the Bay, 1987). The HIV patient may share unrealized aspirations during the life-review process:

> Jim, a 48-year-old gay white male, had been diagnosed with AIDS five years earlier. He had married in his early twenties and subsequently divorced. He had two children, both of whom were adults now. Jim had not discussed the diagnosis with his family as he was fearful of rejection and the lack of support available to them in their home town. He attached much guilt and shame to his diagnosis and ultimately to his homosexuality. He also continued to feel guilty for divorcing his wife—"running away from home"—and not fulfilling the role of good husband and father. More significantly, he felt that he had disappointed his mother. During the life-review process, Jim began to understand that regardless of his life-style, his mother's expectations could never be met adequately. In reflecting about his childhood years with his mother, he realized that he had experienced many episodes of shame and doubt. Jim learned to accept the fact that he had left his wife. He understood that he had been very unhappy and "living a lie." Eventually, he came to understand that he had never abandoned his role as father to his children, and that throughout the years he had provided emotional and financial support and guidance to them. Jim also began to come to terms with his lack of self-worth and low self-esteem conditioned from childhood and early adulthood. At the end stage of his illness, Jim felt at peace with who he had become and the life he had chosen.

Spirituality. Many HIV patients experience a spiritual reawakening during the terminal stages of their illness. This may occur in the middle or ending phase of hospice treatment. Because the spiritual component is an integral part of hospice care, social workers must be knowledgeable about various religious practices and feel comfortable responding to existential concerns. Many HIV patients search for forgiveness and question whether AIDS is a punishment from God for living a homosexual life. Some may attempt to reunite with their church or reconcile their identity with regard to the negative scriptures in the Bible about homosexuality. The social worker must be cautious about whom he refers the patient to for spiritual counseling. Gay-sensitive clergy should be sought. Gay clergy or clergy who actively support the needs of persons with HIV in their congregation or communities are likely to be most supportive of a patient. For many terminal patients, the spiritual search offers release, comfort, and closure in their life.

FINAL PHASE

Suicide. Many hospice patients have suicidal ideation. Patients may fear excessive pain or dementia and cognitive deficits. Patients may also be emotionally and physically exhausted from having fought a long hard battle with AIDS. Caregiver-assisted suicide may be conceived as an option to end suffering by a patient who is too weak to act on his or her own.

Health care professionals are legally obligated to offer healing and comfort to the ill and to "choose life" with their patients. When patients contemplate suicide, caregivers' tendency is to dissuade the patient, minimize such inclinations, or ignore the issue. If the worker acknowledges and validates feelings of suicide, however, the mystery and stigma of this "ultimate act" is removed. As Schoen (1990) suggests, "legitimizing" suicide may be the best prevention. Feelings of hopelessness and fear are allowed to emerge and to be openly discussed. The option of suicide may be situational, a rational decision, or an escape outlet when dying becomes painful and without dignity.

Rational thoughts about suicide challenge hospice workers the most. In such situations, workers must confront issues of legality and ethics within the therapeutic process. Workers must be cognizant of their stance on suicide, both personally and professionally. Social workers are obligated to act according to the tenets of their profession. Workers must support and encourage exploration of such issues with the patient while helping patients find meaning until natural death occurs. These ethical dilemmas must be handled carefully and sensitively by the hospice social worker.

Some patients will successfully commit suicide regardless of interventions or the accuracy of assessment for risk of suicide.

> Larry, a 36-year-old gay white male, had been diagnosed with HIV three years earlier. He had medication-induced diabetes. Larry had lost many friends to HIV and had witnessed end-stage AIDS in many forms. Larry was a fighter and rallied when staff thought his end was near. He had never expressed suicidal thoughts, although he once stated that when his time was near, he would not want to experience the pain or prolonged suffering that he witnessed in his friends who had died. Larry returned from an enjoyable trip visiting with his family. A day later he was found by his home health aide dead from an insulin overdose. He was a brittle diabetic and was well aware that fluctuating insulin levels could be life threatening. He had canceled his last appointment with his worker on the day before his death.

CAREGIVING AND FAMILIES

Because the family is viewed as the unit of care in hospice work, social workers are often faced with multiple treatment issues. The primary caregiver may be the patient's significant other, who often is HIV infected as well. Long-term caregiving can cause undue stress and even weaken the immune system of the caregiver, thus making him or her vulnerable to opportunistic infections. Caregivers face questions of mortality daily, and they may contemplate suicide after the patient's death. In such instances, suicide may seem an acceptable alternative to living their remaining days without their loved one.

The role of caregiving is sometimes perceived by caregivers as a test of their love and faithfulness. Some caregivers are unable or unwilling to accept help from outside sources, despite their need for respite in order to maintain quality of care and their own mental and physical health. Caregiving is frequently shared among primary caregivers and/or friends. In such instances, however, patients may find it stressful to adapt to multiple caregiving styles. This style of caregiving works best when one person is designated as the coordinator of care and when meetings are held frequently to establish shifts, continuity, and consistency in care.

With the AIDS crisis entering its second decade, many caregivers have provided care for more than one friend and have experienced numerous losses. These survivors often wonder who will be left to care for them when they are dying.

Biological families frequently provide daily care or assist with caregiving responsibilities. Depending on the patient's prior relationship with his or her family, the worker may need to help family members resolve longstanding conflicts. Unfortunately, disclosure of diagnosis and sexual preference to biological families may first occur at this stage of illness. Crisis counseling, grief work, HIV education, and family meetings can help family members establish equilibrium.

Some hospices assist patients without caregivers, families, or friends to care for them. In such cases, the hospice team is a welcome sight but not enough to meet the complex needs of patients in the end stage of illness. Hospice volunteers and community AIDS volunteers can be called in to form a circle of support. Home health aides, meal delivery programs, medical van transportation services, lifeline services, attorneys who will make home visits, and visiting clergy help complete this circle of support.

HIV RESIDENCES AND INPATIENT SETTINGS

Supervised housing has become a critical need. Terminal HIV patients may find themselves displaced when caregivers are unable to meet the demands placed upon them or when caregivers are nonexistent. Moreover, the unstable financial situations of many patients force them out of their homes, or their homes cannot be adapted to provide for their comfort and safety. Although the need for HIV residences is great, advocates have encountered several obstacles in establishing residences. Financial support for such residences is often lacking. Local government officials need to be educated about the benefits of providing appropriate housing versus the drawbacks of homelessness or indefinite hospitalizations in county facilities. Clearly, the long-term benefits of providing housing outweigh the start-up costs. Community and neighborhood support is critical in the consideration of a location for a residence. Efforts should be made to solicit support from storekeepers and residents in the immediate area. Such efforts also provide an opportunity to educate citizens about HIV and to dispel misconceptions. After a residence is established, its location should not be told to the general public in order to ensure the well-being and privacy of residents.

In San Francisco, several residential housing models have been developed. The Shanti model, which was designed for the independent HIV patient, maintains a residence staffed on a 24-hour basis to care for end-stage HIV patients. In 1987, Visiting Nurses and Hospice opened Coming Home Hospice, a noninstitutional residence for terminal HIV patients. Hospice by the Bay responded to the acute housing needs of the terminally ill by opening Hodge House in 1989, a four-bed residence for people with AIDS and other terminal illness. Aggregate living not only fulfills the need for housing but is a more cost-effective method of providing 24-hour care.

Finances aside, group living can promote camaraderie and a sense of an alternative family or community for residents. Patients receive critical support by being surrounded by the lives, struggles, and courage of other persons facing end-stage HIV disease. But problems occur as well. Aggregate living is challenging for both residents and staff. Residents must adjust to new living quarters, new roommates, house rules, and staff who provide supervision and structure. New residents might tend to follow house rules as interpreted by older residents, who may be seen as having more authority. Social workers and house staff often must resolve conflicts and act as referees until residents learn to cope with various personalities and styles. Some residents cannot adjust to aggregate living and choose to leave. However, if the resident makes it through this adjustment phase, he or she is generally able to establish a better quality of life.

In the middle stage of illness, residents may flourish in this protective, safe, and secure environment. Their medical needs are attended to by the nurse and aides, and their psychosocial needs are addressed promptly by the social worker. Some residents even experience a "honeymoon" phase, wherein the decreased stress of family living is reflected in a temporary reprieve from severe physical manifestations of the disease.

For some patients, however, this environment may be overwhelming and depressing. Residents may experience sadness and despair as they witness the debilitation of friends. Some patients persevere and develop a deeper appreciation of life as well as a capacity to love and to let go. Relationships between staff and residents may be emotionally heightened as they witness the death of a fellow resident. Witnessing the deaths of others helps some residents define how they wish to die. They may initiate discussion of pain-management issues, who should be present at the time of death, and funeral plans. Social workers and staff must monitor residents closely during these periods and be cognizant of patients' tendency to identify with the experiences of people who are dying around them. A social worker at Hodge House stated,

> The New Year rang in quietly at Hodge House. Christmas was livelier with a good measure of parties, cookies, presents from the Godfathers, a tree that Michael cut down himself, and even Christmas carolers from St. Kevin's. The guys had a resurgence of energy to enjoy the holidays, but by New Year's that had changed. We lost Geoff and Keith on January 5, and Phillip died on the 11th. Tony went into the hospital and the house was lonely and sad (Walker, 1991).

For patients who cannot be managed in a residential setting due to acute nursing needs, a skilled nursing facility or acute-care hospital may be the best and only alternative. Skilled nursing facilities have been slow to accept HIV patients, partially due to their unfamiliarity with the disease, the complexity of treatment needs, lack of training for staff about infectious disease, and the staff ratio required to care adequately for terminal patients in comparison with elderly custodial patients. However, the skilled nursing facilities that do accept HIV patients welcome hospice care.

Hospice services work in conjunction with skilled nursing facility staff. The patient's daily needs are met by the staff at the facility, and the hospice team visits the patient as if the facility were his or her home. The hospice team ensures that pain-management issues are well covered and that IV infusion therapy is received. In addition, the team makes sure that the general physical well-being of the patient is being addressed. When staffing is such that needs of the patient cannot always be met immediately or addressed at the facility, hospice care is able to supply supplemental care. Social work services are often sparse in skilled nursing facilities and the hospice social worker is welcomed.

Sometimes patients feel resentful, isolated, and abandoned when placed in a skilled nursing facility. These feelings must be acknowledged and validated by the social worker. A skilled nursing facility cannot be compared with a person's home. Encouraging patients to review the situation that led to placement helps them understand that placement was necessary. Whenever they can, social workers should encourage patients and caregivers to consider care options other than skilled nursing care.

AIDS phobia and homophobia can present problems in skilled nursing facilities. In caring for HIV patients, these facilities must adjust to serving an entirely different population, a different age group, as well as an illness that is transmittable and life threatening. Hospice staff must work with the facility's administration to provide ongoing education and inservice training to staff.

It can be challenging to work with staff at skilled nursing facilities. Although the hospice team may be stable, patients in a nursing facility are cared for by staff on three shifts. Moreover, what is perceived as "adequate care" for an elderly person may not be adequate for a hospice HIV patient. Pain-management and medication needs can be extensive and staff may not be able to meet these needs adequately.

To the extent possible, the philosophy of hospice care should be integrated into the skilled nursing facility. A home-like environment, use of warm colors, rugs, and allowing patients to bring items from home help humanize an institutional environment. Flexible visiting privileges, phones by the bedside, and overnight provisions for family members and friends of patients also help make patients feel more comfortable.

Lastly, hospice workers must provide support to the staff of skilled nursing facilities. The witnessing of numerous untimely deaths can be emotionally draining for nursing facility staff.

BEREAVEMENT ISSUES

Bereavement care is designed to supplement the family's existing support network and to enhance bereaved persons' capacity to survive the loss and continue with their lives. As Grant (1991) states, "Grief is multidimensional. It is experienced on all levels of the personality—in the heart, the mind, the spirit, and the body. All levels need our nurture, compassion, and patience." Bereavement care helps hospice staff bring closure to an intimate experience shared with families and allows families to reflect on the experience with someone who was involved. Monthly phone calls, home visits by a counselor, grief support groups, memorial services, and bereavement socials allow bereavement to occur in a safe and trusting environment. Bereavement personnel assess who requires immediate attention and when and how to direct interventions. Agency policies and procedures may provide guidelines for risk assessment and the need for standard, urgent, or critical follow-up by telephone or in person. High-risk grief indicators—such as the intensity of the relationship between the bereaved and the patient, the duration of the relationship, recent multiple losses, lack of a support network, psychiatric history, and drug and alcohol use—are important to consider for determining the urgency and type of intervention needed (Hospice by the Bay, 1990). Bereavement intervention strategies such as educating family members about depression and grief and teaching them emotional coping skills, problem-solving skills, and assertiveness skills are valuable adjuncts to standard bereavement counseling (Stanford Hospital Project, 1991).

AIDS bereavement is special in that several factors complicate normal bereavement. AIDS is a highly stigmatized disease, and this stigma is carried by the bereaved. Because homosexual relationships are not acknowledged legally, the loss of a homosexual "spouse" is not recognized. Such stigma may alienate the bereaved from support networks of family and co-workers. Multiple losses from AIDS also result in a diminishing support system of friends. Grieving becomes an ongoing process; each loss serves as a reminder of past losses and likely future losses. If the bereaved person is HIV positive, anticipation of his or her own impending death must be dealt with.

In AIDS bereavement, many persons experience a generalized fear or apprehension of the grieving process. Coping mechanisms become overwhelmed. The bereavement process must address these factors and acknowledge them as specific to AIDS. Support groups for AIDS survivors can diminish the bereaved person's feelings of isolation. Therapists can help restore equilibrium by validating the bereaved person's fear and sense of isolation as a result of multiple losses.

SUPERVISION OF HOSPICE STAFF

Direct hospice work is an extremely challenging and rewarding experience. Persons who are attracted to this field of health care are able to deal with existential issues and accept life on its own cyclical terms. One learns that no death is perfect or that all deaths are perfect when perceived from the perspective of a patient's life. One dies as one has lived. Sharing the moment of a person's last breath is a humbling experience. The hospice experience deeply touches all who participate in it. It can be emotionally devastating and can accentuate one's co-dependent qualities if it is not monitored closely by the worker, fellow team members, and supervisors. The typical professional life span of a direct-service HIV hospice worker is approximately two to three years. When one is exposed repeatedly to the emotional trials of untimely death, one's perspective on life becomes skewed.

To combat burnout and emotional overload, HIV patients should be evenly distributed among all workers. Supervision must be supportive, while serving as a check on the emotional status and motives of workers. Therapeutic techniques should be monitored and clinical tools enhanced. Common countertransference warning signs that supervisors should be sensitive to include overidentification or overinvestment in the patient's health and well-being, feelings of self-worth rising out of treating this population, taking an overactive role in a patient's tasks or as an advocate, and becoming indispensable to a patient and thus fostering dependency (Weitzman, 1990).

Supervision must also allow for anticipatory grieving and bereavement on the part of the worker. Flexibility in work schedule and availability of mental health days are critical. Voluntary support groups in which staff can address bereavement provide a safe haven to share multiple patient losses with fellow team members. These groups help to minimize feelings of isolation. Periodic staff retreats serve as an extension of support and create environments in which staff can socialize in a nonwork setting. Such functions help build teamwork and camaraderie. An educational component can be incorporated into retreats to enhance skills and knowledge about hospice work. Self-exploration exercises, guided meditations, and small group discussions serve to nurture and rejuvenate staff.

CONCLUSION AND RECOMMENDATIONS

Many patients hear of hospice services for the first time when they are referred to programs by their physicians. The medical community has preconceived notions of hospice work, considering it a last resort when no hope exists and death is imminent. Based on these preconceptions, it is no wonder that physicians are hesitant or reluctant to refer patients to hospice programs. For many physicians, a hospice referral connotes failure on the part of the physician or medical science. It also represents the physician's relinquishing control of a patient to another organization. In actuality, though, physicians can determine their level of involvement with the patient and hospice team.

Hospices around the country are making concerted efforts to spread their philosophy of care. Community education and public relations are important elements in a successful hospice program. Speaker bureaus, medical in-service training, seminars, newsletters, and fund-raising events help inform and educate the public. Because hospices are recognizing the need to serve minority clients, outreach in these communities is beginning to occur.

Greene (1984) states, "Helping patients die well takes time and requires the expertise of our interdisciplinary team. Hospice programs have been successful primarily because the team members are unified in their effort and increasingly uniquely qualified to care for the dying patient" (p. 205). We must shed our blinders in the 1990s and help HIV-infected persons to preserve their sense of dignity even in death.

REFERENCES

Aoki, B. (1989). Cross cultural counseling: The extra dimension. In J. W. Dilley, C. Pies, & M. Helquist (Eds.), *Face to face: A guide to AIDS counseling.* San Francisco: AIDS Health Project, University of California, San Francisco.

Byne, W. (1988). Cytomegalovirus. *Treatment Issues: GMHC Newsletter of Experimental AIDS Therapies, 2*(8), 3.

Grant, A. (1991, February). Bereavement: A time of transition. *Hospice by the Bay Winter Newsletter.*

Greene, P. (1984). The pivotal role of the nurse in hospice care. *Cancer Journal for Clinicians, 34*(4), 205.

Hospice by the Bay. (1987). *Volunteer department training materials.* San Francisco: Author.

Hospice by the Bay. (1990). *Bereavement department, assessment tools, policy and procedure.* San Francisco: Author.

Hospice by the Bay. (1991, January). *Provider relations physician packet.* San Francisco: Author.

Kilburn, L. (1988). *A comprehensive guide to organizational development, management, care planning, regulatory compliance, and financial services.* National Hospice Organization, Hospice Operations Manual 174-175. Arlington, VA.

Kübler-Ross, E. (1969). *On death and dying.* New York: Macmillan.

Meyers, H. (1990, September–October). Where are the minorities? *American Journal of Hospice and Palliative Care, 7,* 19.

Napoleone, S. (1988). Inpatient care of persons with AIDS. *Social Casework, 69,* 376-379.

Schoen, K. (1990, November). *AIDS: A clinical update from interdisciplinary team perspectives.* National Hospice Organization Conference, Detroit, MI.

Stanford Hospital Project. (1991, April). *Predictors of depression,* California State Hospice Conference, San Francisco.

Stoddard, S. (1978). *The hospice movement.* New York: Stein and Day.

U.S. Department of Health and Human Services. (1983). *Federal Register, 48*(243). Washington, DC: U.S. Government Printing Office.

Walker, P. (1991, February). News from Hodge House. *Hospice by the Bay Winter Newsletter.*

Weitzman, S. (1990, November). *The therapist as codependent: Dysfunction beyond countertransference.* National Association of Social Workers Conference, Boston.

6

ALTERNATIVE SERVICE ORGANIZATIONS: THE AIDS COMMUNITY

WILBUR A. FINCH, JR.

Ideally, human service organizations would seek to provide services to all who need them within a community. In reality, however, many minority groups are unserved, underserved, or inappropriately served by the established human service system (Hooyman, Fredricksen, & Perlmutter, 1988; Perlmutter, 1988a). With the emergence of AIDS in the United States, a rapidly growing group of people, generally unknown to established agencies, were being identified as needing a broad range of services. At first, this need was limited to members of the gay community, although it would later spread to members of other minority communities. How were these people to be served?

In the early years of the AIDS crisis, it was difficult to mobilize local, state, or federal interest in and support for persons with AIDS, in part because AIDS was considered to be a "gay disease." Because HIV was sexually transmitted, many in the larger society believed that AIDS was the result of a sexually active and promiscuous life-style. The sluggish response of the larger society exacerbated the need for alternative organizations to address the needs of persons with AIDS. Often founded by small groups of concerned people whose friends or partners had contracted AIDS, these organizations offered products and services different from those offered by established agencies serving other needy populations (Rothschild-Whitt, 1979). Their early mission statements frequently embodied a dual purpose: to provide an alternative service to these clients and to seek social change on behalf of those whom they serve (Power, 1986). Mission statements commonly included themes of social justice, social change, and self-empowerment (Perlmutter, 1988a; Wilkerson, 1988; Kanter & Zurcher, 1973). The immediacy of the crisis was stressed and labeling avoided (Morgenbesser, Notkin, McCall, Grossman, & Nachreiner, 1981).

This chapter identifies the changing attributes of these alternative service organizations and discusses how they evolved. Although particular attention is focused on the AIDS community in the Los Angeles area, similar patterns and examples can be found in communities across the nation. The roles of resources, staffing, structure, process, size, and leadership are discussed and the future of these organizations explored.

SERVICE GOALS AND RESOURCES

Initially, funding for most alternative service organizations is not generally provided by traditional funding sources such as United Way or governmental funding bodies (Morgenbesser et al., 1981). As a result, alternative service organizations find themselves in a marginal position economically. Historically, however, the gay and lesbian community has provided financial support to its organizations.

AIDS Project Los Angeles (APLA) is an example of an alternative service organization. Founded in 1982, APLA was the first and is perhaps now the largest of the alternative organizations dedicated to providing multiple human services to persons affected by HIV/AIDS (a "buddy system," housing referrals, transportation, peer support groups, dental services, case management, food services for those too poor or weak to shop, emergency shelter, education, and mental health services). Like most alternative service organizations, this agency arose out of an impassioned discussion among a few friends. These people quickly raised $7,000, and APLA was born (Sadownick, 1988).

Initially, APLA was run primarily by volunteer staff. However, over the years it has sought and received funding from state and local sources, which has altered its structure and made it more bureaucratic in form and process. As a result, its current budget is in excess of $10 million, and it employs approximately 120 persons. The source of an organization's funding, more than any other factor, can alter its structure. Funding often requires a designated division of labor and/or changes in the type of clientele served (Hooyman et al., 1988). Although APLA has retained its use of volunteers, the organization is not as responsive as it once was to the goals and sentiments of early members, who frequently combined social action with service goals. For example, fund raising has increasingly taken precedence over advocating for social change on behalf of the organization's clientele.

Another alternative service organization, Aid for AIDS (AFA), was founded in 1983 in opposition to APLA's growing bureaucratic structure. Its goal was to offer direct financial assistance to persons with AIDS and persons with AIDS-related complex to meet essential needs such as rent, utilities, and food (Sadownick, 1988). In 1987, this organization distributed $317,536 of services, all of which was raised from private donations (Sadownick, 1988). It has retained many of its initial goals and characteristics by limiting public funding to a few salaried positions paid for by the City of West Hollywood.

As AIDS began to expand into other minority communities, APLA's initial goal of serving all AIDS patients became impossible to meet. Narrower priorities were set. Because of this change in focus, minority AIDS activists in the Latino community faulted APLA for channeling government funds into the predominantly white gay community (Martinez, 1987). Similarly, the Reverend Bean, founder of the Minority AIDS Project (MAP), even went so far as to sue the Los Angeles

County Board of Supervisors for failing to gather and distribute money to minority communities (Sadownick, 1988).

As AIDS enters its second decade, alternative organizations to serve minority communities have begun to proliferate. Each defines the problem from its own perspective. Minority AIDS Project was founded in 1985 to provide mental, emotional, and financial support for persons with AIDS and AIDS-related complex. Cara a Cara, founded in 1987, is a prevention and educational program serving the Latino community. Its services include crisis intervention, support groups, and a culturally sensitive speakers bureau. Finally, the Watts Health Foundation opened its office in 1986 to provide outreach to low-income areas in minority communities.

Despite the urgent need for services as well as advocacy, many of the alternative organizations that came into being in response to the AIDS crisis have tended to emphasize fund raising over advocacy goals (Sadownick, 1988). Organizations such as Being Alive, founded in 1985, function as a powerful voice for persons with AIDS, demanding greater accountability from the other AIDS organizations. Most of Being Alive's funds have come from private donations; its services include monthly meetings, advocacy, a monthly newsletter, and a speakers bureau.

The AIDS Coalition to Unleash Power (ACT UP), a national network organization, has devoted its energies to challenging the gross inadequacies of governmental and private-sector responses to AIDS (Sadownick, 1989). Its slogans—"Silence = Death," "Action = Life"—used in acts of protest or civil disobedience, have achieved measurable results such as the release of life-sustaining drugs, a federally funded education program, and the opening of an AIDS ward at Los Angeles County/USC Medical Center, to mention a few. In fact, Sadownick (1989) argues that "ACT UP has forced the gay community to face its continued marginality in politics" (p. 21). This organization continues to maintain its political independence, believing that greater funding can be achieved through demonstrations.

In summary, many alternative service organizations have emerged in response to the AIDS crisis. Over time, some have modified their initial objectives, often because of their increasing reliance upon public funds, developing a greater emphasis on organizational maintenance as opposed to social advocacy. In contrast, other organizations have worked hard to maintain their initial goals and mission.

STAFFING

Traditionally, alternative service organizations have been staffed primarily by volunteers (American Psychiatric Association, 1975). Staff incentives and solidarity derive from the agency's mission and from the act of associating with other agency staff. For example, the Los Angeles Shanti foundation emerged in 1983 as a psychosocial support organization for persons with AIDS or AIDS-related complex and their significant others. The foundation places strong emphasis on personal growth, development, and support of volunteers (Hooyman et al., 1988). By 1988, the foundation had acquired state and local funding to support some hired staff. Private fund raising, however, continued to account for the majority of its resources.

In most of these settings, volunteers may have some professional training but their primary characteristic is identification with the clients being served (Perlmutter, 1988a). Within the Shanti foundation, intensive training, followed by work with clients, weekly supervision and support-group participation, and optional committee work are offered and expected (Hooyman et al., 1988). Belief in the "special" nature of their mission no doubt produces a like-mindedness that increases consensus building among members of these organizations.

In other organizations, issues such as the size of the organization and questions of elitism can produce tensions between volunteers and professionals. Being Alive, for example, is a peer-oriented organization; because members are often HIV positive themselves, the organization has a strong commitment to empowerment. In other words, the staff recruited are personally as well as ideologically committed to the program (Perlmutter, 1988a).

Some organizations have changed their goals and hence staffing patterns over time. The AIDS Hospice Committee began as a volunteer group advocating cost-effective alternatives to hospitalization. Through demonstrations directed at selected members of the Los Angeles County Board of Supervisors, they were eventually able to garner a measure of support for the establishment of hospices in Southern California (Sadownick, 1988). This group later became the AIDS Hospice Foundation when it opened hospices in the south-central Los Angeles and Hollywood areas to care for the terminally ill.

Developing an "army" of volunteers is critical to the successful functioning of these alternative service organizations. A recent study of volunteers in Southern California AIDS organizations found that many of the volunteers were gay men and lesbian women whose demographic characteristics were similar to those of the clients being served (Gabard, 1990). Although the primary motivation of volunteers was "to help people whom government and society had failed to adequately assist" (p. 200), gay volunteers differed from heterosexuals in that they were more likely to work toward a sense of community and prove their worth to the rest of society through their volunteer efforts.

STRUCTURE AND PROCESS

The larger an organization becomes, the more highly structured and formalized it is likely to become. Concomitantly, the process by which decisions are reached becomes more formalized and abbreviated. For example, over time APLA has come to look and function like many traditional social service organizations. On the other hand, other alternative organizations have sought to share power by emphasizing and maintaining a nonhierarchical, collaborative, and egalitarian structural framework (Morgenbesser et al., 1981). Commonly, their rationale for this framework rests upon a belief in democratic, egalitarian values (Power, 1986; Hooyman et al., 1988; Perlmutter, 1988b). For example, Being Alive's mission is to offer peer support while avoiding victimization. Not surprisingly, its members are fearful that the organization may become too large.

In this sense, then, the term "alternative" can refer to both the kinds of services offered as well as the structure through which they are provided (Gummer, 1988). Being Alive functions through teams, each of which has its own coordinator. Democratic action in groups inevitably shifts both time and energy from outcome to process and can be beneficial to participants by providing a sense of empowerment (Wilkerson, 1988).

ACT UP receives no public money and seeks to challenge government and private sector nonresponsiveness to AIDS. Members meet weekly to seek consensus on actions. Every individual has the right to speak and there are no formal leaders (Sadownick, 1989). At some level, ACT UP probably came into being because the majority of alternative service organizations were reluctant to become combative when dealing with the larger society. Although attempting to emphasize the establishment of a new and joyful definition of community, ACT UP members believed that many people would suffer needlessly if members didn't demonstrate their anger publicly. Civil disobedience is not mandatory, and only those with training participate in highly planned activities (Sadownick, 1989).

The concept of *process,* whereby how things get done becomes as important as what gets done, has been emphasized by many alternative service organizations that emerged from the feminist movement (Crow, 1978; Riddle, 1978). For many alternative service organizations in the AIDS community, social processes represent goals in themselves rather than merely the means for obtaining a desired outcome (Kanter & Zurcher, 1973). Thus, Shanti places great emphasis upon learning and the personal growth of volunteers, ACT UP stresses the building of community, and Being Alive seeks to empower its members. The emphasis upon egalitarian values, however, often means that such groups spend an inordinate amount of time on issues of acculturation, evaluation, peer supervision, conflict resolution, and so forth. The term "clan organization" has been coined to describe culturally homogeneous settings, in which members share a common set of values and beliefs about how to coordinate efforts to achieve common objectives. This term is descriptive of alternative service organizations that emphasize the congruence of individual and organizational goals (Gummer, 1988).

SIZE AND TECHNOLOGY OF ORGANIZATIONS

To maintain one-on-one interactions and close relationships among members, many alternative service organizations seek to remain small (Kanter & Zurcher, 1973). Small size allows participatory democracy among members. For example, until recently, Being Alive was small enough that members could meet in one another's homes. Optimal size, however, probably depends on various organizational factors, such as the knowledge of its members and the technology available to the organization. If knowledge and technology can be broadly shared, groups are able to become larger while retaining their participatory characteristics.

A single-purpose group such as ACT UP focuses its energies on planned demonstrations. During regular meetings, knowledge is shared with a growing membership, while the organization's goals remain focused and relatively simple (Rothschild-Whitt, 1979). In contrast, larger organizations, such as APLA, which now offers more than 20 different programs, have had to move toward greater specialization because expertise and knowledge could no longer be shared widely among all members. Aids Project Los Angeles's programs now range from legal to mental health to residential services. Although APLA continues to use more than 1,600 volunteers in their various programs, it has had to relinquish the democratic attributes characteristic of many other alternative service organizations. Consequently, the total membership can no longer respond to issues that affect the organization (Perlmutter, 1988a).

LEADERSHIP

Leadership in alternative service settings is often shared widely among the membership (Selznick, 1957). Sometimes this is accomplished by promoting key values through slogans (such as ACT UP's "Silence = Death"). Personal or psychological methods such as use of support groups also preserve key values of the organization. The training of volunteers provided by Shanti, for example, creates "socially integrating myths" (Selznick, 1957) that infuse daily behavior with broader meaning and purpose. The more central societal change efforts are to the organization, the more important is the individual's personal ideology and value system.

Alternative service organizations, especially when they are just beginning, must deal with periods of economic insecurity, which in turn requires these organizations to take considerable risks and to remain flexible in an unstable environment. For example, in 1985, even APLA experienced a $1 million deficit, which forced cutbacks in client services (Sadownick, 1988). Economic insecurity is even more critical for smaller groups. For example, an "AIDS-Thon" of walkers, runners, skaters, and cyclists recently raised approximately $200,000 for the benefit of 25 marginal organizations that provide specialized services (Pristin, 1991). Such organizations include Aunt Bea's Laundry (which picks up and delivers laundry for people with AIDS), Teatro Viva (a comedy act that seeks to educate gay and bisexual Latinos about safe sex), the East Los Angeles Task Force (which provides care to substance abusers, many of whom are either infected with HIV or are in danger of contracting it), Asian-Pacific Lesbians and Gays (which provides education and referral services for Asians and Pacific Islanders), and PAWS-LA (which provides food and care for the pets of persons with AIDS). Because of their economic instability, many of these organizations are in a constant state of flux and thus require leadership that can tolerate uncertainty.

Leadership in alternative service organizations might best be described as unconventional. Personal ideology and values are critically important for leaders of these organizations (Perlmutter, 1988a). Personal commitment is needed to motivate those who might not involve themselves in risk-taking activities. ACT UP is a good example of this phenomenon. Within two years, ACT UP became the largest AIDS activist organization in Southern California. Clearly, key members had to have a capacity for risk-taking activities that could provoke harassment from civil authorities (Sadownick, 1989).

Passage of the Ryan White Comprehensive AIDS Resources Emergency Act of 1990, which mandates relief to the 16 cities most severely affected by the AIDS crisis, has encouraged leaders in many settings to establish more formal agency networks. The prospect of additional funds has encouraged many organizations to form a consortium for obtaining HIV- and AIDS-related funding. Through this consortium, funding requests have become more formalized. Similarly, ACT UP, at a recent conference of various service organizations examining the inequalities of the health care system in America, added a set of radical proposals to the already complex health care debate (Sadownick, 1991a). Coalition building greatly expands the opportunity for activists and organizations to achieve radical changes in highly entrenched institutions.

PARADOXES

Because of their unique characteristics, alternative service organizations face many contradictions. For example, stabilizing and balancing relationships within the organization ensures continuity (Kanter & Zurcher, 1973). However, too much stability may inhibit organizations from making necessary changes and pursuing goals. Staff turnover generally has a negative impact on alternative organizations, especially smaller organizations. Turnover has been a critical problem for organizations whose members are HIV positive. When members become too sick or frail to continue their work, new staff may affect the service and social goals of the organization. They may lack commitment to the diffusion of knowledge and collective decision making (Power, 1986) and may disrupt personal relationships essential to effective management (Hooyman et al., 1988).

Many alternative service organizations are committed to remaining independent of the traditional human service system. However, their survival as alternative service organizations forces them to depend on other organizations for funds. Some organizations, for example, ACT UP, have successfully avoided becoming dependent. Aid for AIDS has accepted limited public funding for a few staff positions and thus has retained considerable independence.

As previously noted, maintaining a small size is valued by many alternative organizations. However, as the number of HIV/AIDS patients increases, the need for more staff and larger organizations will become evident. Under these circumstances, critical decisions will need to be made. The importance of sharing power within an organization vs. the greater efficiency of an administrative hierarchy will need to be evaluated. The need for expertise and clearer division of roles and responsibilities may further modify the participatory models of many of these organizations. Full collaboration on every decision could become increasingly problematic (Kanter & Zurcher, 1973). However, organizations in which empowerment (Being Alive) and community (ACT UP) values dominate will probably continue to resist such changes.

Strong identification with clients has been a common characteristic of alternative service settings. Socialization of members, either through the adoption of common slogans or through education, places emphasis on the collective well-being of the organization. Pressures on members to conform may limit the ability of alternative organizations to address the needs of a diverse clientele. As occurred with APLA, new services may need to be developed and new staff with specialized skills may need to be recruited, both of which affect the homogeneity of the organization. The expertise garnered in working with one client group may not always be transferable to other at-risk groups.

THE FUTURE

One can speculate about the future of many alternative service organizations should the AIDS crisis eventually be resolved. One possible scenario is that mainstream service organizations would increasingly adopt many service techniques developed in alternative service settings. Or alternative organizations might increasingly accommodate the values of the surrounding community and, like APLA, resemble their mainstream counterparts.

Another possible scenario might be further radicalization. For example, California Governor Pete Wilson's veto of AB 101, a "gay rights bill," stimulated 13 days of demonstrations around the state, which continued on a sporadic basis for some time afterward (Sadownick, 1991a). Certainly, ACT UP's adoption of a national policy for universal health care greatly increases the possibility of collaboration with other groups seeking similar goals (Sadownick, 1991b).

Obtaining funding from external sources may alter the structure of some alternative organizations and, over time, weaken egalitarian values (Rothschild-Whitt, 1979). Organizational structure may increasingly be emphasized when it is beneficial to key agency members who have acquired positions of power.

Finally, some alternative service organizations may disappear simply because their client group no longer exists. Shanti was formed initially to work with the terminally ill; it shifted its focus when the AIDS crisis emerged. This organization could revert to its original mission, although a shift in agency personnel would be likely because many would no longer identify with the client groups being served.

CONCLUSION

This chapter identified and analyzed the attributes of alternative service organization in terms of the many organizations that have emerged to serve the AIDS community in Southern California. The problems these organizations experience in securing necessary funding, their reliance upon volunteers, their efforts to remain small, and their emphasis on process have allowed a culturally homogeneous membership to emerge. At the same time, organizations can be flexible in terms of size if knowledge is shared and technology remains relatively simple. Leadership in these settings is often widely shared among the membership and requires the ability to tolerate periods of economic hardship and a willingness to take risks. In this sense, leadership is unconventional, with greater emphasis placed on ideology and values that support the organization's goals.

Many alternative service organizations were developed initially due to lack of interest in AIDS on the part of government and the unresponsiveness of established social service organizations to problems associated with HIV infection. However, over time, alternative service organizations have had to rely on other organizations for funding, which has in turn resulted in structural modifications and changes in program goals. Also, because many alternative organizations initially addressed the needs and crises of specific minority groups, new organizations have emerged as HIV has spread to new groups. These newer organizations, like those that preceded them, often come into being because a group perceives itself as being underserved or inappropriately served by established organizations. However, as the number of persons with AIDS increases, many alternative service organizations may be unable to respond to the needs of new groups, increasing the pressure on traditional organizations to broaden their services to meet the needs of these new populations.

REFERENCES

American Psychiatric Association. (1975). *The alternative services: Their role in mental health.* Washington, DC: Author.

Crow, G. (1978). The process/product split. *Quest, 4*(4), 15–23.

Gabard, D. (1990). *Retention of volunteers: Factors affecting retention in volunteer associations whose primary mission is to deliver care to adults with AIDS or ARC.* Unpublished doctoral diss., School of Public Administration, University of Southern California.

Gummer, B. (1988). The hospice in transition: Organizational and administrative perspectives. *Administration in Social Work, 12*(2), 31–44.

Hooyman, N. R., Fredricksen, K. I., & Perlmutter, B., (1988). Shanti: An alternative response to the AIDS crisis. *Administration in Social Work, 12*(2), 17–30.

Kanter, R. M., & Zurcher, L. A. (1973). Concluding statement: Evaluating alternatives and alternative valuing. *Journal of Applied Behavioral Science, 9*, 381–397.

Martinez, R. (1987, October 30). AIDS: The crisis in Latino L.A. *LA Weekly*, pp. 10–11.

Morgenbesser, M., Notkin, S., McCall, N., Grossman, B., & Nachreiner, C. (1981). The evolution of three alternative social service agencies. *Catalyst, 11*(3), 71–83.

Perlmutter, F. D. (1988a). Administering alternative social programs. In P. R. Keys & L. H. Ginsberg (Eds.), *New management in human services* (pp. 167–183). Silver Spring, MD: National Association of Social Workers.

Perlmutter, F. D. (1988b). Alternative federated funds: Resourcing for change. *Administration in Social Work, 12*(2), 95–108.

Power, D. M. (1986). Managing organizational problems in alternative service organizations. *Administration in Social Work, 10*(3), 57–69.

Pristin, T. (1991, November 4). AIDS benefit helps smaller organizations. *Los Angeles Times*, pp. 81, 86.

Riddle, D. (1978). Integrating process and product. *Quest, 4*(4), 23–32.

Rothschild-Whitt, J. (1979). Conditions for democracy: Making participatory organizations work. In J. Case & R. C. R. Taylor (Eds.), *Co-ops, communes and collectives* (pp. 215–244). New York: Pantheon Books.

Sadownick, D. (1988, November 25). The AIDS community in Los Angeles: A brutal fight for life. *LA Weekly*, pp. 21–22, 26, 28, 30, 32, 44, 82.

Sadownick, D. (1989, October 6). ACT UP and the politics of AIDS. *LA Weekly*, pp. 20–25.

Sadownick, D. (1991a, November 15). After AB 101. *LA Weekly*, pp. 14–22, 24–26, 28.

Sadownick, D. (1991b, October 18). The movement turns. *LA Weekly*, pp. 15–16.

Selznick, P. (1957). *Leadership in administration.* New York: Harper & Row.

Wilkerson, A. E. (1988). Part 4: Epilogue. *Administration in Social Work, 12*(2), 119–128.

PART 2

SERVICE DELIVERY TO DIVERSE POPULATIONS

7

CONTEXTUAL AND CLINICAL ISSUES IN PROVIDING SERVICES TO GAY MEN

GARY A. LLOYD

This chapter deals with contextual and clinical issues in providing services to gay men. "Clinical" is defined in its broadest sense to include attention both to intrapsychic and interrelational needs of people confronting a lethal disease. Considerable contextual information is presented because of the influence of negative social attitudes toward homosexuality.

Although the "face of AIDS" has changed drastically over the past few years and HIV disease now affects increasing numbers of male and female drug abusers, sexual partners of infected men and women, and children, gay men continue to constitute the largest group of infected and diagnosed cases of HIV disease. In September 1991, the Centers for Disease Control (CDC) reported that 110,678 cumulative AIDS cases (59%) had been reported in which male homosexual/bisexual contact was the exposure category (Centers for Disease Control, 1991). Lesbian women have also been affected by HIV disease, both as partners of gay men in establishing community-based support and treatment services and as persons potentially at risk of HIV infection. (It should be noted that little research has been focused on lesbians and HIV, and no lesbian risk studies have been conducted or sponsored by the Centers for Disease Control.)

The chapter is organized around two focal points: the social and political impact of HIV infection on gay men and clinical interventions that adapt to and reflect the complexity and variability of the progression and manifestations of HIV disease.

The basic assumption underlying the development of this chapter is that homophobia has played, and continues to play, a significant role in the ways gay men, lesbians, health care professionals, and society at large have responded to HIV disease. To the widespread homophobia in the society has been added "AIDS phobia" and perceptions that gay men caused the pandemic. Gay men have experienced HIV-related discrimination from the beginning because of public misperceptions about casual transmission of HIV and "pre-existing punitive attitudes towards those believed to be responsible for the spread of HIV" (Tindall & Tillett, 1990).

SOCIAL AND POLITICAL IMPACT OF HIV ON GAY MEN

The impact of HIV upon gay men (and to a differing degree on lesbian women) has been devastating and far reaching. A stigmatized group has been decimated by a stigmatized and stigmatizing affliction. Thousands of gay men, most of them young, have died. Thousands more are infected and fearful. Most gay men have experienced multiple losses. The entire gay community is marked by a sense of collective mourning, cumulative losses, and continuing grief. The impact ranges from the intense feelings of loss experienced by individuals to fears of setbacks to the movement for civil rights for gay men and lesbian women to anger about the lack of adequate national policies to support services for treatment and support. Many gay men perceive an increase in homophobia because of HIV (Stulberg & Smith, 1988).

The impact of HIV on gay men has been devastating on many counts. Seropositive status may force revelation of sexual orientation. Anticipation of negative familial, workplace, or social response can be extremely stressful. It is well known to HIV-positive gay men that end-stage HIV disease, or AIDS, can be debilitating and disfiguring and is invariably fatal. The life span between infection, appearance of symptoms, and death has lengthened considerably, but there is no cure. This fact alone would be sufficient to demoralize gay men. Of equal weight is the fact that most of the gay men who have died from HIV disease have been young. Before infection with HIV, they were active, healthy men moving into jobs or careers, in school, or making other plans for their adult years. HIV has robbed a generation of young gay men of their futures. The normal course of their life has abruptly changed: young men have died before their parents; men still young enough to believe themselves to be "invulnerable" have succumbed to HIV or found themselves nursing other men their age.

Put another way, the expected developmental course of individuals' lives has been severely disrupted by HIV. The harsh individual, social, and political realities of HIV, however, have also led to major organizing efforts in the gay/lesbian community to develop and expand services. Such efforts have led not only to the development of considerable political strength but to less negative societal reactions to homosexuality as well. These are minor gains, however, when contrasted with widespread loss, discrimination, suffering, and isolation.

HOMOPHOBIA

HIV infection has "prominent social trappings," and "punitive and discriminatory reactions of society to those with HIV infection contribute deeply and fundamentally to the suffering of HIV infected patients" (Rogers & Osborn, 1991, p. 806). The social and political realities of homophobia intensified the impact of HIV disease for gay men. Homophobia (the irrational fear of homosexuals) or heterosexism (the conviction that any expression of sexuality other than heterosexual is "bent" as opposed to "straight") shaped society's response to HIV/AIDS. At their worst, homophobic judgments held that resources were not necessary because gay men deserved punishment for their "deviance" or "perversity." At best, homophobia contributed to the initial failure (only partially corrected over time) of government at all levels to respond to the epidemic with adequate medical and social services. The only bright note in this grim reality is that because of homophobia and neglect, lesbian and gay communities mobilized in unprecedented numbers and ways to develop community-based AIDS service organizations for gay men. As is evident in the histories of other oppressed groups, crisis can inspire collaboration and mutual aid.

Homophobia—both external and internal—is a significant reality for all gay men and lesbian women and may be the most significant reason for unified action. Although references to the "lesbian and gay community" are frequently found in professional journals and the popular media, one should be wary of any inference that sexual orientation is necessarily a basis for group homogeneity. It should be understood that the terms "gay community," "gay/lesbian community," or "lesbian community" are used here solely for convenience and do not adequately reflect—and may actually conceal—the extraordinary diversity among gay men and lesbian women, who mirror the diversity and attitudes of the society within which they live. This "community" is highly diverse with regard to how individuals cope with their sexual orientation and the generally negative social attitudes toward it. Coping may be particularly difficult for people of color from cultures that totally reject homosexuality or from fundamentalist or doctrinaire religious backgrounds that find scriptural reasons to define homosexuality as intrinsically sinful or evil.

Some gay men are "out of the closet" and very active politically, while others fear discrimination if their sexual orientation were to become public knowledge. Some see "coming out" to self and to others as a political statement necessary to combat harassment and discrimination, others view it as a private process of self-acceptance, and still others deny that "coming out" has any meaning at all. Whereas some gay men may don work clothes or suit by day and dress in drag or leather by night, others decry any unconventional or flamboyant behavior because of fear of exposure and ridicule. Many gay men and lesbian women have found support in clubs, homophile churches, and bars, whereas others isolate themselves because of socially reinforced shame or guilt.

Living in a society in which legal and religious systems condemn same-sex orientation has consequences for even the most liberated individuals. Gay men and lesbians are reminded regularly that they are different and unwanted: unwanted for military service, as physicians, as teachers of small children, or for job promotion. Such attitudes have had a strong influence on the gay and lesbian response to HIV. Because of these homophobic attitudes, lesbians who were not infected or sick understood early the social impact of HIV on gay men and the necessity of collaboration to develop health and social services that would not condemn sexual orientation and sexuality.

HIV AND STIGMA

Services to gay men and lesbian women affected by HIV disease are influenced by a complex array of issues and variables. Other than homophobia, primary among those variables is the fact that HIV disease carries a virtually universal stigma. The labeling and social stigma attached to homosexuality have been reinforced and magnified by HIV/AIDS. HIV infection acquired through drug abuse is also highly stigmatizing. When homosexuality, drug abuse, and ethnicity are combined in one person, a triple stigma is almost always evident. Social stigma and labeling may affect the infected person's self-image (already jeopardized by the existence of an intractable and incurable infection) and willingness to use services. Stigma affects whether or when services are developed, how or if they will be used, and the availability and accessibility of medical and psychosocial treatment and support.

GAY MEN AND HIV

The health signs and symptoms that eventually were termed acquired immunodeficiency syndrome (AIDS) and subsequently linked to HIV existed for an unknown period before they were identified and labeled. Called by Osborn (1988, p. 444) a "veritable microbiologic bomb," the retrovirus that severely compromises the human immune system and leaves it open to various opportunistic infections and cancers was spreading in the early to mid-1970s (Burke & Redfield, 1989; Mann, 1988). Sporadic cases of hitherto rarely reported *Pneumocystis carinii* pneumonia and Kaposi's sarcoma (a rare cancer usually found in elderly men) were reported in the United States in 1979. The first cases of what would ultimately be called "AIDS" were recorded briefly in the June 5, 1981, issue of the Centers for Disease Control *Mortality and Morbidity Weekly Report*. More detail about this puzzling disease, which seemed to be confined to clusters of young homosexual men living in urban areas, appeared in the December 10, 1981, issue of the *New England Journal of Medicine* (Relman, 1987; Heyward & Curran, 1988).

Why these rare medical states first afflicted gay men has never been satisfactorily explained. In 1981, it was not yet recognized that HIV could infect heterosexuals and homosexuals alike. It appeared then that gay men were being struck down by a plague that was linked in some undetermined way to their sexual practices or behavior. Because that perception was so strong, these puzzling signs and symptoms were first called gay related immune deficiency. As Altman (1987) observes:

> As the spread of AIDS became linked in the public imagination to the very presence of homosexuals—including lesbians—the gay visibility and affirmation of the past decade allowed for some very nasty scapegoating. AIDS came along just when the old religious, moral and cultural arguments against homosexuality seemed to be collapsing. The 1970's saw a whole series of shifts in the dominant ideology concerning sexuality. . . . Under siege from the rapid changes which were turning homosexuality into a "lifestyle" rather than a "deviance," right-wing moralists sought to shore up traditional condemnations of homosexuality (p. 13).

From the beginning, then, HIV disease was inextricably associated with gay men, social stigma, and homophobia. Interestingly, in reviewing the medical literature from 1981 onward, although homosexual behavior was openly discussed as a critical variable in HIV transmission, homophobia was rarely referred to as a significant influence on or obstacle to the development of adequate and available services, the willingness of physicians and other health care personnel to provide appropriate and sensitive care, or the need for specialized approaches for dealing with gay male patients with HIV.

When compared with the public outcry and the public health attention quickly following the first outbreak of Legionnaire's disease, for example, society's response to HIV was slow and frequently tinged with the sentiment that "they" deserved what they got. Homophobia was a major obstacle to the development of social and medical service centers, the development of a national policy to deal with the ramifications of HIV, and the lack of supportive media attention (Shilts, 1987; Panem, 1988; Perrow & Guillen, 1990).

GAY LIBERATION AND HIV

HIV was beginning to spread about a decade after the June 29, 1969, Stonewall riots in Greenwich Village. This rebellion against police harassment of gay men in the Stonewall bar was viewed by many as the declaration of gay liberation, gay sexual freedom, and gay pride. In the afterglow of the civil rights and sexual revolutions of the 1960s, group cohesiveness generated by the Stonewall riot caused many gay men to view secretiveness and shame as too costly a price to pay for their sexual orientation. For many gay men, gay liberation meant not only freedom to come out of the closet but to engage freely and frequently in all sorts of sexual behavior as well. For those who chose to be sexually active, sexual freedom as well as the spread of sexually transmitted diseases followed in the 1970s. Hepatitis A and B, syphilis, and venereal warts neared epidemic proportions in some large cities. In the late 1970s, infections such as giardiasis and amebiasis became serious health problems. Gorman (1986) states, "A sexual ecology emerged that provided many opportunities for the contraction of infectious disease. However, in the era of antibiotics these conditions were viewed as mere nuisances, the inevitable hazards of a busy sexual lifestyle" (p. 163).

As rumors of HIV spread through the gay community and as gay men began to develop symptoms and die, the sexual liberation of the 1970s was viewed by many gay men as a lethal delusion. Even among "closeted" or cautious gay men who had had few sexual partners, HIV caused fear and doubt. For gay men who were open about their sexual orientation and who had had active sexual lives with many partners, the reality of HIV came as a particularly severe blow. Their sexual revolution abruptly ended in fear of death and cautionary messages about safer sex.

Although gay men on the periphery of, or uninvolved in, gay liberation movements did not have to change their behavior as rapidly as did those who had sampled the freedoms of the sexual revolution, even the most chaste were affected by HIV. For those who struggled with internalized homophobia, the advent of AIDS seemed to indicate that fundamentalist Christians and Jews were right: homosexuals were being punished. Thus AIDS raised the specter of renewed social condemnation and harassment as it rapidly became "a cram course in death" (Holleran, 1988, p. 17).

HIV AND GAY IDENTITY

Because of HIV, both the affective and symbolic meanings of sexual contact and the nonsexual aspects of gay life and "culture" began to change (Gorman, 1986). Most men—gay or heterosexual—do not develop their self-definition solely on the basis of sexual orientation. Sexuality and sexual expression are only part of one's total experience and development of sense of self. For some gay men, however, sexual expression is a critical aspect of identity. When sexual expression results in an incurable and fatal infection, both identity and self-esteem may be threatened. Thus HIV caused fundamental changes in the private lives and public demeanor of many gay men, who were forced to reexamine their values and behaviors.

> A great many people lived a certain life that, within the bounds of what they knew at the time, was reasonably safe. But, like schoolchildren who learn years later that the school they attended was lined with asbestos; or like families who are told, twenty years after buying a house, that they live on a mountain of PCBs, the homosexuals who lived in New York, San Francisco, Los Angeles in the seventies, lived with a devotion to health and appearance that was part of their stereotype, learned afterward that all the while there was an invisible germ circulating in the fluids of their sexual partners that was capable of entering the body; of lying undiscovered, unnoticed, unseen for several years; and then of destroying the system of biological defenses. . . . This plague was retroactive (Holleran, 1988, pp. 17–18).

Responses to the threat of infection and disease varied. In the early days, before multiple losses occurred, denial was a common defense. Some gay men dismissed warnings that their behavior placed them at high risk for contracting HIV/AIDS. Anger was prevalent; for some gay men, AIDS seemed a conspiracy to undo the gay liberation struggle and force everyone back into the closet. Even after the cause of AIDS was discovered and the modes of transmission well documented, some gay men angrily denounced public health officials who moved to close bath houses where men often had many sexual partners in a single night.

As HIV spread and more and more people died, anger and denial gave way to mourning, collective grief, and mobilization of resources. Death of young friends, companions, and lovers became a universal experience. Many grieved, some suffered from survivor's guilt (Boykin, 1991), but none in the entire community remained untouched by HIV.

CLINICAL INTERVENTIONS

THE UNCERTAINTIES OF HIV

Clinical and psychosocial interventions related to HIV vary and change over time because of the unpredictable manifestations and permutations of the conditions caused by the virus. The course of infection is impossible to predict. Although it is virtually inevitable, at this point, that an infected gay man will develop full-blown AIDS or end-stage HIV disease, there is no way of knowing when progression to that stage might occur, whether it will be measured in months or years. Once symptoms appear, they may be episodic and transient or unremitting and incapacitating.

The combination of finality and uncertainty is extremely stressful. Although drug therapies now available can bolster the immune system and some opportunistic infections and dermatological conditions can be treated, infected men are aware of the possibility of wasting syndrome, dementia, or other neurological disorders as well as the possibility of painful conditions affecting all systems of the body. Thus pain is experienced both physically and emotionally because of the various consequences of opportunistic infections, reactions to drugs, dramatic changes in physical capacity and appearance, and anticipatory grief. Seropositive status combined with the social stigma associated with HIV and homophobia can create almost unbearable stress. Over time, this stress is exacerbated by the unpredictable course and episodic nature of the disease process.

Many of the support services developed for gay men are designed to help them cope with stress, manage depression and anxiety, locate and use resources, and maintain a reasonable sense of hope. Providing housing, health, and financial resources to replace losses resulting from job discrimination or income depleted on medical treatment are important service components. Services for gay men must reflect the uncertainties and episodic characteristics of HIV, responding to the needs of the so-called "worried well," asymptomatic HIV-positive gay men, and persons with end-stage HIV disease.

HIV AND THE "WORRIED WELL"

Because HIV infection is so devastating in its symbolic meanings and physical course, even gay men who have not engaged in risk behaviors may be concerned about their well-being. Early in the epidemic, these men were called the "worried well."

In the midst of an epidemic, it may seem unimportant to devote time and resources to people who do not have a history of risk behaviors. However, this group needs services as well. Although some fear may be reduced by shifting attention from "risk groups" to "risk behaviors," many people continue to feel threatened and require intervention. They may exhibit signs of anxiety, depression, shame, guilt, and sexual aversion or dysfunction.

For gay men who are in long-term monogamous relationships or who have been abstinent, social work or clinical intervention may be limited to information about prevention and transmission, psychological bolstering, and connection to support groups. For men who have been careful, in general, but who, perhaps under the influence of alcohol or drugs, have engaged in unprotected sex or shared needles, fear may lead to immobilization and decreased coping skills. A relapse from practicing safer sex is invariably followed by guilt, remorse, and fear. In such instances, the social worker must deal directly with these feelings. If internalized homophobia is involved, self-doubt and self-hatred may contribute to panic states. Even if self-acceptance is evident, intervention must explore emotions, acceptance of the rational fears of the consequences of high-risk behavior, and reinforcement of safer sex practices.

Anticipation of HIV-positive status is common. Even when risk assessment indicates that a "worried well" gay man is at little risk, a social worker may advise testing and conduct a full pretest counseling session. For some men, HIV status becomes an obsession, whereby individuals go from testing site to testing site in a continuing effort to guarantee the accuracy of test results. In such cases, social workers or HIV counselors may need to shift emphasis from HIV status to underlying psychological dynamics that create doubt and the ongoing need for reassurance.

Worried-well individuals are amenable to accepting psychosocial support and HIV-negative test results to the degree that they are able to accept their sexual orientation, have sources of social support, and obtain a sense of identity and control through self-monitoring. Among persons for whom these factors are not present, preoccupation with HIV status can lead to dysfunction in nearly all areas of life.

GAY MEN AND HIV ANTIBODY TESTING

All people who are at perceived or actual risk of HIV must ultimately make a decision about HIV antibody testing. At first glance, deciding whether to take a simple blood test that can reveal HIV antibody status would not seem to be problematic. Since testing became available in 1985, however, many gay men have been ambivalent about learning their HIV status. Testing is resisted because of fear of breaches in confidentiality and subsequent discrimination by health care workers, insurance carriers, employers, and friends and family members. Although such ambivalence has never been fully resolved, resistance to testing has been mitigated somewhat by developments in prophylactic use of drugs to boost the immune system and to slow the progression of infection. Early drug intervention can extend the asymptomatic period and lead to a longer life.

Fear about loss of confidentiality of test results persists. These concerns are continually reinforced by national, state, and local legislative proposals to require mandatory reporting of HIV infection, contact tracing, or quarantine. Although such proposals have not been enacted, they create fear and anxiety about how and whether test results can be kept confidential. Even when gay men follow the advice of social workers or HIV counselors and use only sites that provide anonymous (as opposed to confidential) testing, fear of exposure is frequently expressed.

Fear of exposure stems not only from societal homophobia and discrimination, but from concern about the emotional impact of a positive test result. All people at risk express varying degrees of anxiety, anger, self-recrimination, depression, and worry while they await test results. A positive test result requires major changes in life-style as well as disclosure to others. With disclosure, gay men risk being rejected by lovers, family members, and/or co-workers. In many instances, disclosure of HIV status to family members simultaneously discloses the gay man's sexual orientation as well. In such instances, individuals face the double stigma of homosexuality and HIV-positive status at a time when they are experiencing severe stress, anxiety, and fear about the future. Clinicians hear many catastrophic fantasies (which, for some people, become catastrophic realities) about rejection and dying alone and abandoned.

Clinicians must provide considerable support to clients who are thinking about testing. They must conduct a risk assessment and help clients project how they might deal with a positive test result. The consequences of telling or not telling significant others must be examined and reexamined during the pretesting and posttesting counseling process.

Regardless of the outcome, many clinical issues must be addressed with regard to testing. People who receive a negative test result often express euphoria, which must be tempered by reminders about maintaining their HIV-negative status through safer sex and other precautions. This is particularly important because for some people a negative test result has been taken as license to resume unsafe behaviors. Some gay men continue unsafe practices, returning periodically to anonymous sites for further testing. Such magical thinking allows these clients to continue to practice high-risk behaviors.

If a client reports risk behaviors in the three- to six-month period before testing, future testing is indicated to ensure that the negative test is not a result of the so-called "window period," during which early infection is present but antibodies are not yet detectable through testing. Such recommendations produce anxiety, and clinicians must maintain ongoing contact with and provide psychosocial support for these clients.

Except for some virtually universal responses such as fear of death and disfigurement, it is not possible to predict how gay men will react to the news of an HIV-positive test result. Coping with fear is a highly individual matter. Some men, particularly in the early years of the epidemic, when few support services were available and the life span after diagnosis was very short, withdrew emotionally and physically. Self-isolation is a coping response that should be respected, thus allowing a person to regroup and find ways to cope with this new circumstance.

Many gay men find emotional support as well as a constructive way to release anger and anxiety through political activism or by providing direct assistance to others through coalitions such as Persons Living with AIDS and the AIDS Coalition to Unleash Power (ACT UP). Referral to such groups and other AIDS services organizations can be helpful for persons with positive test findings.

As with all persons who are HIV positive, gay men should be provided with information to reinforce safe behaviors. Although the media have reported that some gay men, such as Patient Zero described by Shilts (1987), knowingly infect others as a kind of retribution for their own infection, most gay men understand that being HIV positive but asymptomatic does not mean they are free of infection and take measures to protect others. The clinician's focus must be on protecting others, but should also emphasize to the client that safer sexual practices or clean drug-injection "works" protect the infected individual from contracting sexually transmitted diseases or other infections that might further damage his already compromised immune system.

HIV-Positive Asymptomatic Gay Men

HIV-positive, asymptomatic gay men require ongoing support from clinicians to make a series of important decisions with far-reaching consequences. The possible outcomes of telling family members and significant others about their HIV status and/or life-style need to be discussed, and relapse into unsafe practices is a continuing concern. They need to prepare for an uncertain future by thinking about possible housing, economic, and social resources needed when symptoms do appear. Wills and durable powers of attorney should be discussed and completed. These practical steps and decisions are difficult for people of all ages but are exponentially more difficult when these decisions must be made by young men with HIV who do not feel sick.

Asymptomatic gay men with HIV must also make decisions about medical treatments and drug therapies. Timely access to medical care, psychosocial support systems, and clinical trials may not be adequate in small cities, low prevalence areas, and rural areas. Inadequate services or lack of access to clinical trials may provoke outbursts of anger, which is often close to the surface in gay men grappling with the implications of their HIV-positive status. Unchanneled anger can create obstacles to obtaining care and place strains upon relationships with caregivers. However, anger can also serve as a motivator for self-care and active seeking of alternative methods of treatment. Seeking knowledge about alternative therapies gives many HIV-positive gay men the sense of being able to control what is happening to them. Taken to the extreme, however, alternative therapies can sabotage conventional treatment. Thus, clinicians need to help clients find balance in their lives and to overcome resistance to conventional services, health care providers, and drug therapies.

Isolation is a major concern. Some HIV-positive men suffer losses in their significant relationships after their HIV status becomes known. Others do not know how or whether to establish nonsexual relationships. Relationships provide valuable support to HIV-positive individuals, although there is always the concern that one of the partners will die and earlier losses will be relived (Martin, 1989).

Gay Men and End-stage HIV

HIV begins with infection, progresses through an asymptomatic period, the development of progressive lymphadenopathy or other signs of immune system disorder, and finally to the breakdown of the body's capacity to resist disease. Among the most common symptoms of full-blown AIDS are *Pneumocystis carinii* pneumonia (PCP), wasting syndrome, and Kaposi's sarcoma (Centers for Disease Control, 1987).

AIDS refers to a condition whereby the immune system cannot protect the body from disease organisms. Some opportunistic infections can be treated with drugs (e.g., aerosolized pentamidine for PCP). Zidovudine (AZT) or the more recently approved dideoxyinosine (ddI), administered alone or with other drugs, may inhibit disease progression or bolster the faltering immune system. However, despite these therapies and the increasing life span of gay men with end-stage symptoms, HIV is fatal. Knowledge of this reality creates severe stress and anxiety as the body begins to show immune system decline.

When symptoms of declining health appear, persons with HIV often relive the losses and sense of abandonment experienced during earlier phases of the disease or at other periods in their life. If they have experienced significant personal losses of friends through death or rejection, the intensity of their feelings when symptoms first appear can be overwhelming. Contingency plans that were made earlier may be reconsidered. They may feel the need to tell more people about their condition and to locate additional medical and psychosocial support services.

Self-control is a critical issue at this stage. Maintaining control over medical treatment and day-to-day living patterns becomes a priority. However, repeated hospitalizations or the need for hospice care, a nursing home, or residence for people with AIDS invariably challenges the individual's ability to control his life. Clinical issues must focus on providing emotional support in the face of multiple losses and diminished self-control, rebellion, refusal to comply with medical directives or the requisites of group living, and anger directed at caregivers.

Changes in physical appearance, particularly when wasting occurs and visible lesions appear, are difficult to accept, especially for young men. Changes in appearance affect self-image as well as patients' willingness to comply with medical treatments and medications.

THEORETICAL PERSPECTIVES

No single theoretical perspective is sufficient for clinicians working with gay men affected by HIV. A person-in-environment paradigm or ecological perspective clearly serves the clinician well in organizing his or her thoughts about the numerous interventions for addressing individual concerns, supporting family members and significant others, locating appropriate resources and benefits, and maintaining contact with health care providers.

HIV-positive gay men's lives are marked by crises. Paradoxically, the knowledge that the effects of a particular crisis can be dealt with and minimized for a time may be stressful in that the issues are not truly resolved, but merely interrupted. Preparing clients for the emotional toll of "continuing crisis" is a key clinical activity.

Cognitive therapeutic approaches can help clients handle anxiety and depression, particularly during the asymptomatic phase. Clinicians must be attuned to suicidal ideation and careful in their evaluation of it. Because of AIDS-related dementia and the interactions of multiple drugs that may disrupt behavior and coping, assessment of mental status or suicidal ideation is often difficult. Psychiatric consultation may be required.

Clinicians must have skills in supporting clients and their support systems through the anticipatory and continuing grief processes. Clinicians must recognize the influence of multiple losses on the outlook of the dying man. Psychological distress increases in proportion to the number of bereavements experienced (Martin,

1988). Although the dynamics of grieving and mourning are universal, HIV brings into play some unique variables. Mourning involves not only responding to the loss of one's own life or that of a loved one, but to losses that have occurred during periods of near-death and remission. Anticipatory grief may be interrupted by yet one more chance, however brief, for life. Grief and mourning may also be affected by the gay man's sexual orientation. If his life-style has been kept secret and if he is alienated from his family, survivors may feel shame about his disclosure, regret that a part of their loved one's life had been hidden from them, or guilt about their treatment of him. Parents may grieve over the loss of family continuity and future grandchildren.

Work related to death, dying, grief, and mourning can create emotional strain for even the most experienced clinician. Thus a clinician who treats gay men with HIV disease should seek out a support group for him- or herself.

HIV is a great social leveler. Even gay men with financial means may ultimately need financial assistance or guidance on how to obtain Social Security, Medicaid, and other benefits. Without such benefits, the individual's capacity for self-control and self-monitoring is seriously impaired.

Intervention Plans

Treatment planning for HIV-positive gay men must be flexible because of the episodic nature of HIV and the fear it engenders. Interventions must take into account the social context of HIV, homophobia, and stigma as well as personal concerns about security and support.

Although emotional support is absolutely essential, it is not always easy to give. Because of the "roller coaster" health and emotional status of persons with HIV, clients often focus their anger on caregivers. Anger and fear of the consequences of anger (e.g., abandonment) frequently coexist. Thus, people with HIV/AIDS require extensive indirect services. Clinicians need to be informed about and utilize (or develop) community and social services to support the multiple needs of these clients.

Gay men are generally willing to develop, support, and use services that are "user friendly." Although initially service organizations were developed through the gay community, organizations today depend upon financial and volunteer support from all levels of society. A clinician does not have to be gay in order to provide services to gay men with HIV. It is essential, however, for clinicians to be aware of their own feelings about sexual orientation. It is essential that clinicians feel comfortable and secure working with gay men and talking about sexual practices.

Although clinical work with gay men with HIV is always complex, it is even more complex when substance abuse is involved. Gay men who use injected drugs and share needles have multiple chances for infection and may express a range of emotions from apathy and despair to rebellion and noncompliance. Clinical work is particularly difficult when the client is actively using drugs. Drug use diminishes compliance with medical and psychosocial interventions and follow-up and may rule out placement in residential facilities as well.

Clinical interventions must take ethnicity and cultural differences into account. In many black and Hispanic communities, for example, homosexuality is considered perverse and the existence of homosexuality may be denied. Clinicians must be aware of cultural attitudes if they are to provide effective services to these communities.

THE FUTURE

Although the number of new AIDS cases being reported in the homosexual/bisexual male category has reached a plateau, complacency must be avoided. Many HIV-positive asymptomatic gay men will become ill over the next several years. Despite the relative success of prevention campaigns to promote safer sex and drug-use precautions, unsafe practices continue, and HIV will continue to be a defining characteristic of life for gay men for many years to come. Many adolescent and young adult gays may now be viewing HIV infection as an affliction of older men. Thus, the sense of invulnerability, which was shattered at the beginning of the epidemic, may once again become a major problem in HIV transmission patterns during the 1990s.

Community-based AIDS service organizations are needed. More important, existing organizations must be expanded during this era of scarce financial resources. Medical and psychosocial services for HIV-positive gay men in all geographical areas of the United States are being stretched to the breaking point. Health care costs are escalating and service provision is diminishing. Such realities will inevitably lead to more case-management services. Although case management is a necessary service, it is not a panacea for already overburdened or inadequate services.

Finally, given the absence of a national policy, integrated programs for prevention, adequate resources, and facilities for treatment and control of HIV disease—as well as the increase in HIV cases among ethnic-minority-group members, women, and children—HIV will negatively affect individuals, families, and society for decades to come. No vaccine or cure is in sight. In the society at large, many middle-class heterosexual people who do not use drugs feel that they have nothing to fear from HIV. Social workers and other HIV counselors will undoubtedly encounter ongoing resistance to additional funding and resources, which may contribute to higher burnout rates among service providers.

This gloomy outlook may be mitigated somewhat by the ongoing responses of gay men to the threat of HIV disease. AIDS services organizations initiated by gay men and lesbian women continue to expand in large urban areas, and new organizations are being developed in smaller communities. Although rural areas are still underserved, steps are being taken to create networks of organizations to address the needs of HIV-positive gay men in rural communities. The service models developed by and for the gay community are models for the development of service-delivery systems for other populations now gravely threatened by HIV disease. Efforts have been made to expand gay-oriented services to include heterosexual men, women, and children. As that trend continues, it is probable that the AIDS service organization model developed by gay men will be supplemented by and adapted to the special needs of other groups so that services will reflect the various populations affected by AIDS.

The heavy toll of HIV disease among gay males has created a community of mourners. Because of the magnitude of losses and the continuing stigma attached both to homosexuality and HIV disease, the pandemic has stimulated political mobilization. The move for civil liberties begun by the Stonewall riot in New York City in 1969 has now evolved into a network of lesbian and gay civil rights and defense organizations throughout the United States, most of which have responded to the many discrimination issues related to HIV disease.

Social workers and other human service professionals practicing with people affected by HIV disease have created peer consultation and supervision groups to assist them both in keeping up with quickly changing knowledge about HIV and in handling multiple losses and supporting necessary grief work. Although there is no happy beginning, middle, or end to the HIV story, the individual and community responses of gay men caring for young, sick men and developing AIDS services organizations serve as a model for responding to critical needs in the absence of public policy and in the face of public denial and/or antipathy.

REFERENCES

Altman, D. (1987). *AIDS in the mind of America.* Garden City, NY: Anchor Books.

Boykin, F. (1991). The AIDS crisis and gay male survivor guilt. *Smith College Studies in Social Work, 61,* 247–259.

Burke, D. S., & Redfield, R. (1989). The stages of HIV infection: A predictable, progressive disease. In N. Rapoza (Ed.), *HIV infection and disease.* Chicago: American Medical Association.

Centers for Disease Control. (1987). Revision of the CDC surveillance case definition for Acquired Immunodeficiency Syndrome. *Mortality and Morbidity Weekly Report, 36*(1S), 3S–14S.

Centers for Disease Control. (1991). *HIV/AIDS surveillance: U.S. AIDS cases reported through August 1991.* Atlanta: Author.

Gorman, M. (1986). The AIDS epidemic in San Francisco: Epidemiology and anthropological perspectives. In R. Craig, R. Stall, & S. M. Gifford (Eds.), *Anthropology and epidemiology.* Dordrecht, The Netherlands: O. Reidel Publishing.

Heyward, W. L., & Curran, J. W. (1988). The epidemiology of AIDS in the U.S. In *The science of AIDS: Readings from the Scientific American magazine* (pp. 40–49). New York: W. H. Freeman.

Holleran, A. (1988). *Ground zero.* New York: New American Library.

Mann, J. (1988). Global AIDS: Epidemiology, impact, projections, global strategy. In *AIDS prevention and control* (pp. 3–13). Oxford: Pergamon Press.

Martin, D. (1989). Human immunodeficiency virus infection and the gay community: Counseling and clinical issues. *Journal of Counseling and Development, 68*(1), 67–72.

Martin, J. (1988). Psychological consequences of AIDS-related bereavement among gay men. *Journal of Counseling and Clinical Psychology, 17,* 856–862.

Osborn, J. (1988). AIDS: Politics and science. *New England Journal of Medicine, 318,* 444–447.

Panem, S. (1988). *The AIDS bureaucracy.* Cambridge, MA: Harvard University Press.

Perrow, C., & Guillen, M. (1990). *The AIDS disaster: The failure of organizations in New York and the nation.* New Haven, CT: Yale University Press.

Relman, A. (1987). *AIDS: Epidemiological and clinical studies.* Boston: Massachusetts Medical Society.

Rogers, D., & Osborn, J. (1991). Another approach to the AIDS epidemic. *New England Journal of Medicine, 325,* 806–808.

Shilts, R. (1987). *And the band played on.* New York: St. Martin's Press.

Stulberg, I., & Smith, M. (1988). Psychosocial impact of the AIDS epidemic on the lives of gay men. *Social Work, 33,* 277–281.

Tindall, B., & Tillett, G. (1990). HIV-related discrimination. *AIDS 1990, 4*(suppl. 1), S251–S256).

8

HIV DISEASE AND SUBSTANCE ABUSE: TWIN EPIDEMICS, MULTIPLE NEEDS

JACK B. STEIN

The combined impact of HIV and substance abuse in America has created formidable stress on the human service system. Social service agencies are expected to do more with fewer resources to meet clients' multiple and complex needs presented by this dual diagnosis. To do so, however, practitioners must learn new ways to adapt their practice skills to the needs of this client population.

This chapter provides an overview of the issues critical to providing quality services to the traditionally underserved population of substance users who are now facing the additional health burdens associated with HIV disease. Specifically, the chapter addresses (1) the link between substance abuse and HIV disease, (2) how social attitudes influence the delivery of services to such a population, (3) key elements to understanding addiction, and (4) recommended treatment goals and counseling strategies.

HIV AND SUBSTANCE ABUSE

Currently, more than 30% of all reported cases of AIDS are directly linked to injection drug use (IDU). It is the second risk factor for HIV infection nationwide and the first risk factor in some urban areas of the country. In the New York/New Jersey metropolitan area, for example, HIV seroprevalence among injection drug users is approximately 60% (National Commission on AIDS, 1991). Furthermore, IDU is the first and fastest growing risk factor for heterosexuals, minorities, women, and children. Of the reported cases among women, 71% are linked directly to IDU or indirectly through sexual contact with an infected drug-using male. Of the reported pediatric cases, 70% are born to mothers infected with HIV through IDU or sex with an HIV-positive male drug user. Among minorities, African Americans and Hispanics collectively account for 44% of all AIDS cases. However, of those cases attributed to IDU (directly or indirectly), African Americans account for 45% and Hispanics 26%. Collectively, more than 70% of cases linked to IDU occur among these two populations (Centers for Disease Control, 1991).

These figures, however, do not fully address the impact of substance abuse on the HIV epidemic. The judgment-impairing qualities of alcohol and noninjection drugs also play an indirect, yet significant, role in HIV transmission. The association between alcohol and high-risk sex has been known for years. Crack (a smoked derivative of cocaine) produces an extremely addictive "high" and is frequently associated with hypersexuality. Moreover, the crack epidemic sweeping the nation closely parallels the rise in syphilis and other sexually transmitted diseases (National Commission on AIDS, 1991). It is only a matter of time before the impact of crack on the HIV epidemic becomes evident, particularly among adolescents.

The inherent immune-suppressing qualities of drugs may also be a potential contributor to HIV-disease progression among individuals already infected with the virus. Continued substance use by an HIV-positive individual may increase viral replication while increasing vulnerability to opportunistic infections associated with HIV (Batki, 1990).

SOCIETAL ATTITUDES

The HIV epidemic has shown how availability of human service programs is often determined more by society's attitudes toward the client population than by the level of needs. If HIV disease were viewed from a value-free perspective, it would be defined solely as a public health problem and interventions would be established accordingly. Instead, policies and services have often been based on political posturing and moral views rather than on sound principles of public health.

Substance abuse, particularly IDU, has never been well tolerated by society. As a group, substance users are seen as incompetent, unable to help themselves, antisocial, and incapable of acting responsibly either as individuals or a community. Subsequently, drug users are often deemed "undeserving" of services compared with other clients. Defining clients as being either deserving or undeserving is of particular significance when resources are limited and budget cutbacks require decisions about who gets served and how.

For years, AIDS activists have sought to secure equal rights and services for all people with HIV disease, as exemplified by the Ryan White CARE Act. Most activists would agree that this struggle for fair treatment is far from over. The combined stigma of HIV and substance abuse allows many clients to fall between the cracks of an uncaring system.

For years, HIV prevention efforts targeting substance users have been thwarted by community disagreement over definitions of "acceptable" prevention messages. Although HIV-prevention campaigns now emphasize the significance of the HIV–substance abuse connection, it is still difficult to arrive at community consensus regarding intervention methods (e.g., needle "exchange" programs), because many people believe that such messages condone drug use.

Antibody testing is another area of concern for clients affected by HIV and substance abuse. From a public health perspective, testing is considered important to motivate individual behavior change and promote early treatment intervention.

However, client advocates argue that widespread testing of disenfranchised populations might actually be counterproductive. Persons affected by the HIV–substance abuse link not only have much to gain from learning their antibody status, but also may have much to lose. Discrimination in employment and health care delivery is still rampant, despite newly established laws to prevent this from occurring. Women are particularly vulnerable to health care discrimination. Women with HIV have a 30% to 50% chance of giving birth to an infected child. Thus, these women must confront difficult choices regarding their reproductive rights and child-care responsibilities (Lloyd, Lipscomb, & Johnson, 1991). Additionally, many women are now being held liable for giving birth to addicted children. How liability will accrue as a result of perinatal HIV transmission is yet to be determined.

Addicted pregnant women or single mothers have traditionally had little access to substance-abuse treatment. Many programs are unable to accommodate the multiple needs presented by female clients. In other instances, women are unable to meet program attendance requirements because of child-care responsibilities. With the added complication of HIV infection, treatment options can severely handicap care delivery to these clients.

UNDERSTANDING ADDICTION

Unfortunately, health care and human service professionals are not above stigmatizing people with HIV/substance-abuse problems. In a representative national random sample of more than 1,000 primary care physicians, nearly 70% believed that they had a responsibility to treat people with HIV (Gerbert, Maguire, Bleecker, Coates, & McPhee, 1991). However, half of the sample also said they would not treat persons with HIV if given a choice. Additionally, a majority indicated that they would rather not treat injection drug users. These data support earlier reports of primary care physicians' unfavorable attitudes toward serving this population.

Service providers have a professional responsibility to overcome personal biases or beliefs that might prevent delivery of quality services to any client in need. To overcome such attitudes, caregivers must be afforded the opportunity to explore the nature of these biases. In many cases, negative attitudes are based on a lack of knowledge and familiarity with particular client attributes. The fear of HIV transmission and the stereotypes of drug users and alcoholics as difficult clients cause many professionals to avoid treating such clients. Professionals who have practice experience working with HIV-infected clients are usually more willing to serve HIV-infected substance users compared with providers who have not had such experiences (Gerbert et al., 1991).

Training and field experience are probably the best means for helping providers to understand the complex dynamics of addiction and to explore any personal biases that may hinder their work with such clients. At a minimum, service providers should understand the following.

1. *A drug is any chemical substance that impairs one's physical, mental, emotional, and social self.* The legal status of a substance has no bearing on its defini-

tion as a drug. For example, alcohol is the most commonly used drug in the United States. There are approximately nine million alcoholics in the Unites States (Lloyd et al., 1991).

2. *Drug dependence can be physical and/or psychological.* Some substances can create an altered physiological state so that, upon discontinuing use, withdrawal symptoms occur. In addition, some substances are psychologically addicting, causing the individual to feel that the substance is necessary to maintain well-being.

3. *Substances are classified according to their effects.*

♦ Stimulants (cocaine, crack, amphetamines)—increased alertness, excitation, euphoria, loss of appetite

♦ Hallucinogens (LSD, peyote)—illusions and hallucinations, poor perception of time and distance

♦ Cannabis (marijuana, hashish)—euphoria, relaxed inhibitions, increased appetite, disoriented behavior

♦ Narcotics (opium, codeine, heroin, methadone)—euphoria, drowsiness, respiratory depression, constricted pupils, nausea

♦ Depressants (barbiturates, benzodiazepines, alcohol)—slurred speech, disorientation)

4. *The etiology of addiction is not fully understood.* Several models, ranging from the moral–legal model to the medical or disease model, have been applied to understand better the cause of substance abuse. Many theorists and practitioners prefer the biopsychosocial model, which holds that any single theory or explanation to explain substance abuse is overly simplistic. This model relies on biological, genetic, psychological, and social factors to describe and explain substance-using behaviors.

5. *Addiction is a significant stressor to the client system.* Stress associated with substance use is often the result of the continuous search to find and financially support a drug habit, the loss of employment and significant others, and the constant avoidance of law-enforcement authorities.

6. *Polysubstance use is widespread.* Individuals who have had an alcohol-abuse disorder are seven times more likely than is the rest of the population to have had a drug-abuse disorder, and vice versa (Goodwin, 1991).

7. *Comorbidity of substance abuse and mental illness is common.* Among individuals who sought treatment for a drug disorder, 64% had had a mental disorder in the previous six months. Of individuals who sought treatment for an alcohol disorder, 55% had a mental disorder; 20% of those who visited a mental health treatment center had a substance-abuse disorder in the past six months (Goodwin, 1991).

8. *Addiction is progressive.* Addiction generally begins with a "recreational" phase. Continued use can eventually lead to compulsive use and ultimately may lead to death if not treated. Although recovery is the goal of treatment, relapse is often viewed as a normal part of the process.

9. *Denial is a common ego defense of substance users.* Denial allows the addict and his or her social system to reject the reality of the addiction. Confronting an indi-

vidual about his or her drug or alcohol use can be interpreted as a direct attack and result in a defensive counterattack, often aimed at family members or caregivers.

10. *Manifested behaviors are merely symptoms of addiction.* Antisocial behaviors, including manipulation, are often observed among substance users. These behaviors, however, are merely symptomatic of the client's addiction. Interventions should focus on the underlying causes of addiction rather than on merely trying to eliminate these behaviors. Assessing the client's strengths and weaknesses, particularly with respect to support systems, is helpful in developing realistic and attainable treatment goals.

COUNSELING SUBSTANCE-ABUSE CLIENTS WITH HIV DISEASE

The HIV epidemic has brought the need for a multidimensional approach to serving clients into sharp focus. In working with substance users with HIV, counselors face the challenge of managing diverse HIV-related concerns while managing chemical dependency and recovery.

Human service providers must learn to integrate the multiple issues presented by HIV and substance abuse into treatment planning and service provision for all clients, regardless of the setting. Providers need to acquire knowledge, examine personal and professional attitudes, and develop new counseling skills. Moreover, professionals need to cooperate as part of multidisciplinary teams to meet the diverse challenges presented by HIV and substance abuse.

Treatment planning for HIV–substance abuse clients requires professionals to examine the following four major treatment-planning areas: (1) HIV awareness and health promotion, (2) psychosocial adjustment, (3) family/other support systems, and (4) community resources (Fischer, Jones, & Stein, 1990). By applying each of these four treatment areas to a three-step planning process, a comprehensive treatment plan can be established for any client with a dual diagnosis of HIV/substance abuse.

Figure 1 illustrates a three-phase process for planning client treatment. Through this process, a "contract" between client and provider is established. This contract should be reviewed and shaped on an ongoing basis to accommodate the episodic nature of HIV and addiction.

HIV AWARENESS AND HEALTH PROMOTION

Regardless of their setting, service providers have an obligation to help a client assess his or her risk of HIV infection and transmission. Using a personalized risk-assessment history, practitioners can help clients initiate plans to modify their

FIGURE 1. THREE-PHASE TREATMENT PROCESS.

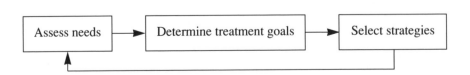

behaviors. Clients' history of drug and alcohol use as well as sexual activity patterns need to be assessed.

- ◆ Type of substance(s) used
- ◆ Approximate dates of first use
- ◆ Route of administration (oral, nasal, injected)
- ◆ Sharing of injection equipment
- ◆ Disinfection of injection equipment
- ◆ Frequency and duration of use
- ◆ Effect of drug use on sexual activity
- ◆ Geographic location where drug use occurred
- ◆ Medical problems related to drug use
- ◆ Substance-abuse treatment experience/history (Lloyd et al., 1991).

Based on the information gathered from this assessment, the client and practitioner are equipped to establish realistic and practical treatment goals. For active substance users, the assessment process presents an important opportunity for seeking treatment for an addiction that may place them at increased risk of HIV infection or disease progression.

Counseling strategies related to HIV awareness and health promotion typically involve ongoing education and behavior modification that build on past client accomplishments and empower further achievements. These goals are often achieved by exploring personal incentives and obstacles, problem solving and planning, skill building, and providing support and reinforcement. Such interventions are particularly important to clients with low self-esteem and poor ego strengths, both of which are characteristics of substance abusers.

PSYCHOSOCIAL ADJUSTMENT

Nichols and Ostrow (1984) describe a model for understanding and responding to the psychosocial distress experienced by substance-abuse clients with HIV. This model suggests three phases of psychosocial adjustment, each of which describes a "typical" response by a substance-abuse client to HIV disease: (1) initial crisis, (2) transition, and (3) acceptance. For clients in the terminal stage of HIV disease, a fourth phase—preparation for death—may occur. The psychosocial responses characterizing each phase may be used to assess "where" client needs lie, thereby allowing the practitioner to formulate appropriate treatment goals and strategies. Client responses will be highly variable and influenced by HIV-disease developmental milestones.

Initial crisis. Triggered by the individual's learning about an HIV-related diagnosis, this phase is characterized by shock and denial. In general, denial is a natural reaction that can serve the important function of helping ease the impact of devastating information. However, addicts may remain "stuck" in this phase for an extended period, which can possibly lead to maladaptive behaviors, such as refusal to seek needed medical attention or continuation of risky behaviors.

Perhaps the most effective counseling response to help clients move beyond this phase involves patience on the part of the counselor and reliance on the trust established between counselor and client. However, while in this state of denial, client-specific HIV issues may be nearly impossible to address. Instead, counseling strategies may best focus on general risk reduction and health-promotion issues that arise during the course of counseling with any client. Other useful approaches involve "normalizing" the client's experience by discussing how difficult it is for others to handle news related to their HIV infection. Over time, however, direct confrontation may be required, particularly in the event that the client persists in engaging in behaviors that are harmful to the client or to others.

Transition phase. As denial subsides, clients enter a transitional phase during which psychosocial reactions can be extreme. Clients are especially accessible to psychosocial intervention during this time. Clients' emotional states range from self-devaluation, fear, depression, and helplessness to escapism, anger, and relapse into risky sexual and drug-using practices. The emotional reactions in this phase are frequently compounded by the emotional vulnerability characteristic of substance users. For example, preexisting depression in addicts may lead to dangerous levels of depression with the introduction of HIV disease. For others, inadequate coping mechanisms may lead to withdrawal and isolation. The possibility of relapse into risky activities is high.

During the roller coaster of reactions and emotions characteristic of the transition phase, treatment goals should aim to maximize overall client functioning. Specifically, this may require providing clients with ample opportunities to ventilate their distress and to receive validation of their responses. Problem solving, priority setting, and developing a peer-support system can be a great help during this period.

Acceptance phase. Some clients are not able to work through the denial and emotional upheaval of the transition phase to achieve acceptance of their condition. For those who do succeed, however, treatment goals should focus on maintaining and modifying life-enhancing achievements in the face of recurrent challenges presented by a dual diagnosis. Like recovery, acceptance of one's HIV disease is a tremendous accomplishment. Also like recovery, it is a precarious process, something to be accomplished one day at a time. New crises are liable to trigger reactions similar to those described in the transition phase. This process is similar to recovery and relapse of addiction. It is no wonder, therefore, that many such individuals find solace in attending self-help meetings that follow the 12-step approach used by Alcoholics Anonymous (AA), but which are adapted to meet the unique needs of persons directly affected by HIV disease.

Preparation for death. Clients in the terminal stages of HIV disease should be given permission to express anything—or nothing—regarding their pending death. The client who has successfully negotiated earlier adjustments to living with AIDS may resolve this grief. For others, the grief is so overwhelming that reverting to drug use seems the only solution.

The overarching goal of this phase is to assist the client in living with dignity until death occurs. Treatment goals include supporting the client's need for grieving over the loss of life, completing unfinished business, and executing wishes upon his or her death. During this phase, the counselor should allow the client to "direct" the events of his or her passing life. For the addict in recovery, unfinished business may be extensive. This may include reconciliations with estranged family, spouses, and friends; arranging care for children; or seeking forgiveness from someone. A counselor's assistance can be crucial in helping prioritize issues for a client and helping devise ways in which to respond.

FAMILY/SIGNIFICANT OTHERS

HIV and substance abuse are significant stressors for family and significant others. Family work is best approached from a systems perspective, which assumes that chemically dependent families, despite unconventional configurations and dysfunctional dynamics, are systems just the same. Many chemically dependent clients, especially those entering treatment, may be loathe to discuss their family and may even deny the existence of ties or their relevance to treatment (Fischer, Jones, & Stein, 1990). The practitioner needs to help clients recognize the relevance of family influences in dealing with addiction and HIV.

In ethnic communities, biological and extended families are often the primary support network for the client. The family provides the context within which the person functions and relates to issues of self-esteem, identity formation, isolation, and role assumptions. Alcohol and drug problems, particularly as they intersect with the sensitive nature of HIV infection, must be framed within the primary value system of that particular community. Hence, effective interventions require appreciation of issues related to gender, hierarchy, decision-making styles, communication patterns, learning styles, and etiquette (Office for Substance Abuse Prevention, 1991).

HIV-specific assessments should focus on the client's need of family support and the family's desire and ability to provide such support. If family dysfunction is severe, the practitioner must decide whether to engage the family in prolonged therapy in the hope of increasing its supportive capacity. If family therapy is undertaken, treatment goals range from short-term goals (e.g., basic education about HIV transmission, prevention, and treatment) to those that require extensive intervention (e.g., helping the family adjust to the psychosocial impact of the client's condition).

Clients should be helped to identify potential support persons who are able and willing to commit themselves to the client's welfare. Practitioners may need to make home visits or invite the family to participate in counseling sessions either with the client or with other families experiencing similar issues.

COMMUNITY RESOURCES

Working with clients affected by both HIV disease and substance abuse is likely to require linkage with every arm of the human service system. However, treatment planning for clients with HIV is severely limited by the lack of HIV-related resources in most communities. This challenge is further handicapped by the additional burden of substance abuse. Most clients with HIV–substance abuse problems are members of disenfranchised groups. Thus, special attention must be focused on broad environmental factors such as poverty, racial discrimination, educational parity, reproductive rights, and child placement. Major counseling goals include identifying and securing needed services while not "overcaring" in a way that minimizes the client's overall functioning. This may best be achieved through a case-management approach that emphasizes close coordination of various community service providers. Care providers are in key positions to advocate for more services. Participation in community coalitions and task forces can be of great help in meeting the needs of substance-abuse clients with HIV.

CONCLUSION

The diverse needs of HIV–substance abuse clients demand that they have access to multiple service systems, including health care, social welfare, mental health, public health, clinical research, and substance-abuse treatment. However, the double stigma associated with HIV and substance abuse often prohibits these clients from accessing needed services. Caregivers must examine their own attitudes toward working with this growing client population, and service agencies must examine policies and procedures that may limit access to services. Flexibility in program rules and regulations may be required to accommodate the multiple stressors faced by these clients.

REFERENCES

Batki, S. (1990, Winter). Substance abuse and AIDS: The need for mental health services. *New Directions for Mental Health Services, 48*, 55–56.

Centers for Disease Control. (1991, September). *HIV/AIDS surveillance*. Atlanta: Author.

Fischer, G., Jones, S., & Stein, J. (1990). *Treatment planning for the client with HIV disease*. Rockville, MD: National Institute on Drug Abuse.

Gerbert, B., Maguire, B., Bleecker, T., Coates, T., & McPhee, S. (1991). Primary care physicians and AIDS. *Journal of the American Medical Association, 266*, 2837–2877.

Goodwin, F. (1991). Identification of dual diagnosis of drug abusers. In *Report from the National Conference on Drug Abuse Research and Practice*. Rockville, MD: National Institute on Drug Abuse.

Lloyd, G., Lipscomb, N. & Johnson, R. (1991). *Social work and the HIV/substance abuse connection*. Rockville, MD: National Institute on Drug Abuse.

National Commission on AIDS. (1991). *Report on the twin epidemics of substance use and HIV*. Washington, DC: U.S. Government Printing Office.

Nichols, S., & Ostrow, D. (1984). *Psychiatric implication of AIDS*. Washington DC: American Psychiatric Press.

Office for Substance Abuse Prevention. (1991). *The future by design: A community framework for preventing alcohol and other drug problems through a systems approach*. Washington, DC: U.S. Government Printing Office.

9

AIDS AND PEOPLE OF COLOR

LUISA MEDRANO AND MICHELE CUVILLY KLOPNER

From the beginning of the AIDS pandemic, ethnic and racial minorities have constituted a large portion of the population infected by HIV. However, epidemiologists, health care providers, and the media have only recently begun to recognize the dramatic needs of these populations. Blacks and Hispanics (Latinos) have been disproportionately affected by HIV, and rate of infection among these minorities has been steadily increasing. For example, blacks and Hispanics (12% and 8% of the population, respectively) make up 20% of the general population in the United States, yet they accounted for 45% of the total AIDS cases reported in 1990 (Centers for Disease Control, 1990).

The rate of infection among black and Hispanic homosexual and bisexual males is two or three times higher than their non-Hispanic white counterparts. Similarly, the same disproportionate rate of infection is evident when one compares white heterosexual and nonwhite heterosexual populations. For example, the rate of infection among heterosexual blacks and Latinos is 20 times higher than that of non-Latino heterosexual whites (Peterson & Marin, 1988; Pares-Avila, Hunt, Hammett, Sifre, Harrold, & Moini, 1989). Heterosexual transmission among Hispanics and blacks is linked to injection drug users and their sexual partners, who are often unaware of their partners' serostatus. Among Hispanics, the infected population includes homosexual and bisexual men who are not injection drug users (53%) and heterosexual male injection drug users (34%) (Marin, 1988).

Compared with non-Hispanic whites, racial and ethnic minorities are experiencing a higher rate of HIV infection. Among women, minority women are the fastest growing group infected by HIV, with blacks making up 52% and Latinos 20% of reported AIDS cases. The two most frequent modes of transmission are injection

Luisa Medrano wrote the sections on Latinos/Hispanics and Asians and Pacific Islanders. Michele Cuvilly Klopner wrote the sections on African Americans and Haitians. Michele Cuvilly Klopner thanks Richard Hermann, Loretta Saint-Louis, and Valerie Stone for their thoughtful comments.

drug use (52%) and being the sexual partner of a drug user (21%) (Amaro, 1988; Diaz, 1991; Quinn, Narain, & Zacarias, 1990). The proportion of AIDS cases in the United States among women of color has increased dramatically from 3% in 1981 to 10% in 1991 (Maldonado, 1991). Between 1985 and 1988, the rate of HIV infection quadrupled among women, a large proportion of whom were women of color in the northeastern United States. Currently, women of color constitute 72% of all women infected with HIV. Alarmingly, in New York City, AIDS is the leading cause of death among black women between the ages of 15 and 44 years and among Latinos 25 to 34 years old. Experts predict that AIDS will be the fifth leading cause of death among women of childbearing age, a statistic that has devastating implications for infants born to infected parents (Chu, Buehler, & Berkelman, 1990).

LATINOS/HISPANICS

DEMOGRAPHIC CHARACTERISTICS

Along geographic lines, the prevalence of HIV infection among Latinos varies according to region. The highest rate of Latino infection occurs in East Coast cities such as New York, Newark, and Boston, followed by West Coast cities such as Los Angeles and San Francisco. In the South, Miami has the highest rate of infection. The prevalence of infection among Latinos in the Northeast is higher than in other regions because of the high concentration of injection drug users (Marin, 1988). In a study comparing Puerto Rican born persons with people in Mexico, Cuba, and other Latin American countries, Selik, Castro, Pappaioanou, and Buehler (1989) found that Puerto Ricans have the highest incidence of infection among Latinos. This high incidence of infection among Puerto Ricans can be explained by the concentration of injection drug users in the Northeast and the frequency of travel between Puerto Rico and the Northeast. Amaro (1987) estimates that every two hours a Latino person is infected with HIV and every four hours a Latino dies from complications related to AIDS.

The statistics on rate of infection among people of color are presented as a brief and shocking sketch of the AIDS epidemic as it touches ethnic and racial communities. However, in order to understand treatment issues for Latino clients, the various cultures that appear in Latino communities need to be explored.

The term Latino/Hispanic is an umbrella term for the various Latin American and Caribbean populations living in the United States: Mexican (61%); Puerto Rican (15%); Cuban (6%); and Central American, South American, and Spanish (18%) (Amaro, 1987). The 20 million Latinos living in the United States represent a mosaic of cultures, races, classes, and languages (De La Vega, 1990). Similarities and differences exist among groups. Generalizations about Latinos as a single group miss subtle and key cultural differences that are useful in understanding the spread of AIDS among Latinos. Clinicians need to understand the important environmental and demographic forces that have shaped their clients' life experiences. Such factors include country of origin, immigrant status, income, level of education, and language. For example, Hispanic women, with the exception of Cuban women, have a median age of 26 years, in contrast with 32 years for the general white population. The factor of younger age, combined with socioeconomic factors such as lower educational achievement and a higher poverty level, place Latinos in general and Latina women in particular at higher risk for infection because these individuals are more likely to experiment with drugs and engage in unsafe sexual behaviors (Amaro, 1987).

In 1979, Latinos were the poorest ethnic group in the United States. Latinos who live in poverty experience poor health conditions and inadequate access to quality health care, which contributes greatly to the spread of AIDS in the Latino population. Latinos who live below the poverty line and are undocumented may choose drug dealing and drug use as a way to cope and survive (Marin, 1990). In a study of attitudes, beliefs, and behaviors among Hispanics in the Northeast and Puerto Rico, Amaro (1990) found that "higher risk sexual and drug-related behaviors were highest among males, those with low education and attainment and those with misconceptions regarding HIV infection and AIDS" (p. 13). Furthermore, when an injection drug user seeks help for a heroin habit, he or she may lack knowledge of available drug-detoxification programs. In fact, adequate prevention programs are scant in Latino communities. Early intervention and treatment are virtually unavailable for Latinos who would like to enter treatment. Only when their illnesses become life threatening do they have access to health care.

Women. Drug abuse, especially injection drug abuse, presents a serious threat to Latina women. Among Latinos, infection by a partner who is an injection drug user is the primary mode of HIV transmission. Prenatal transmission has skyrocketed to 53%, a rate also attributable to injection drug use. In addition, a lack of adequate drug-treatment facilities (consistent with the lack of quality health care overall) to address women's reproductive and prenatal health care needs contributes to the spread of HIV among addicted Latina women (Maldonado, 1991; Worth, 1990; Diaz, 1991).

Sexual abuse further complicates the connection between injection drug use and AIDS transmission in Latina women. Many women who are injection drug users have been raped or experienced incest as children or adolescents; using drugs may be a coping response to their abuse (Worth, 1990). Thus, it is important for clinicians who treat addicted women to obtain a detailed sexual history. However, it is often difficult for Latina women to discuss sexual issues. Clinicians need to approach the subject with sensitivity after a trusting relationship has been established.

Many Latina women find in motherhood the value and fulfillment that are otherwise denied to them within the community. For these reasons, Latinos rarely consider abortion an option even with the presence of maternal HIV infection. Unfortunately, many women learn of their serostatus when their babies become symptomatic and thus do not benefit from early intervention (Scheider, 1988). Moreover, women often do not have access to health care for themselves or their children. Maldonado (1991) reports that 29% of Latino households are headed by women with five or more children and that many of these families are below the poverty line. Clinicians need to be aware of these life circumstances in order best to serve the Latino population by providing information about health care services.

Adolescents. Latino adolescents are at high risk for infection as a result of their failure to use condoms. The pregnancy rate among Latino adolescents is high, which contributes to the high rate of prenatal transmission of AIDS. They make up 18% of AIDS cases reported among 13- to 19-year-olds (Maldonado, 1991).

Culture and behavior. Level of acculturation plays an important role in the prevention as well as treatment of HIV-infected Latinos. Less acculturated individuals (those who speak Spanish and live within a tight circle of family and friends) who live in East Coast and West Coast cities have less knowledge of and more misconceptions about HIV (Amaro, 1990; Rapkin & Erickson, 1990; Marin, 1989). This lack of knowledge stems in large part from the fact that most prevention materials are directed toward the English-speaking population.

Thus, sexual attitudes and behaviors play a role in the AIDS epidemic among Latinos. Despite the "Latin lover" myth, Latino sexuality is private and intimate. Sexual issues are seldom discussed, even between intimate partners. Further, a double standard exists for Latino men and women. Women are expected to remain virginal and naive, their role being purely procreative, with the exception of providing pleasure to their partners. Less acculturated Latino adolescents who seek to join the mainstream community often assume that American women are sexually promiscuous. Latino adolescents are likely to emulate this perceived pattern of sexual behavior, despite the tremendous conflict of such behaviors with the values of their family of origin.

Men, on the other hand, are assumed to be oversexed and "allowed" to have extramarital relationships. Carrier and Magana (1991) state that the oversexed-male myth contributes to frequent use of prostitutes among undocumented laborers. Condoms are used infrequently because of fear of rejection by either the prostitute or the customer. Within the marriage, condom use is rare because condoms are associated with prostitution, extramarital affairs, lack of cleanliness, sexually transmitted disease, and contraception.

When promoting condom use to the Latino community, clinicians, health care workers, and media campaigns should target men and couples (Marin, 1989). Latino women are at a cultural disadvantage in negotiating safe sex practices and sometimes become the targets of physical and verbal abuse when attempting such negotiations. Marin (1990) and Mays and Cochran (1988) suggest the concept of *machismo* can be used to emphasize safety of a man's family. Condom use can be portrayed as a way to reduce the threat of HIV to his family, thus insuring its survival.

Homosexuality and bisexuality are culturally taboo among Latinos. In Spanish, a nonpejorative equivalent for the word "gay" does not exist. Disclosure of homosexuality can result in loss of familial support and alienation from the community. Many Latino males who engage in homosexual encounters do not identify themselves as gay if they take the assertive ("male") role in the encounter (Peterson & Marin, 1988; Carrier & Magana, 1991). Moreover, the stigma associated with condom use in heterosexual encounters also exists in homosexual encounters. Amaro (1991) reported that 65% of bisexual Latino men reported having unprotected sex with a man; 27% of these men reported having unprotected sex with a woman as well.

PRACTICE IMPLICATIONS

Like many minorities, Latinos have been stigmatized by being linked to unemployment, crime, and deviant behavior. Historically, in the United States, they have been denied power. Ironically, substance abuse and AIDS, which obviously contribute to their powerlessness and marginality, have also focused increased public and health care attention on Latinos. Nevertheless, Latinos still face considerable obstacles in obtaining health care and social services.

Few Latinos seek psychotherapy as a way to resolve their problems. Family and friends are generally consulted first. Even if their physician recommends psychological treatment, Latinos are reluctant to seek such help.

After clients' economic (disability, welfare, housing), social (access to services, support groups), and medical needs have been stabilized, clinicians can begin work on psychotherapeutic issues. Latinos do not feel comfortable with formal, institutionalized psychotherapy and tend to respond to the therapist's personality. Successful alliances occur when clients perceive their therapist as a "member of the family" with whom they share their intimate thoughts and feelings. Although Latinos perceive therapists as authority figures and treat them with respect, effective treatment depends on *confianza* (trust), *simpatia* (politeness and respect), and personalism (Marin, 1990). Politeness and respect must take precedence over assertiveness in therapeutic work (Comas-Diaz, 1989). Clients' anger and sexuality need to be explored within a cultural context. Clinicians need to respect clients' religious and folk beliefs; many Latinos rely on *santeria* (intercession of the saints) and *curanderismo* (folk healing) (Comas-Diaz, 1989).

Clinicians must be sensitive to the cultural environment of Latinos in attempting to deal with their economic, physical, and emotional problems. Cultural beliefs play an essential role in the Latino's perception of health and illness, and clinicians need to respect these beliefs. Cultural sensitivity can help clinicians determine the difference between psychopathology and a culturally appropriate response (Comas-Diaz, 1989). In Latino families, it is not uncommon for an individual to live with his or her parents well into adulthood or until marriage. Culturally, such behavior is not considered to be pathological or a sign of acute dependency, in contrast with the Anglo culture in which young adults are expected to leave home at an earlier age.

Sociopolitical empowerment is critical in educating minorities about HIV and AIDS (De La Cancela, 1989). Empowerment is an internal as well as an external process, implying that individuals can determine the course of their own life. Self-determination is subjective in that it requires a sense of self-esteem. It is objective and external in that empowerment is reflected by the individual's interactions within society (Swift & Levin, 1987).

Clinicians need to involve the Latino family and community in their efforts to empower clients. For example, as noted above, the language and images of *machismo* can be reframed to indicate the man's responsibility to use a condom to protect his family (Mays & Cochran, 1988). The Latino sense of community can be employed to motivate Latinos to discuss prevention issues with others (Marin, 1990).

Traditional power differentials in the psychotherapeutic relationship may need to be avoided in work with Latino clients. Freire (1990) states that "people are always capable of looking in a critical way at the world when given the tools to establish a dialogical encounter with others (p. 13)." Clinicians have the opportunity to use psychotherapy as a model of empowerment for Latino clients infected with HIV. Clinicians can serve as advocates for their clients by helping them obtain food, shelter, medical care, and social services. Such efforts serve as a model for clients in their efforts to exercise self-determination and experience empowerment.

Psychotherapy with people of color who are HIV positive must extend beyond exploration of intrapsychic phenomena and object relations. Clinicians need to explore their clients' epidemiological, political, socioeconomic, and cultural background as it affects their lives and communities. To this end, it is important to abandon the goal of adjusting the client to the dominant culture and rather attempt to understand and accept the cultural scripts and values of clients. In so doing, clinicians support the empowerment process.

AFRICAN AMERICANS

EPIDEMIOLOGY

In 1990, the Centers for Disease Control (1990a) reported that more than half of the newly diagnosed AIDS cases in the United States are among nonwhites. Although blacks are only 12% of the population, a disproportionate 30.4%, or 13,186, of these new cases are blacks (Centers for Disease Control, 1991a). Indeed, the risk of AIDS is three times greater for black males than it is for white males, and it is eight times greater for black females than it is for their white counterparts (Selik, Castro, & Pappaioanou, 1988). Most of those affected are between the ages of 30 and 40 years (Centers for Disease Control, 1990b).

Transmission patterns among blacks with HIV are markedly different from those among whites. Racial/ethnic differences in risk are greatest in association with injection drug use by heterosexuals (39.7% among blacks and 6.3% among whites) (Selik et al., 1988).

Among all racial/ethnic groups, homosexual contact between men is the most common route of transmission of HIV (Rogers & Williams, 1987). Among homosexual and bisexual men with AIDS, 44% are black (Centers for Disease Control, 1990b). However, the risk of AIDS in exclusively homosexual men without a history of injection drug use is 1.3 times as great for black men as is it is for white men, and the risk of AIDS among injection-drug-using homosexuals is 2.5 times greater for blacks than it is for whites (Selik et al., 1988).

For blacks infected with HIV through homosexual contact, 30% identify as bisexual rather than as exclusively gay, compared with 14% of whites who identify as bisexual (Rogers & Williams, 1987; Selik et al., 1988). This factor may contribute to the higher incidence of heterosexual transmission among blacks (Rich, 1991). Indeed, the risk of AIDS for women whose sex partner is a bisexual man is 4.6 times as great for black women as it is for white women (Selik et al., 1988).

In both New York State and New Jersey, AIDS is the leading cause of death among black women aged 15 to 44 years (Centers for Disease Control, 1991b). Although black women represent 13.3% of women in the United States, in 1990 they accounted for 51.9% (2,539) of all reported female AIDS cases (Centers for Disease Control, 1991a). Injection drug use is the most common risk factor for black women (60%) (Gayle, Selik, & Chu, 1990). Sexual contact with an injection drug user ranks second in importance (18.3%).

In New York State, AIDS is also the leading cause of death among black children aged one to four years (Centers for Disease Control, 1991b). Black children aged 15 and younger account for 15.4% of children in the United States; however, they represent 54.5% of pediatric AIDS cases (Gayle et al., 1990). Most of these cases are indirectly related to injection drug use, either by perinatal transmission to a fetus from a mother who used injection drugs (45.8%) or a mother whose sex partner used such drugs (14.5%).

Overall death rates have been higher for blacks (29.3 per 100,000, compared with 8.7 per 100,000 for whites) (Centers for Disease Control, 1991b), and early studies suggested that blacks have shorter survival times following AIDS diagnosis (Rothenberger, Woelfel, Stoneburner, Milberg, Parker, & Truman, 1987). However, more recent research has not supported these findings (Lemp, Payne, Neal, Temelso, & Rutherford, 1990; Friedland, Saltzman, Vileno, Freeman, Schrager, & Klein, 1991).

UNDERLYING CAUSES OF PREVALENCE

The disproportionate prevalence of AIDS in blacks is due primarily to behavioral differences and environmental factors. Blacks in the United States have historically experienced limited access to adequate health care, lower living standards, higher unemployment rates, and higher overall mortality rates. Impoverished urban communities are burdened with low literacy, homelessness, and violence.

As a function of these environmental factors, blacks tend to be sicker when they are diagnosed with AIDS and they also tend to delay seeking medical care. Moreover, in clinical settings, women with HIV are identified later than are men in the course of disease, and injection drug users often have poorer underlying health status relative to others who are HIV positive.

Injection drug use appears to be more common in communities plagued by despair and economic uncertainty (Rich, 1991). As these drugs are often injected and as they alter judgment relative to other risk behaviors, they are significantly implicated in the transmission of HIV.

THE LEGACY OF DISEASE MODELS

Within the black community, AIDS represents the confluence of history, culture, politics, and disease. The community's attempt to dissociate itself from AIDS is less a response to AIDS as a medical phenomenon than it is a reaction to the social and political issues generated and reflected by AIDS (Dalton, 1989). Indeed, the black community's response stems from a difficult and tenuous relationship with the larger society. In this regard, it is critical to understand how the parameters of a disease are defined, as those definitions determine intervention-priority target groups and, consequently, bear on the general health and well-being of the larger population.

The black community's reluctance to speak openly about AIDS during the early stages of the epidemic was due, in large measure, to associations that have been made about blacks, disease, and deviance in American society (Hammonds, 1987). Eighty-two percent of adults with AIDS in the black community acquired the virus as a function of behaviors that some find difficult to acknowledge (e.g., homosexuality and drug abuse). Many blacks do not want to be associated with what has been perceived as a gay disease (Dalton, 1989; Hammonds, 1987). This response has its origin in the black community's attempt to contend with the historical construction of sexually transmitted diseases as being the result of the uncontrollable sexual behavior of blacks (Hammonds, 1987). Black institutions, therefore, tend to adopt a conservative stance relative to matters of sexual behavior. With regard to substance abuse, the issues are similar. For blacks to acknowledge substance abuse as a problem is to risk providing evidence to support behavioral stereotypes.

The attempt to break the perceived linkages among blacks, disease, and immorality has exacted a toll on the black community. The existence of black homosexuals is denied to the extent that they are made invisible, and efforts to educate the community and to provide care for those with AIDS are hampered by efforts to appear "respectable" (Hammonds, 1987).

Black Americans are aware of the social, political, economic, and personal prejudices directed against Haitians when AIDS was identified as a disease prevalent among Haitians. Consequently, the black community remains wary of connections made between itself and AIDS. There are misgivings among blacks relative to the curtailment of opportunities for employment, education, and health care due to seropositivity. Thus, concern about the synergy of discrimination based on race, sex, and HIV status is valid (Smith, 1990).

In addition, a legacy of suspicion and mistrust between blacks and the larger society hinders AIDS-prevention efforts. Some blacks believe that AIDS is a conspiracy of whites using biological engineering to eliminate less valued members of society. This view is based on the experience of the community with the 40-year Tuskegee study, in which black males with syphilis were observed without treatment in order to determine the course of the illness, even after the advent of penicillin (Thomas & Quinn, 1991). This study is the longest nontherapeutic experiment on humans in medical history. The resulting rifts between blacks and the scientific community have yet to be healed. Consequently, the lack of interest in AIDS among blacks is also due to the lack of credibility that mainstream institutions (e.g., the media and health care) have within the black community. Blacks are often reluctant to believe that these institutions are genuinely interested in their general welfare independent from the larger society.

Thus, due to the black community's refusal to identify AIDS as a problem relevant to itself, insufficient attention has been accorded to AIDS among blacks. Furthermore, the complex constellation of difficulties that many blacks confront in their daily lives must be acknowledged. For the community, many other problems compete with AIDS for attention.

SPECIAL CLINICAL POPULATIONS

Women and adolescents. Apart from cultural and religious dimensions, social, economic, and political factors influence the sexual behavior patterns of black women. The response of these women to AIDS is determined by the threat that they perceive AIDS poses to them relative to other risks in their lives and by the availability of resources to reduce their risk of exposure (Mays & Cochran, 1988). The attempts of black women to protect themselves against infection are often compromised by their emotional or economic dependence upon their male partners (Peterson & Marin, 1988). Moreover, the unbalanced sex ratio between black men and women (75 single adult men to 100 single adult women) increases the tendency of black women not to jeopardize relationships with their partners. As a result, it is not uncommon for black women to allow themselves to be pressured into unsafe sex practices (Mays & Cochran, 1988). Messages that promote monogamy to reduce the risk of exposure to HIV ignore the fact that 65% of black women are unmarried. Thus, the interpersonal decisions that bear on their HIV-related risks are often based on external, situational contingencies.

Black adults consistently have lower knowledge scores and greater misconceptions about AIDS than do whites (Carghill & Smith, 1990). Studies conducted with adolescent populations indicate that black teens are also less knowledgeable than are their white counterparts about the cause, transmission, and prevention of AIDS (DiClemente, Boyer, & Morales, 1988). Thus, black teens are at greater risk of HIV infection as a result of engaging in unsafe sexual practices due to insufficient information. Increased sexual activity and drug experimentation also increase the risk of HIV infection among adolescents. In this regard, rates for all sexually transmitted diseases are higher among black adolescents (Carghill & Smith, 1990).

Intravenous drug users. Injection drug use represents a pattern of behavior within a specific subculture with its own values and status allocations (Mays & Cochran, 1988). The social setting of drug use and behaviors related to injection may explain the higher HIV seroprevalance rates among blacks. Black injection drug users are more likely to share their needles, syringes, and other drug paraphernalia than are whites (Des Jarlais, Friedman, & Hopkins, 1985). Needle sharing with strangers or acquaintances is more common among blacks (Schoenbaum et al., 1989), thus increasing the risk of transmission (Allen & Curran, 1988). Moreover, sterile needles are not as readily available to blacks, who may also be less able to afford them (Rogers & Williams, 1987).

Blacks have a higher incidence of drug use and because of this may indulge in more risky behaviors. Illicit drug injection coupled with unsafe sex becomes the means of heterosexual transmission of HIV beyond drug users. Given that heterosexual transmission to women can lead to perinatal infection in children, HIV infection in black injection drug users may become a family disease (Craven, Liebman, Fuller, Hagerty, Cooley, Saunders, Steger, & Libman, 1990).

Homosexuality and bisexuality. Due to cultural factors, homosexual men from communities of color tend not to identify as homosexual. Consequently, the extent of homosexual behavior among blacks tends to be underestimated (Mays & Cochran, 1988). Socialization and the limited development of a gay community among men of color may cause these men to be more variable in their sexual behavior than are whites (Peterson & Marin, 1988). For these men, homosexual experience does not compromise their perception of themselves as heterosexual. Hence, bisexual black men may be less likely to identify with gay communities and may not perceive themselves to be at risk for HIV infection.

The adoption of a bisexual life-style among blacks may reflect the intolerance and social difficulties that black homosexuals experience within their communities. The presence of the church in the black community and its fundamentalist position on issues of homosexuality reinforce the perceived lack of acceptance of bisexual and gay men.

PRACTICE IMPLICATIONS

In the delivery of HIV-related services to the black community, the disease cannot be divorced from the framework within which it finds expression. For proposed interventions to have maximal contextual relevance, they must take into account differences in the occurrence and transmission patterns of AIDS among blacks and the behavioral, social, and economic reasons for these differences (Rogers & Williams, 1987). It is also critical that practitioners understand the types of adaptive coping strategies utilized by blacks.

Interventions on both the individual and group (i.e., family, community) levels must be oriented toward teaching personal accountability and respect for the value of others. Mays and Cochran (1988) suggested that intervention strategies focus on the individual as a responsible member of a social organization. For blacks, cooperation is a more powerful motivator of behavior change than is emphasis on individual action (Mays & Cochran, 1988). Such a model is based on the principle of shared social responsibility as opposed to the principle of individual preservation.

AIDS affects black women in their capacity as caregivers. Intervention efforts need to be directed toward these women as they play a central role in controlling the spread of HIV in their community. In so doing, however, interventions must acknowledge and address the social realities of black women from individual, cultural, economic, and sociopolitical perspectives.

Service providers are often distrustful of injection drug users. It is important, however, that addiction be recognized as a medical and psychosocial disease (Craven et al., 1990). Rich (1991) suggested that substance abuse should always be considered as a primary diagnosis. Ongoing and untreated substance abuse not only compromises compliance with medical treatment, it also increases morbidity and the risks of mortality. For patients engaging in psychotherapy, it is critical to address drug-use issues so as to secure appropriate treatment options.

It is imperative that families of black persons with AIDS be allowed to be involved in the care of their loved ones. The treatment options presented by these families must also be seen as valuable. For example, a strong and valued tradition among blacks is to tend to the needs of the sick within the family, as opposed to accessing institutional care. Thus, hospice care may not be sought by a black patient and his or her family in the terminal stages of illness. Within other black families, however, diagnosis may lead to the loss of critical support at a time of intense need. In these instances, the inability to accept disclosures of homosexuality, bisexuality, or drug use may lead to abandonment and alienation.

Black homosexual/bisexual men are often isolated and discriminated against within their own community. The church may not extend support. The potential role of the black church must not be overlooked, however. Religious institutions, long a primary source of authority in the black community, are able to provide assistance to those who are HIV infected and their families as well as assist those who are attempting to protect themselves against infection. Importantly, prevention and treatment messages to black men must be addressed to men who perceive themselves as heterosexual, despite their episodic homosexual practices.

In view of the prevalence rates of HIV infection in their community, blacks are disproportionately underrepresented in clinical trials (Smith, 1991). Increased participation of black women and injection drug users in these trials is needed. However, potential candidates for these trials are often reluctant to self-refer due to the black community's distrust of trials and skepticism of the medical establishment (El-Sadr & Capps, 1992). Moreover, many blacks experience barriers to participation, including their limited access to health care and the unlikelihood of trials being held in impoverished, urban areas.

The failure to narrow the chasm between the health status of blacks and whites is the result of glaring inequities and social disparities. Nonetheless, the need for blacks to confront AIDS-related issues within their communities does not obviate the need for dialogue with others. In view of the complexities of the AIDS pandemic, it is important that providers and service recipients communicate across cultural and social differences.

HAITIANS

EPIDEMIOLOGY

Based on the number of cases per 100,000 population, Haiti is among the world's 20 nations most affected by AIDS (Farmer, 1990a). The HIV seroprevalence rate in asymptomatic adult cohorts in Haiti is 9% in urban areas and 3% in rural areas (Pape & Johnson, 1988). Rates are comparable for men and women. In a country that can ill afford another health burden, AIDS has indeed become a source of considerable suffering (Farmer, 1990a).

Epidemiological patterns of HIV infection among Haitians suggest that for both males and females the most frequent route of transmission is heterosexual contact. Researchers studying Haitians with AIDS in Haiti found that 23% of patients reported bisexuality as a risk behavior, 11% reported being blood-transfusion recipients, and 1% reported being injection drug users (Pape et al., 1990). Among those reporting bisexual transmission in this sample, many were male prostitutes who had had contact with North American tourists (Farmer, 1990b). The Collaborative Study Group of AIDS in Haitian-Americans (1987) also found that among Haitians with AIDS in the United States, homosexuality, bisexuality, injection drug use, and blood transfusion do not play as significant a role in the transmission of HIV as does heterosexual contact.

HAITIAN MIGRATION: AN OVERVIEW

In order to discuss the personal, familial, social, and political implications of HIV infection in the Haitian diaspora, it is important to describe the process of the migration as it is experienced by Haitians in the United States. Although many characteristics of Haitian migration distinguish it from other migratory patterns, the phenomenon of Haitian migration may be examined within the larger context of the migration of black peoples from the West Indies and the Caribbean basin.

The French were the last Europeans in St. Domingue, as Haiti was called during its colonial history. In 1804, through a revolt of slaves who had been brought by Europeans to St. Domingue from Africa, Haiti became the second republic in the Western hemisphere and the first free black country in the world.

Migratory movements of Haitians to the United States predate the independence of either country (Laguerre, 1980). Migration in the nineteenth century was not significant due to the factor of racial discrimination in the United States. The first wave of migration in the twentieth century dates to the American occupation of Haiti from 1915 to 1934 (Fontaine, 1983; Laguerre, 1980).

In more recent decades, the United States has been the major receiving country for emigrating Haitians (Allman, 1982). An undetermined number of Haitian immigrants are undocumented, and because the figures for these migrants are speculative, accurate data on the total number of Haitians in this country at this time are difficult to obtain. Allman (1982) suggests that one adjust for underenumeration and illegal migrants and control for factors of mortality, new births, return migration, and out-migration in attempting to achieve an estimate of the Haitian population. Based on these considerations, N. Glick Schiller estimates that approximately 940,000 Haitians are in the United States (personal communication, June 1, 1992). More than a decade ago, the states with the largest concentrations of Haitians were New York, Florida, New Jersey, Illinois, and Massachusetts (Laguerre, 1980). Community specialists indicate that the geographic concentrations of Haitians remain unchanged. New York City has more than 250,000 Haitians and is the largest Haitian community in the United States. On the basis of these numbers, it is clear that Haitians are one of the largest West Indian populations in North America (Laguerre, 1980). (To put this in perspective, the population of Haiti is estimated at 6 million. Hence, the number of Haitians living as expatriates equals approximately one-sixth of the country's current population.) It is estimated that most of these immigrants are young, with a mean age of 29 years, and that 59% of them are female (Stepick & Portes, 1986).

In both the preemigration context and in the country of resettlement, considerable intraethnic diversity exists within the Haitian population. The heterogeneity in the sociodemographic profile of Haitian immigrants is generally reflective of the dissimilarity of experience among different waves of migrants. Haitian arrivals to this country during the late 1950s and 1960s were typically from the urban middle and upper classes (Fontaine, 1983). Rural Haitians have constituted the majority of the arrivals since 1972 (Laguerre, 1980).

The recent wave of Haitian immigrants consists mostly of semiskilled, domestic, and agrarian workers (Laguerre, 1980). The primary determinants of the initial outmigration for these recent arrivals have been the existing economic and political orders in Haiti (MacEoin & Riley, 1982). The motivation for migration is also fostered by the desire for family reunification (Stafford, 1987).

PSYCHOSOCIAL CHALLENGES AND ADAPTATIONS

The experience of the migration among Haitians is defined in large measure by parameters established by the United States Immigration and Naturalization Service. The migration process described by Sluzki (1979) has relevance to Haitians and may be discussed within these parameters. In this model, migration consists of a continuum of discrete but interdependent stages that trigger different types of challenges and that require different cognitive, affective, and behavioral adaptations.

The first of these stages is the preparatory stage, which begins with the commitment to migrate. Among Haitians, the decision regarding who will migrate is not one that is made autonomously on an individual level, but rather it is centered in group-based strategies wherein the critical consideration is who is best able to accomplish the migration process successfully. The extended kin network is typically involved in this process, and it is at this point that the structure of the Haitian family begins to change. The hope is that the pioneer immigrant, that is, the first one to leave, will be able to lay the groundwork for others to follow. From there, a chain migration develops, whereby relatives in the United States assist others in Haiti to emigrate (Stafford, 1987). Due to the indefinite separations many couples experience as a result of a partner's migration, one or both partners may seek other companions until the couple are reunited.

The second stage is the actual act of migration. For Haitians, migration can take a variety of forms. It may involve submitting applications for necessary visas (which is in itself a complex task) and entering the new country through lawful means or it can be perilous and fraught with difficulty, as is the case for those who not only risk their lives at sea but who also face possible internment upon arrival.

The third stage of the migration is a period that is characterized by efforts to satisfy basic needs. Here, survival becomes the first priority. When employed, Haitians generally occupy unskilled and service-industry positions that afford them little security (Stafford, 1987). Moreover, they are often subject to discrimination in their search for employment and while employed due to various factors, most notably their lack of skills relevant to an industrialized society, their lack of fluency in English, and, for some, lack of documented-immigrant status.

Other difficulties that Haitians confront during the third stage of migration include lack of orientation to an urban setting and lack of access to general health care, particularly family planning and prenatal care. Illegal-alien status and lack of experience with health care institutions in the country of origin also result in underutilization of available health care in the United States. Other concerns of the Haitian immigrant include crowded, unsafe living conditions that facilitate the spread of opportunistic infections such as tuberculosis. Illiteracy is frequently observed among many Haitians who are recent arrivals as they have had little experience with institutional educational systems. Against this backdrop of sociocultural history, politics, and the demands of resettlement and acculturation in the diaspora, AIDS among Haitians in the United States may be examined and understood.

RESPONSES TO THE POLITICAL CONSTRUCTION OF DISEASE

Haiti's role in the AIDS pandemic has been unique (Farmer, 1990b). In 1983, the Centers for Disease Control (CDC) categorized Haitians as a group at high risk for AIDS. This categorization suggested to some in the scientific and political communities that AIDS had originated in Haiti. This was the first time in the history of modern medicine that a nation was associated with a pathological condition.

Scientific basis for this attribution was lacking. Indeed, Farmer (1990b) described this classification as one of "bad science" (p. 72). The use of culturally insensitive instruments had failed to identify behaviors now known to place individuals at risk for HIV infection. Consequently, Haitians were singled out by virtue of their ethnic and cultural features (Viera, 1985). With considerable pressure applied by the Haitian community, in 1985, the Centers for Disease Control (CDC) removed Haitians from its list of risk groups (Farmer, 1990b). However, the Food and Drug Administration did not reverse its ban on Haitians as potential blood donors until 1990. The stigma nonetheless persists, and the repercussions have been tremendous. AIDS has had a more negative impact on Haiti's international image than have political repression and intense poverty (Abbott, 1988). Although the CDC has removed Haitians from its list of high-risk groups, the category has yet to be removed from the list established in the popular imagination (Farmer 1990b). Anti-Haitian backlash has been felt in cities throughout North America. Farmer (1990b) documented the discrimination experienced by Haitians as a function of AIDS in the areas of employment, housing, education, health care, and commerce.

As a result of the disastrous consequences of the initial attribution of blame, the Haitian community delayed acknowledging the toll that AIDS has exacted upon its members. The community's denial slowed efforts to combat the spread of the disease as it indirectly discouraged prevention and education efforts. In this regard, however, the constellation of other difficulties that besiege the Haitian community must also be recognized. For Haitians, AIDS is but one more problem with which they must contend in the adaptation and acculturation processes.

AIDS AND RACISM

In the United States, the perception often held by the larger society is that blacks are an indistinguishable, homogeneous mass. However, black immigrants are keenly aware of the cultural differences that separate them from one another and from whites. In this regard, Bryce-Laporte (1972) discussed the "double invisibility" of the black immigrant, whereby the black immigrant is invisible to whites because he or she is black and invisible to other blacks because she or he is foreign born.

In the case of Haitians, the process of integration into a stratified society is compounded by race and by the individual and collective response to the experience of race in the United States. Haitians go from majority status in their country of origin to identification as a "racial minority." Consequently, discussions of AIDS among Haitians must clearly acknowledge factors of race and racism.

THE CONTEXTUAL FRAMEWORK OF INTERVENTION

A given group's cultural characteristics and value systems influence its concepts of disease and illness. The critical issue here is understanding how and by whom a situation or a problem is defined. Among Haitians, the community's understanding of AIDS not only determines the degree to which it avails itself of services, but it also determines compliance with recommended treatment regimens as well as the potential course of illness.

In a review of Haitian ethnomedicine, Laguerre (1984) states that rural Haitians believe that illness can be of natural or supernatural origin. Natural illnesses are thought to be of short duration, whereas supernatural illnesses appear suddenly and without previous discomfort. Few Haitians of lower socioeconomic status adhere to the germ theory of disease as an explanation for illness (Laguerre, 1984). Hence, Haitian patients tend to perform self-diagnosis and to adopt a rather critical stance toward alternative understandings of etiology and symptomatology.

For many Haitians, two related but distinguishable AIDS entities can be identified: (1) AIDS the infectious disease and (2) AIDS that is brought on by unnatural causes (Farmer, 1990b). Protective measures are thought to be helpful against the former, but useless against the latter. Some Haitians believe that magical intervention is effective against the unnatural form of the disease, thereby making it the less virulent of the two. The natural, infectious version of the illness, however, is considered to be universally fatal (Farmer, 1990b).

131

A Haitian person with AIDS may, therefore, seek more traditional forms of care, as such forms of care are thought to be more valid and reliable. The range of treatment options available to patients is thereby increased. They may seek the assistance of a medical provider, a voodoo priest, an herbalist, prayer, or any combination of these. The option selected is determined by the perceived cause of illness. The factors predictive of the options chosen are social class, residential background in Haiti (rural vs. urban), and education. As the disease progresses, it is not unusual for patients to shift in their attribution models and in their conceptual understanding of illness.

In both of these disease paradigms, however, blaming the victim is an uncommon response to AIDS (Farmer & Kleinman, 1989). In the Haitian world view, personal accountability is not valued as much as is the primacy of social relations (Farmer & Kleinman, 1989). Indeed, in Haitian metapsychology, external locus of control is emphasized. Consistent with this sociocentric world view, the self is defined in relation to a collective of related and unrelated family members. In this model, socialization is accomplished by reference to the field, that is, it is achieved by inducing shame as opposed to guilt.

GENDER-ROLE ISSUES

Following migration, Haitian women in the United States find themselves in a more pluralistic society in which they have greater means available to them for self-definition (Buchanan, 1979). They achieve greater self-reliance in contrast with the role that they occupied in a traditionally matrifocal, but patriarchal, society. However, the benefits they derive from economic gains are often offset by the pragmatic demands of social roles and the cultural definitions of those roles (Buchanan, 1979). Thus, despite possible gains outside the home, observable behaviors and responsibilities within the home remain unchanged.

Traditional sociocultural role expectations determine how males and females view themselves and each other as well as the value that they attach to themselves and each other. Hence, Haitian women tend to continue to defer to men in sexual matters. Communication between males and females regarding sexuality is not culturally syntonic.

As potential spouses, Haitian women are considered desirable if they are perceived as being sexually inexperienced. Women who assume responsibility in sexual matters are thought to be of less strict moral standards and, therefore, are considered undesirable. Thus, a woman who is prepared for sex (e.g., one who initiates the use of a condom) goes beyond her defined role, the potential result of which is rejection. Moreover, Haitian men, at times, are reluctant to suggest use of a condom, as doing so may be perceived as lack of interest in a committed, long-term relationship with their sexual partner. It is not uncommon for Haitian men to engage in sexual activity outside marriage as an assertion of their virility to themselves and to others.

AIDS AS A FAMILY DISEASE

Among Haitians, AIDS is a family disease. When Haitian pioneer immigrants come to this country, they carry not only their own personal hopes, but also the hopes of others who have been left behind. In large measure, the ability to migrate is due to the commitments and sacrifices of others. Thus, immigrants have a great sense of indebtedness to and personal responsibility for those who remain, and the remittances sent by expatriates are often critical to a family's survival.

When an immigrant contracts AIDS, his or her illness is synonymous with failure. The experience of illness is shameful in that one fails not only oneself but also those dependent upon the immigrant to improve their own life circumstances. Indeed, the immigrant's illness impedes both the remittance process and the process of migration sponsorship leading to family reunification. Also, AIDS among Haitians is a family disease in the sense that often partners and children become ill as well and thus must confront the challenges of living with AIDS.

In times of difficulty, Haitians traditionally seek assistance from their kin networks. However, recent immigrants do not have extended-family support at a time of critical need, as family reunification is often impeded by lack of official or permanent legal documentation. Moreover, because of the stigma attached to AIDS in the Haitian community, many HIV-infected Haitians do not disclose their status, even to those with whom they are close. As they are unaccustomed to seeking help outside of their customary networks, Haitians with AIDS are often isolated. As their disease progresses, many Haitians entertain thoughts of returning to Haiti to see their families. However, many may be denied reentry as a result of their legal or HIV status. Thus, Haitians with AIDS must decide whether to remain in the United States where they are afforded prolonged, sustained health care or to return to Haiti where they may die among loved ones.

PRACTICE IMPLICATIONS

Haitians often delay seeking treatment. For some, delay is the result of denial and misunderstanding; others fear that utilization of public health care programs will compromise regularization of their alien status. Ethnic and cultural barriers to service utilization also exist in that the numbers of bicultural and trilingual (English, French, Haitian Creole) providers are insufficient to address the needs of Haitians.

In providing services cross-culturally, it is critical that providers be ethnically accountable at all times. When working with Haitians, providers must acknowledge the patient's conceptual system by formulating treatment plans *with*, not *for*, the patient that neither contradict nor violate that conceptual system and that convey respect for it. It is also important to integrate adaptive indigenous structures in the treatment plan for patients who request such services when these resources are available. For example, with patients who are engaged in psychotherapy and who are also receiving traditional medical care, it may be appropriate to support them in their wish to avail themselves of the services of an herbalist or a folk healer.

The sociopolitical context of Haitians in the United States creates extensive unmet social needs that affect the types of problems with which patients present. Case management and indirect service activities are important elements in the care of these patients. Extensive networking and advocacy are required to secure critical collateral services.

The provision of cross-cultural services requires self-awareness relative to one's own attitudes, ideal and actual norms, and sense of social organization. An awareness of these psychosocial elements of culture is often difficult to achieve. Providers have much to learn from their patients, who must be considered the experts regarding their needs. Haitians must be encouraged to speak within their own community about AIDS. Providers acknowledge differences based on national, ethnic, and cultural origin so as not to obscure the variety, depth, and richness of patients' experiences.

It has been noted that AIDS moves along the fault lines of our society (Bateson & Goldsby, 1988). It is a disease that reflects our social and global inequities. In the development of effective AIDS prevention and intervention programs for Haitians, we must address the cultural, contextual, and environmental factors that impinge on the functioning of the Haitian community.

ASIANS AND PACIFIC ISLANDERS

It was not until 1988 that the Centers for Disease Control created a category in its surveillance reports for Asian/Pacific Islander AIDS cases. Before that time, the reported cases were so few that they were included in the "other" category together with American Indians and Alaskan natives, making up to 1% of reported cases.

Even today, the fact that Asians and Pacific Islanders are lumped together is detrimental for realistic surveillance, further overlooking dangerous trends of infection among these groups. Although Asians and Pacific Islanders still represent a small percentage (0.6%) of AIDS cases, the rate of infection among them doubles approximately every 10 months (National AIDS Network, 1989). On the West Coast (particularly San Francisco and Los Angeles), where a larger concentration of these groups is found, the Asian/Pacific Islander population growth rate exceeds that of all other minority groups in the nation. It is projected that by the year 2000, this group will represent 15% of the nation's total population growth, compared with an 11% increase of the nation's general population (Lee & Fong, 1990).

This rapid growth, together with the diversity of cultures and languages represented in the Asian/Pacific Islander grouping, presents special challenges to HIV/AIDS prevention and intervention efforts. Forty-three distinct Asian/Pacific Islander groups from 40 countries and territories who speak more than 100 languages and dialects are in the United States (Lee & Fong, 1990; Mandel & Kitane, 1989; Jue & Kain, 1989).

Little research is available to calculate the prevalence of HIV infection by ethnicity among Asians and Pacific Islanders. With words of caution, Lee and Fong (1990) present a San Francisco study in which Filipinos accounted for 46% of the prevalence of HIV infection among Asians and Pacific Islanders, followed by Chinese (20%), Japanese (19%), Polynesian/Hawaiian (7%), and Vietnamese (4%). More epidemiological studies are needed that take ethnicity and immigration variables into consideration.

In terms of modes of transmission, Asians and Pacific Islanders tend to have higher incidence of HIV infection among men who have sex with men: 75% homosexual/bisexual, 4% injection-drug use, and 8% blood transfusion before 1985. Interestingly, transmission among people older than 50 has accounted for 14% of those infected with HIV. Another aspect that sets these communities apart from whites and even other minorities, is that 1% of Asian/Pacific Islander men compared with 35% of Asian/Pacific Islander women contract HIV through heterosexual activity (Lee & Fong, 1990).

In an in-depth analysis of the cultural factors involved in the underreporting of AIDS cases, Gock (in press) found that Asians and Pacific Islanders fear shame and loss of face. Fear of disgrace to the family may lead people to lie about or never disclose their condition. This intense sense of loyalty and affiliation causes some individuals to choose between dying in isolation or suffering the rejection of family and community. Asians and Pacific Islanders' emphasis on family and procreation makes homosexuality an unacceptable behavior. Thus, married and bisexual men may maintain homosexual contacts secretly (Jue, 1990) in an effort to protect themselves and their families from stigmatization. In many Asian and Pacific Island cultures, discussions about illness and death, as well as about sex, are taboo. Illness and death are avoided because talking about them is thought to create a self-fulfilling prophecy. Also, illness may be viewed as a punishment from the ancestors for having offended them (Lee & Fong, 1990).

A strong intraethnic group identification supports Asians and Pacific Islanders' belief that if they do not have sex with persons from other ethnic groups, especially whites, they can avoid infection (National AIDS Network, 1989). In addition to their denials, misconceptions, and lack of information, Many Asians and Pacific Islanders still believe that HIV/AIDS is a white, gay men's disease. Many native Asians view homosexuality as a decadent Western influence. However, with the process of acculturation, some families have begun to understand and accept the homosexual preference of a family member (Wu & Pak, 1989).

Because of the diversity of these communities and their strong cultural beliefs, clinicians face immense challenges in providing adequate services to Asians and Pacific Islanders. Cultural norms, socioeconomic background, educational level, and acculturation stage, of course, are important factors in work with any minority group. To provide effective treatment for Asians and Pacific Islanders, therapists need to understand the role of shame and reverence for family and tradition. Asians and Pacific Islanders, as well as other minorities, take pride in caring for their own. The family and the community provide a safety net to hold and help their members. Psychotherapy, for many Asians and Pacific Islanders, increases their sense of shame and isolation. Moreover, many Asians and Pacific Islanders believe that psychotherapy is for Westerners and that only "crazy people" use such services. In work with these clients, clinicians should anticipate resistance to therapy. If translators are used, clients need to be assured that confidentiality will be maintained.

When assessing premorbid conditions, it is important to keep in mind that no group is immune to alcohol and drug abuse, domestic violence, or sexual abuse. Careful and sensitive inquiry should be conducted to evaluate the client's need for substance-abuse treatment or shelter. Asian/Pacific Islander women, like many minority women, lack information about AIDS. This lack of knowledge is reinforced by the cultural script that women should not know about sex or be assertive about safer sex practices. Condom use, according to Jue and Kain (1989), is associated with prostitution and uncleanliness. Therefore, women may feel that asking their husbands or boyfriends to use condoms may jeopardize their relationship. Moreover, many minority women rely on their partners for economic and emotional support; becoming assertive about safer sex practices may put them at risk of abandonment or abuse.

Often patients need help with concrete services, such as medical referrals and welfare benefits. Such assistance helps develop a trusting relationship by empowering the client. After clients' medical and physical needs are met, clinicians can begin to conduct more in-depth psychological work. Issues of disclosure of serostatus and sexual orientation to the family should be explored carefully. With disclosure, when, how, how much information, and to whom information should be directed are important factors, as is the issue of whether the patient will return home to die with family or stay away with little or no support. For women with HIV/AIDS, their role as caretaker to partner and children makes disclosure to children and family especially complicated, raising the issue of the children's placement or adoption.

Jue (1990) discusses how somatization in Asians and Hispanics makes it difficult to differentiate between illness-related symptomatology and psychosomatic complaints. For many minorities, somatization is the voice of feelings that need to be explored during the psychotherapeutic process. Clinicians need to be flexible if they are to understand clients' dynamics without pathologizing these dynamics by judging clients with the dominant culture's norms. Normalcy and the "appropriate" healing process should be determined in light of the cultural, ethnic, and social background of the individual.

REFERENCES

Abbott, E. (1988). *Haiti: The Duvaliers and their legacy.* New York: MacGraw-Hill.

Allen, J., & Curran, J. (1988). Prevention of AIDS and HIV infection: Needs and priorities for epidemiologic research. *American Journal of Public Health, 78,* 381–386.

Allman, J. (1982). Haitian migration: 30 years assessed. *Migration Today, 10*(1), 6–12.

Amaro, H. (1987, September). *Hispanic women and AIDS: Considerations for prevention and research.* Paper presented at an NIMH/NIDA Research Workshop, Women and AIDS: Promoting Healthy Behaviors, Bethesda, MD.

Amaro, H. (1988). Considerations for prevention of HIV infection among women. *Psychology of Women Quarterly, 12,* 429–443.

Amaro, H. (1991). *AIDS/HIV related knowledge, attitudes, beliefs and behaviors among Hispan-*

ics in the Northeast and Puerto Rico. Unpublished manuscript, School of Public Health, Boston University.

Bateson, M. C., & Goldsby, R. (1988). *Thinking AIDS: The social response to the biological threat.* Reading, MA: Addison-Wesley.

Bryce-Laporte, R. (1972). Black immigrants: The experience of invisibility and inequality. *Journal of Black Studies, 1*(3), 29–56.

Buchanan, S. (1979). Haitian women in New York City. *Migration Today, 7*(4), 19–25, 39.

Carghill, V., & Smith, M. (1990). HIV disease and the African-American community. In P. Cohen, M. Sande, & P. Volberbing (Eds.), *AIDS knowledge base.* Waltham, MA: Medical Publishing Group.

Carrier, J. M., & Magana, J. R. (1991). Use of ethnosexual data on men of Mexican origin for HIV/AIDS prevention programs. *Journal of Sex Research, 28,* 189–202.

Centers for Disease Control. (1990a). *AIDS in racial and ethnic minorities* [Slide Series L-238(6)]. Atlanta, GA: Author.

Centers for Disease Control. (1990b). *HIV/AIDS surveillance report* (December 1990). Atlanta, GA: Author.

Centers for Disease Control. (1991a). The HIV epidemic: The first ten years. *Morbidity and Mortality Weekly Report, 40,* 357–369.

Centers for Disease Control. (1991b). Mortality attributable to HIV infection/AIDS-United States, 1981–1990. *Morbidity and Mortality Weekly Report, 40*(3), 41–44.

Chu, S. Y., Buehler, J. W., & Berkelman, R. (1990). Impact of the human immunodeficiency virus epidemic on mortality in women of reproductive age, United States. *Journal of the American Medical Association, 264,* 225–229.

Collaborative Study Group of AIDS in Haitian-Americans. (1987). Risk factors for AIDS among Haitians residing in the United States: Evidence of heterosexual transmission. *Journal of the American Medical Association, 257,* 635–639.

Comas-Diaz, L. (1989). Culturally relevant issues and treatment implications for Hispanics. In D. A. Koslow & E. P. Salett (Eds.), *Crossing cultures in mental health.* Washington, DC: SIETAR International.

Craven, D., Liebman, H., Fuller, J., Hagerty, C., Cooley, T., Saunders, C., Steger., K., & Libman, H. (1990). AIDS in intravenous drug users: Issues related to enrollment in clinical trials. *Journal of Acquired Immune Deficiency Syndromes, 3*(Suppl. 2), S45–S50.

Dalton, H. (1989). AIDS in blackface. *Daedalus, 118*(3), 205–227.

De La Cancela, V. (1989). Minority AIDS prevention: Moving beyond cultural perspectives towards sociopolitical empowerment. *AIDS Education and Prevention, 1*(2), 141–153.

De La Vega, E. (1990). Considerations for reaching the Latino populations with sexuality and HIV/AIDS information and education. *SIECUS Report, 18*(3), 1–8.

Des Jarlais, D., Abdul-Quader, A., Minkoff, H., & Tross, S. Crack use and multiple AIDS risk behaviors. *Journal of Acquired Immune Deficiency Syndromes, 4,* 446–447.

Des Jarlais, D., Friedman, S., & Hopkins, W. (1985). Risk reduction for the acquired immunodeficiency syndrome among intravenous drug users. *Annals of Internal Medicine, 103,* 755–759.

Diaz, E. (1991). Public policy, women, and HIV disease. *SIECUS Report, 19*(2), 4–5.

DiClemente, R., Boyer, C., & Morales, E. (1988). Minorities and AIDS: Knowledge, attitudes, and misconceptions among black and Latino adolescents. *American Journal of Public Health, 78,* 55–57.

El-Sadr, W., & Capps, L. (1992). The challenge of minority recruitment in clinical trials for AIDS. *Journal of the American Medical Association, 267,* 954–957.

Farmer, P. (1990a). Sending sickness: Sorcery, politics, and changing concepts of AIDS in rural Haiti. *Medical Anthropology Quarterly, 4*(1), 6–27.

Farmer, P. (1990b). AIDS and accusation: Haiti and the geography of blame. In D. Feldman (Ed.), *AIDS and culture: The human factor.* New York: Praeger.

Farmer, P., & Kleinman, A. (1989). AIDS as human suffering. *Daedalus, 118*(2), 135–160.

Fontaine, P. (1983). Haitian immigrants in Boston: A commentary. In R. Bryce-Laporte & D. Mortimer (Eds.), *Caribbean immigration to the United States.* Washington, DC: Smithsonian Institution, Research Institute on Immigration and Ethnic Studies.

Freire, P. (1990). *Pedagogy of the oppressed.* New York: Continuum Publishing.

Friedland, G., Saltzman, B., Vileno, J., Freeman, K., Schrager, L., & Klein, R. (1991). Survival differences in patients with AIDS. *Journal of Acquired Immune Deficiency Syndromes, 4,* 144–153.

Gayle, J., Selik, R., & Chu, S. (1990). Surveillance for AIDS and HIV infection among black and Hispanic children and women of childbearing age, 1981–1989. *Morbidity and Mortality Weekly Report, 39*(SS-3), 23–30.

Gock, S. T. (in press). No longer immune: AIDS and the Asian Pacific communities. In D. Takevchi & N. Zane (Eds.), *Asian and Pacific Islander American health issues.* San Francisco, CA: Asian Pacific Health Forum.

Hammonds, E. (1987). Race, sex, AIDS: The construction of 'other.' *Radical America, 20*(6), 28–36.

Jue, S. (1990, January). AIDS and the Asian Pacific community. *Newsletter of the Asian Pacific AIDS Task Force,* pp. 1–2, 4.

Jue, S., & Kain, C. D. (1989). Culturally sensitive AIDS counseling. In C. Kain (Ed.), *No longer immune: A counselor's guide to AIDS* (pp. 131–148). Alexandria, VA: American Association for Counseling and Development.

Laguerre, M. (1980). Haitians in the United States. In S. Thernstrom, A. Orlov, & O. Handlin (Eds.), *Harvard encyclopedia of American ethnic groups.* Cambridge, MA: Harvard University Press.

Laguerre, M. (1984). *American odyssey: Haitians in New York City.* Ithaca, NY: Cornell University Press.

Lee, A. D., & Fong, K. (1990, February–March). HIV/AIDS and the Asian and Pacific Islander community. *SIECUS Report, 18*(3), 16–22.

Lemp, G., Payne, S., Neal, D., Temelso, T., & Rutherford, G. (1990). Survival trends for patients with AIDS. *Journal of the American Medical Association, 263,* 402–406.

MacEoin, G., & Riley, N. (1982). *No promised land: American refugee policies and the rule of law.* Boston: Oxfam America.

Maldonado, M. (1991). Latinos and HIV/AIDS, implications for the 90s. *SIECUS Report, 19*(2), 11–15.

Mandel, J. S., & Kitane, K. J. (1989, spring). San Francisco looks at AIDS in Southeast Asia. *Multicultural Inquiry and Research on AIDS, 3*(2), 1–2, 7.

Marin, B. (1990). Hispanic culture: Implications for AIDS prevention. In J. Boswell, R. Hexter, & J. Reinisch (Eds.), *Sexuality and disease: Metaphors, perceptions and behavior in the AIDS era.* New York: Oxford University Press.

Marin, G. (1988, August). *AIDS intervention issues among Hispanics.* Paper presented at the American Psychological Association Conference, Atlanta, GA.

Marin, G. (1989). AIDS prevention among Hispanics: Needs, risk behaviors, and cultural values. *Public Health Reports, 104,* 411–415.

Marin, G., & Marin, B. (1989). *Perceived credibility of various channels and sources of AIDS information among Hispanics.* (Technical Report #3). San Francisco: Center for Prevention Studies, University of California, San Francisco.

Mays, V. M., & Cochran, S. D. (1988). Issues in the perception of AIDS risk and risk reduction activities by black and Hispanic/Latina women. *American Psychologist, 43,* 949–957.

National AIDS Network. (1989). The many faces of Asian AIDS. *NAN Multi-Cultural Notes on AIDS Education and Services, 2*(3), 1–2.

Pape, J., & Johnson, W. (1988). Epidemiology of AIDS in the Caribbean. *Bailliere's Clinical Tropical Medicine and Communicable Diseases, 3*(1), 31–42.

Pape, J., Stanback, E., Pamphile, M., Boncy, M., Deschamps, M., Verdier, R., Beaulieu, M., Blattner, W., Liautaud, B., & Johnson, W. (1990). Prevalence of HIV infection and high-risk activities in Haiti. *Journal of Acquired Immune Deficiency Syndromes, 3,* 995–1001.

Pares-Avila, J. A., Hunt, D. E., Hammett, T., Sifre, S., Harrold, L., & Moini, S. (1989, November). *AIDS prevention among female sexual partners of I.V. drug users in Puerto Rico.* Paper presented at NIDA/NIMH technical review workshop, Facilitating HIV-related Behavior Change among Latinos and Native Americans, Albuquerque, NM.

Peterson, J. L., & Marin, G. (1988). Issues in the prevention of AIDS among black and Hispanic men. *American Psychologist, 43*, 871–877.

Quinn, T. C., Narain, J. P., & Zacarias, F. R. (1990). AIDS in the Americas: A public health priority for the region. *AIDS, 4*, 709–724.

Rapkin, A. D., & Erickson, P. I. (1990). Differences in knowledge of and risk factors for AIDS between Hispanic and non-Hispanic women attending an urban family planning clinic. *AIDS, 4*, 889–899.

Rich, J. (1991). HIV infection in communities of color. In H. Libman & R. Witzburg (Eds.), *Clinical manual for the care of the adult patient with HIV infection (supplement).* Sherborn, MA: ADLB Publications.

Rogers, M., & Williams, W. (1987). AIDS in blacks and Hispanics: Implications for prevention. *Issues in Science and Technology, 10*, 12–16.

Rothenberg, R., Woelfel, M., Stoneburner, R., Milberg, J., Parker, R., & Truman, B. (1987). Survival with the acquired immunodeficiency syndrome. *New England Journal of Medicine, 317*, 1297–1302.

Scheider, B. E. (1988). Gender, sexuality and AIDS. In R. A. Berk, (Ed.) *Social responses and consequences in the social impact of AIDS in the U.S.* Cambridge, MA: ABT Books.

Schoenbaum, E., Hartel, D., Selwyn, P., Klein, R., Davenny, K., Rogers, M., Feiner, C., & Friedland, G. (1989). Risk factors for human immunodeficiency virus infection in intravenous drug users. *New England Journal of Medicine, 321*, 874–879.

Selik, M., Castro, K., & Pappaioanou, M. (1988). Racial/ethnic differences in the risk of AIDS in the United States. *American Journal of Public Health, 78*, 1539–1545.

Selik, R. M., Castro, K. G., Pappaioanou, M., & Buehler, J. W. (1989). Birthplace and the risk of AIDS among Hispanics in the United States. *American Journal of Public Health, 79*, 836–839.

Sluzki, C. (1979). Migration and family conflict. *Family Process, 18*, 379–390.

Smith, M. (1990, December). *Statement of Mark D. Smith, M.D., M.B.A.* Paper presented at a meeting of the National Commission on the Acquired Immune Deficiency Syndrome, Baltimore, MD.

Smith, M. (1991). Zidovudine: Does it work for everyone? *Journal of the American Medical Association, 266*, 2750–2751.

Stafford, S. (1987). The Haitians: The cultural meaning of race and ethnicity. In N. Foner (Ed.), *New immigrants in New York.* New York: Columbia University Press.

Stepick, A., & Portes, A. (1986). Flight into despair: A profile of Haitian refugees in South Florida. *International Migration Review, 20*, 329–350.

Swift, C., & Levin, G. (1987). Empowerment: An emerging mental health technology. *Journal of Primary Prevention, 8*(1–2), 71–94.

Thomas, S., & Quinn, S. (1991). The Tuskegee syphilis study, 1932–1972: Implications for HIV education and AIDS risk education programs in the black community. *American Journal of Public Health, 81*, 1498–1504.

Viera, J. (1985). The Haitian link. In V. Gong (Ed.), *Understanding AIDS: A comprehensive guide.* New Brunswick, NJ: Rutgers University Press.

Worth, D. (1990). Minority women and AIDS: Culture, race and gender. In T. Feldman (Ed.), *Culture and AIDS.* New York: Praeger.

Wu, S., & Pak, S. (1989, Spring). The hidden minority, perspectives on being Asian and gay. *Harvard East Wind Magazine, 2*(2), 22–25.

10

WOMEN AND HIV

DINA ROSEN AND WENDY BLANK

The roles of women in the HIV pandemic have changed considerably since the early 1980s. Their roles must be looked at from both a systemic and interpersonal perspective. From a systemic point of view, it is important to consider the harsh realities of women's political, social, and economic status in our society. From an individual, interpersonal point of view, we must consider how women view themselves and how they relate and are expected to relate to others. In a society that places great emphasis on wellness and productivity, all people faced with terminal illness deal with feelings of stigma, lowered self-esteem, loss, and depression as well as economic hardships. For women with HIV, these issues are magnified.

Historically, women have assumed the caregiver role. They have cared for children, prepared the meals, and "made the home" (Lerner, 1981). Although gender roles have changed and expanded over the past two decades, women continue to fulfill traditional roles while assuming other roles such as breadwinner. Fulfilling traditional roles has resulted in women being more financially dependent, isolated, and less able to access medical care, social support, and information about health services. However, the chronicity, symptomatology, and stigmatization of HIV affect a woman's ability to fulfill these roles and expectations.

During the past 11 years, by reason of women's traditional role as caregivers, mothers have cared for gay sons and infected children, lesbian women have cared for their gay brothers, and wives have cared for ill husbands. But women are now faced with the additional reality that they are among the fastest growing group of individuals infected with HIV. The AIDS cases that we see today result from infections that occurred 5 to 10 years ago (Noble, 1991). The World Health Organization estimates that during the 1990s, 3 million women and children will die from AIDS. In 1981 women accounted for 3% of people infected with AIDS in the United States; by 1990 the percentage of women infected had risen to 11.5% (Pearl, 1990). Between 1989 and 1990, the number of women with AIDS increased by 34%, compared with a 22% increase among men.

In 1991 AIDS is expected to be one of the five leading causes of death among U.S. women between the ages of 15 and 44 years. Moreover, HIV disease disproportionally affects ethnic minority women. Black and Hispanic women make up only 17% of all U.S. women but represent 73%, with Blacks comprising 52% and Hispanics 21%, of all reported AIDS cases among women (Noble, 1991, pp. 1–2).

These statistics are alarming; yet many experts believe that women are underrepresented because of errors in the epidemiological reporting from the Centers for Disease Control (CDC). Because the gay male population was first identified as being infected with symptomatic HIV disease, the criteria established to define an "AIDS" case was based on case definitions for males. According to the Women's Treatment and Research Agenda (a work in progress) medical professionals were not and still are not adequately trained to identify physical manifestations of HIV disease in women. Guidelines have not been established to include infections specific to women for case definition of AIDS. Pelvic inflammatory disease (PID), chronic vaginal candidiasis (vaginal yeast infection), chlamydia, and human papillomavirus (HPV) are a few of the manifestations of HIV that are specific to women. Because the CDC does not recognize women's specific opportunistic infections or include an HIV-positive female with cervical cancer among those defined with AIDS, women are not accurately represented in national statistics on AIDS (Chu, Buehler, & Berkelman, 1990).

As an infected population, women continue to be underrepresented in national and international data. Little documentation on women and HIV has been recorded in the past four years. Statistics show a rapid increase in AIDS in women despite poor diagnostic measures. Transmission risks and education geared toward women about these risks are severely underresearched. Virtually nothing is known about woman-to-woman transmission of the virus, although documented cases do exist (Denenberg, 1990). Women at risk have come to the attention of HIV service providers by reason of the high incidence of babies infected with HIV and because of women's reproductive issues rather than from concern for the infected women themselves.

Historical factors complicate these issues. Women are less likely to seek medical attention and often delay seeking medical treatments because of perceived familial priorities or financial limitations (Perez, 1991). When women do seek treatment, their medical and emotional concerns are often minimized by health care providers, who may perceive women as hysterical or overreactive (Benson & Maier, 1990). This can be viewed as a systemic problem. However, individual problems such as lack of assertiveness and self-empowerment are common among women, especially minority and impoverished women.

S, a 21-year-old African American woman living in the housing projects of south central Los Angeles, had always had financial problems. She had three children (ages 5, 3, and 1) and was married. She had tested positive for HIV one year previously, after suffering from pneumonia. S was an injection drug and crack cocaine user, as was her husband. She had not told anyone about her HIV infection until she entered a women's group. In fact, S was not sure what it meant to be

HIV positive, except that she did not feel good most of the time. She did not have any idea how the HIV virus was transmitted. S felt isolated, alone, and scared. She reported symptoms of panic attacks, yet remained firm about not disclosing her HIV status to her close-knit, extended family. S considered having another child. Her physicians did not spend time explaining the issues of HIV with her and she reported that she was treated in a demeaning way. She did not receive treatment for symptoms that were treatable.

POPULATION DESCRIPTION

Professionals need to understand the population when beginning clinical work with women infected with HIV. As professionals, we are trained to recognize population-specific needs and concerns. When dealing with HIV disease and women, issues of race, gender, and economic status play key roles. In addition, specific medical issues and access to adequate health and emotional care also play important roles.

It is also important for professionals to be aware of the historical development of HIV disease epidemiology when interacting with HIV-positive women on an interpersonal level. Early in the pandemic, attention was focused on male homosexuals, who had the highest rate of HIV infection, followed soon by injection drug users. Later, prostitutes were also identified as being at high risk. And finally, as of 1990, sexual partners of injection drug users and bisexual men were identified as being at high risk (National Institute of Allergy and Infectious Diseases, 1990). Thus, concern about high-risk groups has evolved into concern about high-risk behaviors, the later approach being more inclusive, especially for women. Attitudes and stereotypes about persons who engage in high-risk behaviors affect the perceptions of care providers and the women whom they serve. Unfortunately, HIV-positive women have also bought into these stereotypes. They report feeling isolated, alone, shameful, and guilty for having contracted the virus: "I feel I'm the only woman in this city who is infected." "I can't tell anyone I'm infected. What would they think?" "I'll never be able to date or have sex again." "Who is going to look after my children?" "Who will care for my aging mother?" "I have just enough money to get by now; what happens if I get sick?" "Everyone asks me when I cleaned up. When I tell them I never used needles they look at me like I'm a whore."

In our clinical work with women infected with HIV, we have identified two distinct future-focused groups as well as a third, less future-focused group of disenfranchised individuals.

The first future-focused group places a high value on the role of wife and mother—women who believed they would meet "Mr. Right," get married, have children, raise a family, and retire to a good and happy life. Minority women place a strong emphasis on the family as the primary social unit. Fertility and childbearing strengthen a woman's status and are complicated by HIV infection (Marin, 1991). HIV disease might be assumed to influence women's choices regarding pregnancy and childbearing, but HIV-infected women and their seronegative counterparts with similar demographic backgrounds become pregnant at similar rates. Even when counseled, 50% of HIV-infected women choose to continue their pregnancy (Obstetrics and Gynecology Clinics of North America, 1990).

The second group values career and success. These women spend much time and effort becoming educated and work long and hard to advance in the professional world, with hopes of financial independence, personal autonomy, well-being, and longevity.

HIV has had a drastic effect on women in both groups. For those in the first group, childbearing becomes a life-and-death issue. Not only is having children a moral dilemma, in that 30% of children born to an HIV-positive woman will contract the virus, it is also a medical dilemma in that pregnancy and birthing are physically debilitating to a woman who is already medically compromised. The care and well-being of her newborn, even if it is not infected, and of any children born previous to the infection are major concerns and a major source of stress.

The lives of career-oriented women are radically altered as well. These women tend to be future oriented with long-range goals. Their identity is strongly tied into what they are doing and where they are going. Their HIV status creates issues of loss of identity, loss of future goals, and fear of disclosure and judgment about their HIV status. After women become symptomatic, they must deal with insurance issues, discrimination, and ability to perform work-related duties.

Disenfranchised women with AIDS are even more isolated than are women in the other two groups. The "invisibility" of this group makes it difficult for them to find treatments and interventions. They tend to be blamed for having contracted the virus. They are stigmatized by society and seen as promiscuous, immoral, uneducable, irresponsible, and criminal (Denenberg, 1990). These women must also deal with primary issues of drug addiction, homelessness, and prostitution before they can focus on taking care of themselves and on their HIV status. This population is not perceived as future oriented or as contributing to society. They face greater struggles on many fronts because they are less educated and less information is available to them. They have difficulty accessing the health care system and they lack support systems in the community. When working with disenfranchised populations, professionals need to be aware of these barriers.

Women with HIV face many unique problems when compared with their male counterparts or children with HIV. Denenberg (1990) reports that women, on average, live 16 weeks from the date of their diagnosis of AIDS, whereas white gay men live 21 months. Diagnosis of full-blown AIDS comes late in the course of their illness because of women's difficulty and delay in accessing health care resources. Women are underdiagnosed and subject to organ-specific diseases and conditions that the CDC has not yet specified as constituting an AIDS diagnosis. Women are misdiagnosed because they are not viewed as being likely to have HIV disease and professionals are not trained adequately to detect its signs and symptoms in women.

Sociopolitical issues also affect women with HIV disease. Women are systematically excluded from experimental drug trials because of fears that they will become pregnant (Denenberg, 1990). Moreover, women do not have equal access to drug and alcohol treatment programs. Women are poorer than men are and bear the majority of child-rearing responsibilities. Women tend to have inadequate or no health insurance. And finally, fewer AIDS service agencies and support services are designed to meet the special needs of women.

Lesbian women deserve a special note. The health care community and lesbians alike do not believe that lesbians are at risk for AIDS. In part, this is due to AIDS being characterized as a male homosexual disease. Moreover, lesbians have been told that they have the lowest risk for contracting sexually transmitted diseases. More important, the CDC and those who maintain records on the number of AIDS cases have not gathered information on infected lesbians. Lesbians may be misdiagnosed or diagnosed even later in the course of HIV infection than are other women (Cole & Cooper, 1991). In addition, many believe that lesbian women do not frequently engage in sexual activity and that their activity is confined to woman-to-woman sex. However, it is estimated that 75% of self-identified lesbian women have had sexual contact with men and that 32% of these women engaged in vaginal and anal intercourse with gay and bisexual men (Cole & Cooper, 1991). Such misconceptions are another example of the need to shift focus from high-risk groups to high-risk behaviors, underscoring the fact that all women are at risk.

> J, a 34-year-old Caucasian lesbian, has a history of injection drug use as well as multiple sex partners, including both women and men. J became pregnant two years ago with her second child, and at that time tested positive for HIV antibodies. At first, J went on a drug binge. Eventually, however, she discontinued her drug use with the aid of Narcotics Anonymous. After a difficult pregnancy and delivery, her daughter has tested HIV negative for the past 12 months. The child is in a foster-care placement specializing in HIV-positive children. J did not feel that she could care adequately for the child, given her own health status. She is, however, involved in a committed, monogamous relationship with another woman. J has become active in grass-roots organizing regarding HIV disease.

Adult men and women with HIV share many issues: shame, guilt, and isolation. Fears of transmitting the virus to others, prolonged and painful illness, death and dying, and loss of financial security are common among men and women with HIV. The stigmatization of persons with HIV/AIDS leads to isolation, fear of intimacy, and feeling like a pariah. Denial is a common coping skill for everyone infected. Although denial can help persons cope with their diagnosis, it can also prevent individuals from accessing health care or support services.

Grief and loss issues affect everyone with HIV. Life goals are drastically altered. Adults must change their activities and revise their future plans. Women who are future oriented must adopt a new perspective on their lives. Disenfranchised women must focus on survival, their diagnosis further diminishing hope in their lives.

PRESENTING CONCERNS AND ASSESSMENT ISSUES

Women with HIV need support, advocacy, and education. Because supportive services are lacking, women seek counseling and therapeutic interventions for numerous psychological problems and issues. Women feel isolated, distrustful, depressed, fearful, anxious, and angry at themselves and the systems that do not meet their needs. They seek supportive therapy and counseling to address and work through issues in an effort to improve their coping skills and enhance their quality of life.

Women with HIV seek assistance in negotiating various systems; thus an ecological approach to assessment is required. Counseling with regard to identifying and seeking the assistance of public benefits is important because many of these women have few financial resources. Disability benefits are available, but the application process can be confusing and exhausting and, without a diagnosis of AIDS, nearly impossible to obtain. Medical care specific to women with HIV is difficult to find. Thus, women need referrals to sensitive health care providers who are knowledgeable about infections and symptoms specific to women. Transportation concerns are common among women, as is child care. Women have problems negotiating school systems for HIV-infected children. School systems are generally unprepared and without HIV policies. The custodial laws are constantly in flux, and women must become aware of their legal rights to maintain custody of their children throughout their illnesses as well as plan for their children's care after death. The educational system can present challenges to children with HIV due to the stigma, fear, and lack of education about HIV infection. Professionals need to advocate on behalf of clients for children's services.

> C, a 25-year-old middle-class Caucasian woman, had married three years ago and had a child. When her daughter was one year old, the child began to get sick. At that time, both C and her daughter tested HIV positive; C's husband is HIV negative. Fortunately, C's family was very supportive, although she frequently needs to explain why she cannot fulfill all the duties requested of her. Because their financial resources are scarce, the family lives with C's mother. C spends many hours taking herself and her daughter to the many doctors they must see. They live on the outskirts of the city and both of them tire easily. C has had a great deal of difficulty enrolling her daughter in preschool due to her HIV status. After numerous tries, and with the assistance of many advocates and professionals, they have finally found a preschool with an AIDS policy.

Good HIV education for women is sorely lacking and should be routinely assessed. Because many women lack knowledge about HIV, service providers need to assume the role of health educator. Thus, professionals must remain current on health and benefit changes as well as the clinical aspects of HIV disease.

Theoretically, an interpersonal/systemic model works well with women with HIV. This theoretical perspective takes into consideration the biophysical, cognitive/perceptual, emotional/psychodynamic, behavioral, cultural, and motivational factors that affect the functioning of individuals. The state of a woman's health affects virtually every aspect of her functioning and should be taken into consideration when assessing needs. This theoretical framework allows women with HIV to deal with their misconceptions, self-concept, judgments, and sense of reality on an interpersonal level (Hepworth & Larson, 1986).

An interpersonal/systemic model allows clinicians to address individual needs while viewing the woman within the context of her situation. This framework provides a structure from which the professional can develop therapeutic interventions (Rodway, 1986). It is important to consider not only the physical symptoms of HIV but also the external factors that both affect and are affected by the HIV infection, for example, a closed-minded family system, an unresponsive support system, a discriminating work environment. After an interpersonal-needs assessment has been completed, focus can be shifted to identifying external systems that affect an HIV-positive woman, for example, child care, the workplace, accessing health care and public benefits, drug treatment, and housing. A comprehensive biopsychosocial assessment to evaluate medical status, psychological coping skills, support systems, and emotional stability is an appropriate starting point. Assessment must also consider familial relationships, child rearing, childbearing, family-of-origin issues, substance abuse, and socioeconomic issues.

INTERVENTIONS

A systemic practice approach allows for different modes of intervention (Rodway, 1986). Intervention plans for HIV-infected women must be eclectic and responsive to the clients' ever-changing circumstances.

After identifying the direct needs of the client, the service provider must make appropriate HIV-sensitive referrals. Most HIV-positive women are not aware of available services and require education and information. Connecting the client with an HIV women's support group helps her understand that she is not alone. In such groups, she can reach out to others and overcome her own internalized AIDS phobia and stereotypes.

Service providers must make sure that referral sources are in fact HIV sensitive. They must make outreach efforts and provide education to representatives of community resources and public social services. In some instances, the service provider needs to develop such services.

The referral/assessment process helps to define the appropriate roles and limitations of the clinician. Depending on their available support systems, level of coping, and medical status, some women have a broad spectrum of needs. Some women may require multiple interventions; others have fewer needs and require minimal interventions. Regardless, clinicians must provide a nonjudgmental, safe environment where the woman can vent her feelings, share her fears, and gain the strength to cope with the judgmental and stigmatizing systems that she will encounter.

Specific treatment interventions vary, depending on the client's presenting problems. Stress-reduction techniques should be taught to all persons with HIV regardless of their stage of illness. Guided imagery allows women to relax while getting in touch with their own ability to heal themselves. Meditation helps clients slow the mind and focus on pleasant and relaxing thoughts. Deep breathing, which can be practiced anywhere at anytime, helps women who are working or are in stressful situations for prolonged periods to slow down and get back in touch with their bodies. Clinicians need to teach women these basic skills.

For women who have been recently tested and diagnosed as HIV positive but who exhibit no symptoms, clinicians should assume the role of supportive educator by providing realistic expectations of the disease process and ways in which they can best maintain their health. The clinician needs to help the woman explore her feelings while empathizing with her shame, guilt, fear, and depressions.

For a symptomatic woman, interventions should be geared toward improving coping strategies by reinforcing appropriate behaviors, encouraging her to access appropriate health care, and helping her deal with her relationships. Self-empowerment and assertiveness training are very important. Assertiveness training improves self-esteem. Using "I see . . . I feel . . . I want . . . " expressions is an effective technique. The "I see . . . " expression allows the woman to share her perceptions of her situation. The "I feel . . . " expression helps her share how she feels about her situation. And the "I want . . . " expression allows her to identify what she would like done about the situation. For example,

> J, a patient of Dr. R, did not receive the time and attention from her physician that she wanted. After discussing this concern with her clinician, during her next doctor's appointment, she said, "Dr. R, when I come for an office visit I see you rush in and rush out without spending much time with me. I feel unattended to, unimportant, and hurt by these actions. I would like you to plan to spend time with me and answer any questions I may have." Since then, Dr. R has spent more time with her. Thus J began to receive the quality of care she deserved because she expressed her feelings in a direct, honest, assertive manner.

For those in end-stage disease, death and dying issues are paramount. Women may develop an increasing dependency on clinicians during this stage. Women's support groups can play a key role in providing a safe and supportive environment. The end stage is difficult. Clinicians must maintain boundaries, yet traditional helping approaches may no longer meet the client's needs. Clinicians may have to make home or hospital visits. Such visits should be planned in advance, time limited, and as frequent as is appropriate. Clinicians should be wary of breaking routines or patterns of service at this point so that the client does not develop an unrealistic dependency on the clinician. Too much dependency can alienate the support system already in place. If other support systems are not available, clinicians must determine the extent of their involvement. Consulting with other professionals regarding level of involvement and maintaining professional distance is helpful.

The roles of service providers are influenced by clients' needs. Clinicians become advocates when dealing with medical, legal, financial, and substance-abuse-treatment resources. Their role may shift to educator about the disease process, gynecological manifestations, signs and symptoms of illness, and safer-sex practices. When an eclectic, concrete approach to service provision is utilized, women are typically very receptive to services. Initially, many women find it difficult to access services because of their shame, guilt, fear of judgment, stigma, and the general lack of female-specific services available. Clinicians need to provide relevant and accurate information and be nonjudgmental. Once women are introduced into a service system that is nonjudgmental and able to provide support and assistance, women are appreciative of the services they have received and tend to seek services.

In addition to concrete assistance, service providers need to create an environment that is welcoming, reassuring, nonjudgmental, nonstigmatizing, and supportive. For example,

> K, a 24-year-old white, single woman who was diagnosed as HIV positive after having a test "just for the hell of it," reported that she did not believe she was in a high-risk group, although now she sees her high-risk behavior. K had had several sexual partners, and her physician believed that she was infected in her late teens.
>
> K contacted a clinician after she was told that the clinician was sensitive to women's issues and was very knowledgeable about HIV/AIDS. She had learned that she was HIV positive only two weeks earlier, had little information, and was frightened. The clinician provided basic information about available resources for support and assistance as well as appropriate medical referrals. K expressed concern about gynecological problems that she was experiencing. In addition, she had heard that the antiviral medications that had been prescribed for her were toxic for women. After providing information and recommending resources, K agreed to attend a women's support group.
>
> Here, the role of the clinician switched from educator to therapist. The group focused on support and sharing HIV/AIDS issues and the impact of HIV on participants and those around them. Although K learned a great deal from group members, she continued to depend on the clinician for individual support and guidance outside the group.
>
> K requested that the clinician meet with her family, which was visiting from out of town. Thus, the clinician's role became that of family therapist. An extraordinary level of trust has developed between K and the clinician. K states that this is due to the fact that the clinician was not only supportive but knowledgeable about resources and well-connected in the community. K also stated that after talking to several male clinicians who were "difficult to connect with," she finally found a female clinician with whom she felt much more comfortable.

Ethnicity, culture, and social class become less of an issue in the helping process due to the general lack of services for HIV-infected women. Because women are stigmatized and generally remain closeted with regard to their HIV infection, they are able to develop bonds when they disclose to one another. However, it is often useful and necessary to address ethnic, cultural, and class differences with clients. By acknowledging differences, service providers relate to the client's perception of her problems and needs (Engel, 1984). Moreover, knowledge of the client's culture helps build trust throughout the course of the helping relationship. Also, the client's culture and class influence her response to illness as well as her general health-seeking behaviors (Aoki, 1989).

In working with women with HIV, boundary issues are often confusing. Service providers struggle with their level of involvement and the frustrating ambiguities regarding touching and hugging, giving advice, and working with extended-family and friendship networks. Professional training emphasizes maintaining objectivity and professional distance. But service providers may have difficulty making sense out of the uncertainty of HIV disease and the appropriate therapeutic approach to take. Providers may have been directly affected by HIV/AIDS in their personal life. Overidentification can detract from clinicians' ability to help (Caldarola & Silven, 1989). Clinicians' feelings of attachment, care, and concern for their clients must be recognized and validated. A client's guilt, shame, and isolation, as well as feelings of being dirty, poisonous, and toxic, can be addressed verbally as well as nonverbally by means of appropriate touching. Such methods are somewhat contradictory to the traditional "rules" of the helping professions (Namir & Sherman, 1989).

Countertransference issues include fear of contagion, death, and dying; a sense of powerlessness; need for professional omnipotence; and anger (Dunkel & Hatfield, 1986). Clinicians need to address these issues before a beneficial therapeutic process can occur. Clinicians should seek consultation, support from peers and supervisors, and education regarding HIV-specific concerns. If these issues are not addressed, providers' discomfort and clients' resistance to painful issues may steer them toward "quick fix" solutions (Caldarola & Silven, 1989). Additionally, if clients sense unresolved feelings and fears on the part of the clinician, negative transference will occur and a trusting relationship will never develop. Thus, service providers must develop healthy coping strategies and outlets for their feelings before they can effectively assist clients with HIV.

CONCLUSION

It is essential that women's needs with regard to HIV be brought into public consciousness. Women with HIV disease need to become "visible," and stereotypes must be destroyed. The role of women in the AIDS pandemic has changed dramatically. Whereas early on women were perceived as care providers to the ill, the incidence of women with HIV is rising at an alarming rate. The majority of these women are poor, uneducated, and members of minority groups. Their access to health care is restricted, and they lack knowledge of risk behaviors and HIV in general. The health care profession has neglected the special needs and issues of women with HIV disease. The HIV pandemic has exposed the inefficacy of the public health care system in general and its care of women in particular. Educational materials need to focus on women and their risk factors. More women-specific services need to be provided. Women must be included in clinical trials, and the definition of AIDS needs to be broadened to include women-specific infections. The political, social, and economic status of women must be improved, and service providers must approach women with HIV in a nonjudgmental, nonstigmatizing way.

REFERENCES

Aoki, B. K. (1989). Cross cultural counseling: The extra dimension. In J. W. Dilley, C. Pies, & M. Helquist (Eds.), *Face to face: A guide to AIDS counseling* (pp. 26–33). San Francisco: AIDS Health Project, University of California, San Francisco.

Benson, D. J. D., & Maier, C. (1990). Challenges facing women with HIV. *FOCUS: A Guide to AIDS Research and Counseling, 6*(1), 1–2.

Caldarola, T. J., & Silven, D. (1989). The HIV-positive client. In J. W. Dilley, C. Pies, & M. Helquist (Eds.), *Face to face: A guide to AIDS counseling* (pp. 15–25). San Francisco: AIDS Health Project, University of California, San Francisco.

Chu, S., Buehler, J., & Berkelman, R. (1990). Impact of the human immunodeficiency virus epidemic on mortality in women of reproductive age, United States. *Journal of the American*

Medical Association, 264, 225–229.

Cole, R., & Cooper, S. (1991, January). Lesbian exclusion from HIV/AIDS education. *SIECUS Report, 19*(2), pp. 114–117.

Denenberg, R. (1990). Unique aspects of HIV infection in women. In *Women, AIDS, and activism.* Boston: South End Press.

Dunkel, J., & Hatfield, S. (1986). Countertransference issues in working with persons with AIDS. *Social Work, 31,* 114–117.

Engel, G. L. (1984). The need for a new medical model: A challenge for biomedicine. In J. E. Mezzich & C. E. Berganza (Eds.), *Culture and psychopathology* (pp. 47–48). New York: Columbia University Press.

Hepworth, D. H., & Larsen, J. A. (1986). *Direct social work practice theory and skills.* Chicago: Dorsey Press.

Lerner, H. E. (1981). Early origins of envy and devaluation of women: Implications for sex-role stereotypes. In E. Howell & M. Bayes (Eds.), *Women and mental health* (pp. 26–40). New York: Basic Books.

Marin, B. V. (1991). Hispanic culture: Effects on prevention and care. *FOCUS: A Guide to AIDS Research and Counseling, 6*(4), 1–2.

Namir, S., & Sherman, S. (1989). Coping with countertransference. In C. Kain (Ed.), *No longer immune: A counselor's guide to AIDS* (pp. 266–268). Alexandria, VA: American Association for Counseling and Development.

National Institute of Allergy and Infectious Diseases. (1990, December). AIDS epidemiology branch seeks answers to critical questions concerning AIDS in women and their children. *NIAID Research on Women and HIV.* Bethesda, MD: Author.

Noble, G. (1991, April). Women and AIDS: The growing crisis: Update. *CDC HIV/AIDS Prevention Newsletter,* pp. 1–2.

Obstetrics and Gynecology Clinics of North America. (1990, September). *Reproductive decisions and HIV.* State University of New York Health Science Center at Brooklyn, Brooklyn, NY.

Pearl, D. (1990, November 30). AIDS spreads more rapidly among women. *Wall Street Journal,* pp. B1, B4.

Perez, E. (1991, December). Why women wait to be tested for HIV infection. *SIECUS Report, 19*(2), pp. 6–7.

Rodway, M. (1986). Systems theory. In F. J. Turner (Ed.), *Social work treatment: Interlocking theoretical approaches* (pp. 518–520). New York: Free Press.

11

CHILDREN AND AIDS

GEORGE LEWERT

In December 1982, the Centers for Disease Control (1982) reported for the second consecutive week unexplained immunodeficiency and opportunistic infections in infants in New York, New Jersey, and California. The report described 22 children with an inherited immune defect that had not previously been seen. It later became apparent that these reports were the first official announcement of the arrival of a new infectious agent in children: human immunodeficiency virus (HIV).

Today, 10 years after this report, we are faced with meeting the needs of growing numbers of children and their families affected by HIV. These families place increasing demands on our social and medical care systems. The needs of this population are indeed immense; human service providers can and must adapt traditional skills and develop new ones to meet these needs.

BACKGROUND

Beginning in 1982, pediatricians practicing in urban areas such as Newark, New Jersey, New York City, and Miami, Florida, began to realize that the newly identified immune deficiency syndrome was not confined to homosexual men and injection drug users (Koop, 1990). Infants and children presented with symptoms and illness suggestive of the same infection, including what is now called AIDS. After experiencing initial difficulty separating these children from patients with other immunological illnesses, in 1984, researchers discovered HIV (Novello & Wise, 1990) and began to realize the true potential of HIV infection in children (Faloon, Eddy, Weiner, & Pizzo, 1989). However, it was not until 1984 that "pediatric AIDS" was provisionally defined by the Centers for Disease Control (1984) in their official surveillance report. The definition of AIDS as it applies to children was revised in 1987 due to the different range of symptoms experienced by HIV-infected children as compared with adults (Centers for Disease Control, 1987).

Initially, children, most notably young hemophiliacs treated with the clotting factors derived from pooled blood products, were considered at risk for contracting

HIV via transfusion of HIV-infected blood and receipt of other blood products. Since 1985, however, blood has been routinely tested for HIV antibodies, which has led to a blood supply that is virtually free of HIV.

By far the vast majority of infected children (nearly 85%) acquire the virus from their mother before or at birth (Centers for Disease Control, 1991). Such transmission is variously called vertical, intrauterine, transplacental, perinatal, and congenital, reflecting uncertainty about how and when transmission from mother to child occurs. The efficiency of vertical transmission is not clearly understood yet, but studies estimate that 25% to 45% of children born to HIV-infected mothers will become infected with HIV themselves (Andiman, Simpson, Olson, Dember, Silva, & Miller, 1990). So far no definitive predictors of risk to an infant born to an infected mother are known; thus each child must be evaluated for infection. In fact, due to the child's possession of passive HIV antibodies from the mother, the HIV antibody test is not a reliable predictor of infection status. It is not until the child is 15 to 18 months old that a positive HIV test can demonstrate HIV infection with certainty in the absence of major infections indicative of HIV/AIDS (Faloon et al., 1989).

Cases have been documented of children infected through the ingestion of breast milk from mothers infected by the virus after their child's birth (Hutman, 1990). This has led to recommendations that women with or at high risk for HIV refrain from breast feeding if infant formula is readily available.

Sexual abuse is another mode of potential infection of children. Little conclusive data are available on the number of children who have been infected in this way (Gutman et al., 1991). High-risk groups include runaways who are victimized via prostitution and/or injection drug use.

The racial and geographic distribution of infected children mirrors that of infected women. For example, in New York State, HIV/AIDS is the leading cause of death among black women aged 15–44 and is the second leading cause of death among black children aged 1–4 (Centers for Disease Control, 1991).

Most HIV-infected children live in the inner city and in areas where there are high concentrations of injection drug use (Rogers, 1987). The majority of infected children (77%) are black and Hispanic (Centers for Disease Control, 1991). Because these children come from families ravaged by drug abuse and poverty, their lives are further complicated by social, psychological, and financial burdens. These families have few resources to cope with the overwhelming demands of a chronic and life-threatening illness such as HIV/AIDS.

CHARACTERISTICS OF INFECTED CHILDREN AND FAMILIES

Families with few resources and multiple problems are faced with overwhelming stress upon diagnosis of HIV. Such a diagnosis may overwhelm an already vulnerable family structure and result in a parent's relapse into drug use, abandonment by a partner/spouse, and/or emotional chaos or paralysis leading to the breakdown or dissolution of the family unit. The infected child may be abandoned and uninfected siblings placed in foster care or with extended-family members.

Although the emotional dynamics of caring for an HIV-infected child are similar to those experienced by families who face other life-threatening illnesses, other factors add to the stress surrounding an HIV diagnosis. Most affected families are single-parent households living at the extreme margins of society. The families are barely able to meet minimal survival standards for housing, income, health insurance, nutrition, and education. Compliance with complex and demanding treatment regimens requires considerable family organization and stability, characteristics not commonly found in such families. These families typically use medical facilities only in a medical crisis, thus preventing early diagnosis (Mitchell & Heagarty, 1990). Families affected by HIV/ AIDS may have one or more members with a past or present history of drug use. Family violence and child abuse are not uncommon (Lewert, 1988; Deren, 1986).

Cultural beliefs of many black and Hispanic families may be influenced by indigenous, nonmedical healers, well-intentioned grandparents, or other members of the community. Their influence should be explored in order to ensure compliance with prescribed medical regimens (Mitchell & Heagarty, 1990). Challenging firmly held cultural belief systems is not productive and is likely to alienate family members. Rather, these beliefs need to be integrated into treatment.

Depression is often a precipitating factor in parental drug use and is commonly found in psychosocially and economically deprived families at greatest risk for HIV infection (Septimus, 1989). Although many women are becoming infected via their male sex partners (Howe, 1990; Marte & Anastos, 1990), women are also threatened with HIV transmission through the smoking of "crack" cocaine. Sexual favors may be exchanged for the drug, thus exposing these women to HIV via multiple sex partners (Des Jarlais & Friedman, 1988a; Des Jarlais & Friedman 1988b; Fullilove, Fullilove, Bowser, & Gross, 1990).

The hopelessness of multigenerational poverty is compounded by an HIV diagnosis. Families who must face the mortality of a child and other family members while dealing with the debilitating effects of poverty are often unable to find the internal and external resources with which to combat their problems. Moreover, the stigma of HIV diagnosis is an omnipresent burden suffered by both persons with AIDS and their caregivers.

THE IMPACT OF HIV DIAGNOSIS

The interval from HIV infection to the onset of symptoms is often shorter in children who are infected congenitally than it is in those infected by transfusion (Oxtoby, 1990). It is also shorter in children than it is in adults. Therefore, the child is likely to be the first symptomatic family member. In many families, diagnosis of the child leads to diagnosis of parents and siblings. A child's diagnosis sends a shock wave through the entire family, threatening its present and future integrity. Parents may experience disbelief and numbness, impairing their ability to understand fully the ramifications of their child's illness and its implications for other family members. Disbelief is sometimes reinforced by the absence of symptoms in the child if the child is not severely ill or visibly symptomatic when the diagnosis is made.

155

The family is extremely vulnerable during this period. Past or present drug use, bisexuality, or promiscuity may be revealed upon diagnosis (Lewert, 1990a). Additionally, the family has not yet established a trusting relationship with the hospital multidisciplinary care team, which is essential to them in coping with the physical and psychological demands of HIV.

LIVING AND COPING WITH HIV

The first task for all members of the care team is to establish a trusting relationship with the family. Care providers need to offer empathy, information, and hope so that families can endure and integrate the diagnosis and its ramifications into their lives. For one parent, hope may be encouraged by the sight of other children with HIV in apparent good health who are older than her newly diagnosed infant. Another parent may find hope in a new drug or treatment regimen.

Initially, hope can be inspired through education about the manifestations of HIV infection. Misinformation and misplaced fears surrounding HIV/AIDS must be corrected. New treatments offer hope for increased life expectancy and quality of life; the perception that HIV diagnosis is an immediate death sentence is not necessarily true.

Moving a family into a comprehensive care and helping network demonstrates nurturance and support, which the family may have never experienced before in any setting. Obtaining concrete support services such as home care, day care, special schooling, financial help, improved housing, psychological or psychiatric services, group support, and recreational activities convince families that the caregiving team's interest is genuine and worthy of the family's trust.

Most people are aware of the ostracism and stigma surrounding HIV/AIDS. Children are no exception. Parents are faced with the difficult problem of determining whom they can trust among family and friends with the knowledge of the diagnosis. Helping professionals should assist them with this task by considering with the parents who should be told and how they should be told. Those rare parents who do not fear societal response to their child should be sensitized to the possible ramifications of public disclosure for the child, which unfortunately remain quite real.

INTERVENTION

Various strategies should be followed to maximize the coping abilities of the family upon diagnosis. Although intervention should be child centered, it must also be family based, because HIV infection in children, as with other chronic and life-threatening childhood illnesses, has a profound effect on the family unit.

INFANTS AND TODDLERS

Children from birth to two to three years of age are unable to understand the meaning of chronic illness or death. Thus, their experience of the illness will be defined by the reactions of their parents or caregivers. Although children will react physically to the pain and suffering caused by treatment, emotionally they respond to separations caused by hospitalization as well as the availability and nurturing abilities of parents if cared for at home. Some parents become overwhelmed by fear for their child's life and may withdraw from the child when he or she becomes acutely ill or welcome hospitalization because their care responsibilities are alleviated. Parents need to be provided with information and encouraged to provide consistent nurturance to the child.

PRESCHOOL-AGE CHILDREN

As children grow older, they develop a better sense of the meaning of their illness and become familiar with their routine of care. They may anticipate the pain of hospital visits or stays.

Preschool children benefit from a discussion of what they can expect when visiting the doctor or when they are hospitalized (McCue, 1980). Providing the child with a doctor's kit and appropriate books allow him or her to play out fears and confront anxieties. Children receiving gamma globulin infusions may enjoy using tape and IV tubing on a doll to replicate their experience of the treatment. Children enjoy role-reversal games, for example, the social worker becoming the tearful patient and the child the reassuring, or perhaps frightening, nurse or doctor. Such play may reveal a child's fear of IV needles or blood drawing as well as how he or she may prefer to be soothed. Play also provides a child some control over his or her situation and thus has considerable therapeutic value.

SCHOOL-AGE CHILDREN AND PREADOLESCENTS

School-age children present greater challenges to the team and to the parent. These children are more acutely aware of how their illness and treatments make them different from their peers or uninfected siblings. Because many parents wish to keep their child's diagnosis a secret, the child may be bewildered by the need for secrecy.

A child interprets both the spoken and unspoken expressions of parents. Despite the perceptions of some parents that their child is unaware of the nature of his or her illness, children's revelations tell us otherwise.

> One eight-year-old child who had lost both parents to AIDS but hadn't been told about his own diagnosis reminded his foster mother that he was due to take his medication (AZT). His foster mother asked why he was so concerned, as she seldom forgot to give it to him. He said, "Daddy didn't take his medication and he died. I don't want to die like Daddy."

His response convinced his foster mother that she needed to discuss his illness with him in more detail.

Withholding information from school-age children presents additional burdens for both the child and parent and is a difficult issue to resolve. The issue becomes more complicated if siblings or others in the household cannot be completely trusted with disclosure of the diagnosis. Most school-age children who are told about their illness do not share the information with others if they are given adequate reasons for not doing so. On the other hand, keeping a secret from other family members and friends may cause them to feel ashamed of their illness. Children may experience social isolation and discrimination after their seropositivity is revealed. Although public knowledge of HIV has improved, many families with HIV are not willing to risk stigmatization.

Some children and families have been able to share an HIV diagnosis with their community and school, resulting in proactive educational efforts that anticipate and address common fears and concerns related to risk of transmission (Grady, 1988). Regrettably, sharing information is the exception rather than the rule (Woodard, 1990; Navarro, 1991). Parents may be confused when faced with a caring schoolteacher who expresses concern about the child's numerous absences from school. They wish to respond truthfully to such compassion but often fabricate an explanation or minimize their child's medical problems. Sometimes children are not given medications during the school day in order to maintain secrecy (Navarro, 1991).

Studies of children with life-threatening illnesses indicate that they understand the concept of death at a younger age than do their healthy counterparts (Koocher & O'Malley, 1981). Many children with HIV have experienced the loss of one or both parents, a sibling, or important others in their family. Thus the need to share information about the disease is a difficult issue to ignore. Decisions regarding whether to share information and how much information should be shared must occur with the input of parents or other involved family members. The pros and cons of sharing information must be discussed, and the family should make the final decision. This process is ongoing as the child's and family's needs change.

If the diagnosis is disclosed to the child, he or she needs a substantial support network that clearly communicates how the infection was transmitted and gives assurance that the parent (if vertically transmitted) or hospital (if transfusion related) did not intend to cause the infection. The child needs help dealing with a wide range of questions and feelings that follow disclosure. Some children want to know if they can be cured or whether they will die. Such issues must be addressed according to the child's cognitive abilities. Children may begin to piece together past events and begin to understand the cause of their numerous other infections, hospitalizations, and treatments. Paradoxically, such knowledge can bring relief. Sometimes children do not respond immediately to or ask questions about their illness. They may do so at a later point in time. If the parents do not agree with disclosure, they should be urged to disclose as much about the symptoms of HIV and treatments as possible in order to maximize the child's participation and sense of control in the treatment process (Lewert, 1990b). To illustrate, one eight-year-old's mother did not feel comfortable disclosing the diagnosis to the child but was able to disclose the diagnosis of a severe cardiomyopathy and its effects on his level of activity. Such information helped the child become aware of physiological warning signs that could prevent a crisis.

Most parents worry about their child's ability to carry on with his or her life, fearing that the child will become depressed and unable to maintain a normal level of functioning. Although these are valid concerns, they also reflect the parents' difficulty facing the truth *with* their child. Usually parents feel responsible and guilty regardless of whether HIV was transmitted via transfusion or perinatally. They may have a tenuous hold on their anger and barely suppressed feelings of powerlessness; disclosure threatens their ability to control these emotions.

Thus a strong and supportive network needs to be established for the parent or caregiver as well as for the child. Professionals must anticipate and plan for a full range of psychological effects on the child and family members. The health care team must prepare the parent for eventual disclosure or perhaps be actively involved in disclosing the diagnosis with the parent.

Parents of children who have been vertically infected feel especially guilty. The children need to understand that their parents' role in transmitting the disease was inadvertent, so that the children do not blame their parents for causing their illness.

> One nine-year-old child who had not been told of the diagnosis was felt to be aware of it anyway. This issue was discussed with her mother and grandmother. The mother was struggling to cope with her own HIV infection and did not feel capable of actively participating in the disclosure process. However, she agreed that her child should be told. The health care team disclosed the diagnosis to the child in the presence of her grandmother and a nurse with whom the child had developed a "big sister" relationship. Since disclosure, the child has continued to do well physically and emotionally.

Despite this and other successes with disclosure, the issue needs to be studied further to gauge children's long-term adjustment to living with knowledge of HIV diagnosis.

ADOLESCENTS

The latency period of HIV is not clearly understood, but some vertically infected children reach adolescence. Also, children with hemophilia or children who were infected due to other health conditions that required a blood transfusion prior to 1985 make up the population of adolescents with AIDS. Some adolescents contract HIV through injection drug use or through homosexual activity. Many adolescents contract HIV but are not diagnosed until early adulthood, due to the latency period of HIV (Hein, 1989). Children with a preexisting condition such as hemophilia or sickle-cell disease must cope with two life-threatening conditions.

Regardless of how they were infected, HIV-infected adolescents face a unique set of challenges. During adolescence, children commonly feel a sense of invulnerability. Authority is challenged, and peer support and approval are sought (Septimus & Weiner, 1990). An HIV diagnosis challenges the child's sense of invulnerability and can make compliance with treatment especially difficult. The child may rage against the diagnosis and manifestations of the disease. Peer relationships may be extremely difficult, causing the child to become overly dependent on the family or treatment team. The likelihood of sexual experimentation makes disclosure a vital issue to resolve. Issues of responsibility and safer sex practices must be addressed and alternative sexual expressions explored.

CLINICAL INTERVENTIONS

PARENTS

Although HIV pretest counseling may begin to prepare a parent for the possible diagnosis of a child with HIV, no amount of anticipatory counseling can truly prepare parents for confirmation that their child is infected. The crisis the diagnosis precipitates is usually, but not always, apparent in that numbness and disbelief may occur, often followed by extreme sadness and fear of imminent death of the child and other family members. At this point, anticipatory grieving begins.

This period is critical for the family and interdisciplinary team. Caregivers must project calmness, caring, and competence in their ability to care for the child and other family members. The parent's ability to trust team members will enable them to endure this initial crisis. Parents need to be educated about HIV and to have any misinformation corrected. Because HIV/AIDS is so often simply equated with death, professionals need to inform parents about the spectrum of HIV disease as well as new treatments that improve the duration and quality of life.

At the core of all interventions, especially during the initial phase, must lie hope. Without hope, parents may succumb to despair and helplessness. Hope and optimism must be felt and strongly projected by all members of the treatment team.

Hope and a relationship of trust with one or more members of the treatment team minimize the risk of parental denial and/or avoidance of follow-up treatment for their child (Wooley & Stein, 1989). Hope and trust can also minimize the possibility of relapse into drug abuse as well as intervention of child protection services due to medical neglect (Boland, Tasker, Evans, & Keresztes, 1987). To complicate matters, arrangements may have to be made for parent(s) to begin their own regimen of medical assessment and care.

Although the reactions of parents and families differ, most parents are able to move from the shock and panic of initial diagnosis to acceptance of the diagnosis within two to six weeks. Understanding the way in which a parent copes with the initial diagnosis is the first step in the psychosocial assessment and is vital to understanding family dynamics, premorbid functioning, current strengths and vulnerabilities, and how the the diagnosis is likely to alter family functioning. This assessment should be ongoing; as the level of trust and need varies, so will the amount and type of information that should be shared. Information about present or past family dysfunction, such as drug and alcohol use, psychiatric problems, and family violence, is essential to gauging the capabilities of parents and to formulating clinical interventions and referrals to outside sources of support that will build or preserve family functioning.

Other family needs may be more basic, but certainly no less important. First, a family must have adequate medical insurance and a means of getting to and from their medical provider. Ensuring that families receive the maximum income support they are entitled to receive and providing home care, visiting nurse services, referral of the infected child and/or siblings to day-care programs help lessen the parents' burden. Geographical areas with high prevalence of children with HIV/AIDS may have specialized programs for children; in areas without specialized services, programs that serve children with other disabilities may be a good resource.

Among the many models of potential engagement of the HIV-infected child and family, individual counseling is usually the point of entry. Parents, infected children, well siblings, and other involved family members have unique perspectives and needs that are usually treated best through individual counseling.

Children need the opportunity to express themselves in words and in play according to their age and capabilities. Healthy siblings must also be helped to understand and cope with the changes and losses taking place within the family. Older children may be engaged verbally, either formally or informally. Younger children may be better able to express their fears and traumas through play. Children of all ages have a strong need to protect their families from the pain and trauma that they experience, especially if they perceive their parents as struggling emotionally with the child's, as well as their own, HIV infection.

Although many children have concerns and fears related to death and dying, they often respond to nonverbal cues from family members that abort or preclude discussion. For example, one 10-year-old girl from a family who had not discussed her diagnosis pretended in her play that the daughter of a farmer could not do her chores because she was resting in the hay loft as a result of her sickness. The farmer, his wife, and the son continued their work but were very worried about her. Another mother was shocked when her teenage daughter told her that she knew her eight-year-old brother had AIDS. The daughter had kept this "secret" for two years, explaining that she didn't want to anger or upset her mother because she could tell her mother was worried and upset enough.

Parents need to address issues that are equally difficult. Relationships developed during the less emotionally laden period can lay the groundwork for the more sensitive and emotionally difficult issues now facing parents. Most parents need to plan for custody of their child(ren) following their own death and may need assistance in how to approach relatives or friends. Conversely, they may need to decide how aggressively they wish the medical staff to treat their child in the end stages of illness. In advanced illness, discussion of funeral arrangements and other preparations for death must also be considered.

Although many HIV-infected families may not be structured in a conventional manner, couple and family counseling should be utilized when possible. Due to unresolved blame, guilt, anger, lack of support, fears of contagion, loss of health and functioning, and death, families and interpersonal relationships undergo severe stress (Septimus & Weiner, 1990). Diagnosis may have unmasked secrets that may resurface after the parents or family have reestablished some stability. For example, one woman learned that she and her son had contracted HIV from her husband, who had unknowingly infected her. She discovered his injection drug use at the same time. She was angry and resentful, and the marriage eventually dissolved.

Educating other family members about HIV and the stress it adds to familial interactions is necessary for promoting understanding and empathy among family members. Usually a crisis can be addressed by channeling the collective resources of the family toward a solution, even if only a temporary one. Unfortunately, many couples and families avoid or deny the various issues and problems HIV presents. Relationships may be restructured to allow members to function temporarily and tenuously. The level of family disorganization and dysfunction must be carefully considered before attempting to use such treatment modalities. Active drug or alcohol abusers must be evaluated for potential abuse, violence, or psychosis.

GROUPS

The extreme isolation experienced by most parents caring for an HIV-infected child make group support a useful treatment modality for this population. The fear of discovery and resulting stigma create anxiety in most parents. In group work, parents know that their situation is shared by all group members, which creates a safe environment where parents can let down their guard and share their fears, concerns, and needs (Chesler & Barbarin, 1987).

In groups, parents can share their knowledge and experience regarding child care, school, medical treatments, or emotional upheavals. Issues of anger, disbelief, strained familial relationships, and sadness or their own fears are common themes. The death of a child or parent may be a cathartic, sometimes overwhelming, experience for all group members.

Parent support groups are usually hospital based, although community service providers may also sponsor such group meetings. Not all parents desire or are able to tolerate group work and may take shelter in denial and avoidance, which are more easily sustained in isolation from others. Other parents may talk informally with similarly affected parents in waiting areas, which serves as an unstructured, yet nevertheless important, group experience. Although parents and other family members should be encouraged to participate in available groups, they should not feel forced to do so. The relationships developed within a formal or informal group can be extended into the personal lives of parents with the development of telephone support networks and child-care exchanges (Spiegel & Mayers, 1991).

CASE MANAGEMENT

Past distrust of social and government agencies creates obstacles in constructing new linkages for these families. Parents may be accustomed to the frequent demands and contacts of multiple service providers, ranging from welfare and drug treatment to child protective services and special supplemental food programs for women, infants, and children. Workers from these agencies may be perceived as demanding and uncaring, and parents may enter into relationships with the hospital or community care team with the same negative perceptions and expectations. Although additional demands will inevitably be placed on parents and families as a result of their child's (and their own) health care needs, social workers have opportunity to develop a trusting relationship with parents by assuming a case-management role.

Using the case-management approach, one social worker ideally should follow a child wherever he or she is within the hospital system (inpatient or outpatient). The hospital system may be the least familiar and most intimidating to parents. Having a reliable guide eases worry.

With his or her knowledge of resources and advocacy skills, the case manager can act as an advocate by coordinating the Byzantine world of community entitlement programs and psychosocial support services to produce tangible services such as day care, additional income, and home care, thus reducing the burden on parents and families. Such efforts with tangible outcomes build trust and confidence and encourage parents to tackle the more difficult and complex issues that may lie ahead.

DRUG AND ALCOHOL ABUSE

Many families have one or more members who are present or past abusers of drugs or alcohol. Parents who are struggling with an active addiction may need encouragement and assistance to enroll in an inpatient or outpatient rehabilitation program. A spouse of an active user of drugs or alcohol faces a higher risk of physical and/or emotional abuse (Bailey, 1969). Women and families at risk may need referral and relocation to a battered women's shelter as well as specialized counseling. Should a parent be emotionally unable to protect children at risk, child protection authorities should be notified.

CHILD PROTECTION

Child protective services can often pose troubling conflicts to the social worker and treatment team. Some parents are on the borderline between providing minimum care and neglecting their child's needs. Although medical follow-up and compliance with prescribed treatment may be in question, the medical team may lack evidence that the child is not being given prescribed medications. Acting in the child's best interest often involves the careful weighing of the parent's physical and emotional limitations posed by illness or preexisting problems. Sometimes, providing additional support and preventive services can forestall a child protection report. Whenever parental behavior borders on neglect or abuse, the concerns and options available to the worker and the parent must be discussed so collaboration on a remedial plan can occur. Regrettably, the demands on the parent are sometimes too great and cannot be overcome. When no other family resource is available to care for the child(ren), temporary or permanent foster-care placement must occur.

FOSTER CARE

Without dedicated and caring foster parents and specialized transitional facilities, many HIV-infected children would languish in hospital wards without ever receiving the attention, stimulation, and love so essential to them. Foster parents dedicated to the care of HIV-infected children are unheralded and largely invisible, except to those who care for and support them and their foster children. The overwhelming majority of foster parents are excellent caregivers who often form strong emotional attachments to the children. Many foster parents assume all the pain and anguish of a biological parent, without being accorded the same rights and privileges. Many treatment decisions, including the enrollment of their foster child in a clinical treatment trial, may not be theirs to make (Martin & Sacks, 1990). Consequently, they may require the same type of interventions as any other parent, such as help with grieving the losses caused by the illness of the child and coping with frustrations within the foster care or other human service systems.

LEGAL ISSUES

Parents may find it difficult to face planning for the future needs of their children. It is important to raise legal issues early in order to encourage them to think about a will, child custody, power of attorney, or appointing a health care proxy. The social worker should have a working knowledge of these and other basic legal services important to HIV-infected families so they can explain them in an unintimidating way. Early knowledge and planning can avert a crisis from occurring at a later point when physical, mental, or emotional impairment may preclude parents' ability to exercise good judgment in such matters.

Parents can be encouraged to investigate legal issues by framing such matters as being in the best interest of their child(ren). A well-prepared plan minimizes unnecessary disruptions and enhances the parent's sense of control. It may even preclude the need for foster care, as surrogate parents can be identified if enough time and effort are devoted to the task.

In many communities free legal services are available to HIV-infected individuals. Some services have been incorporated into hospital-based teams (Weimer, Patterson, & Johnson, 1991). Elsewhere, other legal aid services may exist or be developed with law schools or legal firms on a *pro bono* basis.

OTHER RESOURCES

Other resources available to children and families affected by HIV have been modeled after services for children with other chronic or life-threatening illnesses. For example, summer camps offer a child and family a temporary respite from everyday burdens by providing organized activities in a pleasant environment that contrasts with the inner-city neighborhoods where most families with HIV live. Camp Sunburst in Petaluma, California, has been a pioneer in providing such services, offering a camp experience not only for HIV-infected children but for parents and siblings as well. In such settings, parents and children are able to deal with the ramifications of HIV outside the hospital environment. Although the number of camps providing sessions for HIV-infected children is increasing, demand continues to exceed supply.

Organizations such as Make-A-Wish and the Starlight Foundation, among others, provide children with the opportunity to have a wish fulfilled, ranging from a trip to Disney World, going on a shopping spree, or meeting a sports or entertainment idol. Such resources allow the child and family temporarily to escape the burdens of illness.

Some areas in the country with a high prevalence of HIV have developed organizations that serve HIV-infected children specifically. New York City has two organizations that plan holiday and birthday parties; provide Christmas gifts; organize recreational activities; provide families with needed supplies, equipment, and furniture not otherwise obtainable; and train volunteers for hospitals and other institutions that serve HIV-infected children.

DEATH AND BEREAVEMENT

Avoidance and denial are perhaps the two most common defenses employed by individuals and families affected by HIV. Often, the imminence of death causes families to seek the services of social workers for the first time (Easson, 1970). At this time, significant others may ask or be told about the HIV diagnosis. Parents may need to decide if they wish their child to die at home or in the hospital as well as how aggressively they want their child to be treated if the child is suffering and death is inevitable. Planning and paying for funeral arrangements may have been postponed, and parents may need help making arrangements. Sometimes the parents' and family's needs do not become evident until after the death of the child. Many parents lose their sense of purpose, especially if they have been their child's nurse and companion throughout the illness. The parents' own sense of mortality may be acutely experienced, particularly if they are infected. Loss of a child can lead to depression, regression to drug or alcohol use, or to suicidal ideation. Therefore, it is essential that workers maintain contact with the parents after the death of the child to help them deal with the pain of their loss and to redefine their goals and purpose. Even after their child's death, the fear of stigmatization may make them reluctant to disclose the cause of their child's death to members of their extended family or the community, thus adding an additional burden to grief.

EMOTIONAL STRESS ON STAFF

The overwhelming needs of HIV-infected children and their families are an emotional minefield for psychosocial professionals. Facing the illness and eventual death of a parent and child simultaneously, while dealing with the multiple needs of other family members, can be overwhelming. After the worker connects with the family, family members' needs may multiply. Workers may feel frustrated and resentful if the family does not provide adequate care for their child by missing appointments, not complying with prescribed treatments, or engaging in behaviors that are destructive to themselves or to others.

Workers need to be attuned to the disparate characteristics of this population and be able to share their emotional responses with colleagues, either informally or within a formal staff support group. A supportive milieu is essential to the professional's stamina and effectiveness in work with HIV-infected children and families.

The rewards of helping courageous parents and children make the struggles worthwhile. Battles can be won and gains achieved in the family's war against HIV. Even in the losses, workers have the rare opportunity to witness the power of the human spirit in the face of overwhelming catastrophe.

THE FUTURE

We can be sure of only two things regarding the future of HIV-infected children and their families: (1) they will increase to 10 million children infected worldwide by the year 2000 (Press release, 1990) and (2) they will require comprehensive psychosocial care from dedicated, skilled, and compassionate providers (World Health Organization, 1991).

Despite the immensity and complexity of their needs, HIV-infected children and their families can discover hope and empowerment in the face of HIV. Positive changes can be effected in their lives. Proven practice methods developed to assist children and families affected by other chronic and terminal illnesses can be adapted to the special needs of pediatric HIV infection, which must be viewed predominantly as a family illness.

Each child and family poses a unique test to the worker. The worker may need to wade through the weaknesses of the family in order to find its strengths, then devote his or her efforts to convincing family members that they do in fact have strengths that can be built upon. Although success may be difficult to determine, one sure measure is the ability of the family and worker to find meaning, hope, and joy in lives that are compromised but not condemned by HIV.

REFERENCES

Andiman, W., Simpson, B., Olson, B., Dember, L., Silva, T., & Miller, G. (1990). Rate of transmission of human immunodeficiency virus type 1 infection from mother to child and short-term outcome of neonatal infection. *American Journal of Diseases of Children, 144,* 758–766.

Bailey, M. (1969). *Alcoholism and family casework.* New York City Affiliate, National Council on Alcoholism, New York.

Boland, M., Tasker, M., Evans, P., & Keresztes, J. (1987, Winter). Helping children with AIDS: The role of the child welfare worker. *Public Welfare, 45,* 23–29.

Centers for Disease Control. (1982). Unexplained immunodeficiency and opportunistic infections in infants: New York, New Jersey, California. *Morbidity and Mortality Weekly Report, 31,* 665–667.

Centers for Disease Control. (1984). Education and foster care of children with human T-lymphotropic virus type lympadenopathy associated virus. *Morbidity and Mortality Weekly Report, 32,* 688–691.

Centers for Disease Control. (1987). Classification system for human immunodeficiency virus (HIV) infection in children under 13 years. *Morbidity and Mortality Weekly Report, 36,* 225–230.

Centers for Disease Control. (1991). Mortality attributable to HIV infection/AIDS. *Morbidity and Mortality Weekly Report, 40,* 40–44.

Centers for Disease Control. (1991, February). *HIV/AIDS surveillance report, United States, 1981–1990.* Atlanta: Author.

Chesler, M., & Barbarin, O. (1987). Childhood cancer and the family. New York: Brunner/Mazel.

Deren, S. (1986). Children of substance abusers: A review of the literature. *Journal of Substance Abuse Treatment, 3,* 77–94.

Des Jarlais, D., & Friedman, S. (1988a). HIV infection among persons who inject illicit drugs: Problems and prospects. *Journal of Immune Deficiency Syndromes, 1,* 267–273.

Des Jarlais, D., & Friedman, S. (1988b). The psychology of preventing AIDS among intravenous drug users. *American Psychologist, 43*, 865–870.

Easson, W. (1970). *The dying child: The management of the child or adolescent who is dying.* Springfield, IL: Charles C Thomas.

Faloon, J., Eddy, J., Weiner, L., & Pizzo, P. (1989). Human immunodeficiency virus in children. *Pediatrics, 114*, 1–26.

Fullilove, R., Fullilove, M., Bowser, B., & Gross, S. (1990). Risk of sexually transmitted disease among black adolescent crack users in Oakland and San Francisco, California. *Journal of the American Medical Association, 263*, 851–855.

Grady, M. (1988, January). Helping schools to cope with AIDS. *Medical Aspects of Human Sexuality, 22*(1), 21–34.

Gutman, L., St. Claire, K., Weedy, C., Herman-Giddens, M., Lane, B., Niemeyer, J., & McKinney, R. (1991). Human immunodeficiency virus transmission by child sexual abuse. *American Journal of Diseases of Children, 145*, 137–141.

Hein, K. (1989). AIDS in adolescence: Exploring the challenge. *Journal of Adolescent Health Care, 10*(3), 10–35.

Howe, E. (1990). Societal and clinical approaches to preventing pediatric AIDS: Some ethical considerations. *AIDS and Public Policy Journal, 5*(1), 9–16.

Hutman, S. (1990). The current status of pediatric AIDS: Diagnosis, treatment, prevention and research. *AIDS Patient Care, 4*(4), 7–11.

Koocher, G., & O'Malley, J. (1981). *The Damocles syndrome.* New York: McGraw-Hill.

Koop, C. (1990). Foreword. In P. Pizzo & C. Wilfert (Eds.), *Pediatric AIDS: The challenge of HIV infection in infants, children and adolescents.* Baltimore: Williams and Wilkins.

Lewert, G. (1988). Children and AIDS. *Social Casework, 69*, 348–354.

Lewert, G. (1990a). Psychosocial needs of HIV-infected children and their families. *Pediatric AIDS and HIV Infection: Fetus to Adolescent, 1*(6), 141–144.

Lewert, G. (1990b, February). *Uncharted territory: Meeting the needs of the HIV infected preadolescent and their families* (abstract). Sixth Annual National Pediatric AIDS Conference, Washington, DC.

Marte, C., & Anastos, K. (1990, Spring). Women—the missing persons in the AIDS epidemic. *Health/PAC Bulletin*, 11–19.

Martin, J., & Sacks, H. (1990). Do HIV infected children in foster care have access to clinical trials of new treatments. *AIDS and Public Policy Journal, 5*(1), 3–8.

McCue, K. (1980). Preparing children for medical procedures. In J. Kellerman (Ed.), *Psychological aspects of childhood cancer.* Springfield, IL: Charles C Thomas.

Mitchell, J., & Heagarty, M. (1990). Special considerations for minorities. In P. Pizzo & C. Wilfert (Eds.), *Pediatric AIDS: The challenge of HIV infection in infants, children and adolescents.* Baltimore: Williams and Wilkins.

Navarro, M. (1991, March 28). Children with a secret (spelled AIDS). *New York Times*, p. A1.

Novello, A., & Wise, P. (1990). Public policy issues. In P. Pizzo & C. Wilfert (Eds.), *Pediatric AIDS: The challenge of HIV infection in infants, children and adolescents.* Baltimore: Williams and Wilkins.

Oxtoby, M. (1990). Perinatally acquired HIV infection. In P. Pizzo & C. Wilfert (Eds.), *Pediatric AIDS: The challenge of HIV infection in infants, children and adolescents.* Baltimore: Williams and Wilkins.

Press release. (1990, September 25). World Health Organization, Geneva, Switzerland.

Rogers, M. (1987). *Transmission of human immunodeficiency virus infection in the United States: Report of the Surgeon General's workshop on children with HIV infection and their families.* Washington, DC: U.S. Government Printing Office.

Septimus, A. (1989). Psychosocial aspects of caring for families of infants infected with human immunodeficiency virus. *Seminars in Perinatalogy, 13*(1), 49–54.

Septimus, A., & Weiner, L. (1990). Psychosocial considerations and support for the child and family. In P. Pizzo & C. Wilfert (Eds.), *Pediatric AIDS: The challenge of HIV infection in* *infants, children and adolescents*. Baltimore: Williams and Wilkins.

Spiegel, L., & Mayers, A. (1991). Psychosocial aspects of AIDS in children and adolescents. *Childhood AIDS, Pediatric Clinics of North America, 38*(1), 153–167.

Weimer, D., Patterson, J., & Johnson, J. (1991, February). *Legal services for pediatric AIDS patients and their families* (abstract). Sixth Annual National Pediatric AIDS Conference. Washington, DC.

Woodard, C. (1990, September 15). Parents threaten to picket AIDS boy's school. *New York Newsday*, p. 3.

Wooley, H., & Stein, A. (1989). Imparting the diagnosis of life threatening illness in children. *British Medical Journal, 298*, 1623–1626.

World Health Organization. (1991, May). *In point of fact. Global program on AIDS* (Report no. 74). Geneva, Switzerland: Author.

12

ADOLESCENTS, HIV, AND AIDS

JULIA N. PENNBRIDGE, MARVIN BELZER, ARLENE SCHNEIR, AND RICHARD G. MACKENZIE

We should not be surprised to learn that HIV infection is spreading through the adolescent population. Although HIV was once considered to be a disease of gay white men and injection drug users, it is now recognized that HIV can infect anyone whose behaviors expose him or her to it. In October 1986, Surgeon General C. Everett Koop stated, "Adolescents and preadolescents are those whose behavior we wish to especially influence because of their vulnerability when they are exploring their sexuality (heterosexual and homosexual) and perhaps experimenting with drugs" (U.S. Department of Health and Human Services, 1986, p. 4). This "call to arms" led to substantial federal, state, and local dollars being spent on prevention education for adolescents. Although preventive interventions are appropriate, concern regarding adolescents must extend beyond prevention to include both treatment and care. Although relatively few adolescents have AIDS, we must not downplay both present and future impact of the disease. AIDS is now the seventh leading cause of death in adolescents 15 to 24 years old (Novello, 1988).

In response to the growing concern about HIV infection among adolescents, the Division of Adolescent Medicine at Childrens Hospital Los Angeles established its Risk Reduction Program in 1989. The Risk Reduction Program provides comprehensive outpatient and inpatient medical care, health education, case management, and psychosocial services to HIV-infected adolescents; these same services, along with HIV-antibody testing and medical assessment, are provided to youth at risk. Since the program began, we have identified and served 40 HIV-positive youth and many more youth at risk. Characteristics of the HIV-positive population receiving services have changed since the program began. Initially, our patients were predominantly lower-risk young people whose serostatus had been identified through various mandatory testing programs (amnesty, military, and Job Corps). At present, as we had originally anticipated, our patients' risk profiles more closely resemble those of infected adults. This chapter is based on the experiences we have gained providing services to these young people.

Experience has shown that we can better understand and provide better care for HIV-positive young people when we view them as adolescents first and HIV-infected individuals second. Consequently, after setting the stage by discussing the epidemiology of HIV among adolescents and young adults, adolescent development, followed by the impact of HIV infection on adolescent development, will be discussed. Although normal adolescent development must be the context for service delivery, HIV-positive adolescents manifest their issues in even more idiosyncratic ways. They require services that acknowledge that they are individuals with a life-threatening disease. Finally, assessment, initial interventions, and longer-term intervention are discussed.

EPIDEMIOLOGY

Sexual exploration is a normal part of adolescent development and the proportions of sexually active teens have gradually increased during the 1970s and 1980s (Hofferth, Kahn, & Baldwin, 1987; U.S. Department of Health and Human Services, 1988). Survey data indicate that approximately 60% of male teens (Sonenstein, Pleck, & Ku, 1989) and 50% of female teens initiate intercourse by age 19 (Zelnik & Kantner, 1980). An even higher proportion of never-married metropolitan youth— 86% of the males and 78% of the females—have experienced intercourse by age 19 (U.S. Department of Health and Human Services, 1988). Although sexual activity among teenagers is increasing, the proportion of youth regularly using condoms (which reduces transmission of HIV) remains low (15%–31%) (Keller, Bartlett, Schleifer, Johnson, Pinner, & Delaney, 1991; Hingson, Strunin, Berlin, & Heeren, 1990; Zelnik & Kantner, 1980). High rates of teenage pregnancy and dramatic increases in sexually transmitted diseases (STDs) also indicate the prevalence of unprotected intercourse (Shafer, Irwin, & Sweet, 1982).

Adolescent experimentation with drugs also fosters the spread of HIV. Although it is not known how many adolescents share needles, it is known that adolescents are using classes of drugs that are commonly injected. Many adolescents drink alcohol, smoke marijuana, and snort cocaine (Johnston, 1991). Although not directly transmitting HIV, these substances impair judgment and increase the likelihood of unprotected intercourse.

Normal adolescent development can include sexual exploration and drug experimentation, but we have no definite data on how these behaviors have affected the spread of HIV among adolescents. However, two sources of data on the epidemiology of HIV in teens are available: (1) the Centers for Disease Control (CDC) numbers on reported AIDS cases and (2) seroprevalence studies conducted on subpopulations of adolescents.

REPORTED AIDS CASES

As of April 31, 1991, 670 cases of AIDS among 13- to 19-year-olds had been reported to the CDC. This figure represented 0.4% of all AIDS cases reported to that agency. Also by April 31, 1991, 34,334 cases of AIDS among 20- to 29-year-olds had been reported, which represented 20% of all reported AIDS cases. Because the natural progression of HIV to AIDS takes approximately 10 years (Rutherford et al., 1990), one can assume that most of these 20- to 29-year-olds became infected during their adolescence. In 1987, the male-to-female ratio of AIDS in adolescents was 5:1. By February 1991 it had reached 3:1, whereas the adult ratio at this time was 8.5:1. These ratios indicate that HIV is disproportionately infecting adolescent women. Minority adolescents are also disproportionately represented, with African Americans accounting for 36% and Hispanics 18% of all reported AIDS cases in adolescents, although these populations make up only 14% and 8%, respectively, of the U.S. adolescent population.

Patterns of HIV transmission are changing and will continue to change. Between November 1989 and October 1990, the largest group of adolescents with AIDS were those with hemophilia or coagulation disorders (31%). Other modes of transmission were as follows: 18% through male homosexual/bisexual contact, 10% through injection drug use, 23% through heterosexual contact, 7% through receiving blood transfusions, and 12% undetermined. Because the blood supply became much safer in 1985, the incidence of AIDS cases is expected to drop among patients with coagulation disorders and those receiving blood transfusions during the next decade. However, the number of AIDS cases due to other modes of transmission is likely to increase. Indeed, for the year ending October 1989, 12% of reported AIDS cases were attributed to heterosexual contact. By October 1990, this percentage had increased to 23%. Thus heterosexual contact will become the leading cause of new AIDS cases in adolescents.

Seroprevalence Studies

Whereas the reported AIDS cases reflect the patterns of infection from the previous 5 to 15 years, they do not accurately indicate who is currently HIV infected. Accurate assessment of the prevalence of HIV among adolescents would require a random survey of the entire U.S. adolescent population. Obviously, this is not possible. Estimates can be made only from seroprevalence studies of specific adolescent subpopulations.

Between October 1985 and March 1989, more than one million people younger than 20 years old were tested for HIV antibodies when they applied to enter the military (Kelley, Miller, Pomerantz, Wann, Brundage, & Burke, 1990). In this large sample, 35 individuals out of every 100,000 tested positive (prevalence .35 per 1,000). The prevalence among females was .32 per 1,000. Higher prevalences were found based on geography and ethnicity. Urban teens in Maryland, Texas, New York, and the District of Columbia showed a prevalence rate greater than 2 per 1,000 (Burke et al., 1990). The prevalence among African American youth was 1.06 per 1,000, among Hispanic youth .31 per 1,000, and among white youth .18 per 1,000. These rates probably underestimate the true prevalence among these groups because males engaging in homosexual behaviors and injection drug users are discouraged from applying to the military.

Several other adolescent seroprevalence studies have been conducted (Burke et al., 1990; Kelley et al., 1990; Shalwitz, Goulart, Dunnigan, & Flannery, 1990; Stricof, Novick, & Kennedy, 1990) that capture particularly well the complexities in the epidemiology of HIV and AIDS in adolescents. The three subpopulations considered are youth seeking services from STD clinics, Job Corps applicants, and runaway and homeless youth.

Between 1988 and 1989, specimens sent to the CDC from STD clinics around the nation showed a median rate of infection to be 13 per 1,000 in males and 6 per 1,000 in females in youth between 15 and 24 years of age. The ranges of these rates (0 to 46 per 1,000 in adolescents 15 to 19 years old and 0 to 304 per 1,000 in young adults 20 to 24 years old) suggest the complexity of this situation even more powerfully (Wendall, Onorato, Allen, McCray, & Sweeney, 1990).

The Job Corps, a federally funded training program for disadvantaged out-of-school youth, tested 137,209 16- to 21-year-olds between 1987 and 1990. The seroprevalence rate was 3.7 per 1,000 for males and 3.2 per 1,000 for females (St. Louis, Conway, Haymen, Miller, Peterson, & Dondero, 1991). Testing showed a gradual increase in seroprevalance by age (8.9 per 1,000 21-year-olds were infected). Minority youth were disproportionately infected, with a seroprevalence of 5.3 per 1,000 among African Americans, 2.6 per 1,000 among Hispanics, and 1.2 per 1,000 among whites. Geographically, the northeast and southeast had the highest rates of infection, with a seroprevalence rate of 11 per 1,000 in Washington, D.C., 9 per 1,000 in Florida, and 8.2 per 1,000 in New York, compared with 2.9 per 1,000 in California.

Runaway and homeless youth often engage in high-risk behaviors simply to survive. It is hardly surprising, therefore, that a study of this population in New York revealed a seroprevalence of 53 per 1,000 among 16- to 20-year-olds. The male-to-female ratio among this group was 1.42:1 (Stricof, Kennedy, Nattell, Weisfuse, & Novick, 1991). Other studies have identified relatively high seroprevalence rates among homeless-youth populations. These higher rates have been linked to histories of injection drug use, male homosexual behaviors, crack use, prostitution, and histories of STDs (Rotheram-Borus et al., in press; Stricof et al., 1990).

Clearly, seroprevalence rates among adolescents vary widely. Currently, the highest rates are found in the northeast and southeast areas of the nation, with urban African Americans and Hispanics disproportionately affected. Nevertheless, young people visiting STD clinics, runaway and homeless youth, and poor youth are also at high risk. Given this overview and the difficulty of assigning specific risk to specific groups, all adolescents, including female adolescents, must be considered at risk for contracting HIV.

ADOLESCENT DEVELOPMENT

Adolescents infected with HIV face an array of issues that are compounded and confounded by the adolescent development process itself. Adolescent development is dynamic, often unpredictable, and idiosyncratic. Each adolescent follows his or her own course, each phase of which involves distinct attitudes and behaviors. It is useful to conceptualize adolescence in three phases: early (ages 12–14), middle (ages 15–17), and late (ages 18–21) (Neinstein, 1990).

During the early phase, adolescents may experience wide mood swings. They lose interest in family activities and develop intense relationships with same-sex friends. They become preoccupied with themselves and their changing bodies and also uncertain about their appearance. They need more privacy and want to make their own decisions, yet cannot always make appropriate decisions.

During the middle phase, adolescents identify most strongly with their peers and conflicts with parents peak. They begin to accept their bodies, seek to make themselves more attractive, and increase their sexual activity and experimentation. Increased intellectual and emotional abilities parallel feelings of omnipotence and increased risk-taking behaviors.

Late adolescence usually brings a reacceptance of parental values as the peer group becomes less important. Pubertal changes are accepted and more time is spent in intimate relationships. With a clearer sense of their individuality, young people during late adolescence refine their moral, religious, and sexual values and become more able to compromise and to set personal limits.

This tri-phase view of adolescent development is commonly used by adolescent medicine practitioners (see Neinstein, 1990; Mehr, 1981). In the following sections, adolescent development is referred to in general terms. It is constructive to consider adolescent behavior in terms of several distinct tasks that must be completed during this life phase as well as to consider the completion of these tasks within several constraints imposed by biological, social, and economic factors. The primary tasks of adolescence include the following: (1) to develop and define a sexual identity, (2) to become an autonomous individual, and (3) to formulate a plan for the future. Factors constraining the completion of these tasks include cognitive development (concrete vs. abstract thinking) and the myth of invulnerability, low self-esteem, depression, the importance of peers, and family dysfunction.

Sexual identity. The hormonal and physiological changes during puberty force adolescents to confront their sexuality. They may be confused about their sexual orientation and become isolated and depressed if they perceive themselves to be different from their peers and may engage in considerable sexual experimentation in an effort to be like and liked by their peers. The development of a close peer group is very important to adolescents, who will frequently risk the anger of parents in order to gain the acceptance of peers. During this sexual-experimentation phase, the "myth of invulnerability" can have particularly negative consequences (Hernandez & Smith, 1990; McCleary, 1988). Professionals working with adolescents (and adults too) confront this myth each time they hear the words "I'll be all right; it won't happen to me." Adolescents may feel impervious to harm and ignore the potentially negative consequences of their behaviors. Teens will admit that they do not use condoms, while believing that an STD "can't happen to me." This belief may remain inviolate even after they have contracted gonorrhea or syphilis.

173

Adolescents who see themselves as different, who do not easily develop a close and supportive peer group, can become isolated and depressed, and their self-esteem may plummet. Even those who identify with a peer group have periods of feeling unaccepted; their self-esteem, too, may drop precipitously. In either case, to negotiate successfully the task of defining their sexual identities, adolescents need role models, a positive self-image, and a supportive and loving family.

Separation/individuation. This adolescent task requires that the established bonds between adolescents and their families be broken and restructured. Even when these bonds exist and are healthy, the process can be turbulent and painful for both adolescents and their families. If the bonds do not exist or are unhealthy, the process becomes more difficult and painful for the adolescent. The need to be like friends and to be accepted by them can become desperate and lead to experimentation with sex and drugs. Sexual activity and drug use, then, can symbolize the rejection of parental values and reinforce the adolescent's sense of self as a distinct individual. During the process of individuation, the importance of family and adults decreases. Adolescents may see themselves in opposition to adults and thus discount or not listen to what adults say. They may believe that adults are not experts on how to be adolescents, that adults have *de facto* "sold out." Many adolescents believe that only other adolescents can really understand them and be trusted.

Future planning. This adolescent task comes to the fore in late adolescence when, beginning to see themselves as separate individuals, adolescents must decide how they want to live as adults. Family circumstances impinge directly upon this task by defining opportunities and shaping expectations. The process of career planning requires a future orientation and the willingness to think through the consequences of specific actions. Youth who have experienced racism, sexism, and poverty or who have serious psychological or drug-use problems may be pessimistic about their future opportunities. The obstacles to their success can be too overwhelming for them to be willing to risk planning for the future.

THE IMPACT OF HIV INFECTION ON ADOLESCENT DEVELOPMENT

An HIV-positive diagnosis for adolescents can thwart their attempts to complete the tasks of adolescence. Infected adolescents see themselves as different from other adolescents and may be less inclined to consider their future. The developmental barriers experienced by HIV-positive adolescents vary with their developmental phase. In addition to the developmental phase of the adolescent, three other factors should be considered: service-provider expectations, family issues, and societal response to the diagnosis. Service providers and the families of HIV-positive adolescents must appreciate the unique processes of adolescence if they are to provide effective service and support. Societal factors must be considered because the marginal status of adolescents within the larger society presents special legal and service-access issues for those treating HIV-positive teens.

ADOLESCENT PHASES

It is interesting to consider HIV infection in terms of the early, middle, and late phases of adolescence. Currently, HIV-positive 12- to 14-year-olds are most likely to have been infected through blood products. Generally, those in early adolescence who confront life-threatening illnesses regress both cognitively and emotionally. Common behavioral manifestations of this regression include school failure, fighting with peers, and conflicts with authority figures. Thus, the whole family may require support and anticipatory guidance. Service providers will face additional challenges if children who acquired HIV perinatally survive to adolescence.

Experience suggests that teens 15 to 17 years of age have more difficulty accepting an HIV-positive diagnosis than do older teens. Adolescents in the middle phase are more likely to run away from home or a shelter and to discontinue their medical treatment. They find it extremely difficult to come to terms with their diagnosis and to change risky behaviors. For example, a 15-year-old male who was infected through injection drug use ran away from home and residential placements many times. He terminated and reinstituted medical treatment at least three different times. His girl friend knew he was HIV positive; however, despite personal contacts with a social worker, the young woman was unwilling to come in for testing. The patient has been very resistant to discussing safer sex practices and reports that he and his partner neither talk about nor plan their sexual encounters.

Older adolescents appear to accept more easily their HIV-positive diagnosis than do adolescents in the middle phase and often seek out testing for themselves. Even if their living situation is unstable, they are more likely to comply with treatment and are more willing to discuss and to try to change their risk behaviors. For example, a 19-year-old male who was homeless, a drug abuser, and involved in prostitution when he was tested got a job, found an apartment, and stopped using drugs. He reported being able to discuss his HIV status with potential sex partners and claimed to be practicing safer sex.

INDIVIDUAL CHARACTERISTICS

Sexual identity. At a time when they are recognizing and beginning to explore sexuality, HIV-positive adolescents are told not to engage in some sexual behaviors and to make all sexual activity safer. Some young people view their diagnosis as a punishment for premarital or homosexual activity, and many adolescents respond initially to their diagnosis by claiming that they will never have sex again. This statement, however, may merely be a predictor of how honestly they will report sexual activity rather than a measure of their future sexual behavior.

The adoption of safer sexual practices is difficult for all HIV-positive people. However, the HIV-positive adolescent experiences additional barriers to safer sexual activity. Teenagers generally do not plan their sexual encounters. Moreover, the HIV-positive adolescent must overcome lack of access to condoms, inability to discuss condom use with his or her partners, embarrassment, and so forth.

The adolescent myth of invulnerability is not shattered by an HIV diagnosis. Adolescents who know that they are HIV positive and who have been educated about the effects of the disease may still deny the possibility that they will ever become ill with an HIV-related illness. Similarly, they may not believe that they will pass the virus to their sexual or drug-using partners. Such denial, though a powerful coping mechanism in some cases, can interfere with adolescents' willingness to undergo necessary medical treatment and diminish their motivation to engage in safer behaviors. The fact that many of their peers engage in the same high-risk behaviors supports their denial.

Some young people react to an HIV-positive diagnosis by becoming depressed or anxious, which can lead to various acting-out behaviors. For example, a 16-year-old girl responded to her diagnosis by having unprotected sex with several young people, both males and females. Her behavior culminated in hospitalization for acute herpes infection. A 19-year-old male became extremely depressed after learning of his serostatus. He constantly thought about suicide and at one point planned to drive his car off a cliff.

Separation/individuation. Although HIV-positive youth wish to depend on their peers, their diagnosis may deprive them of close peer relationships and thus compound the problems of individuation. As they seek to separate from parents, they may be rejected by friends who learn of their HIV status or they may withdraw from peer groups because they are concerned about potential responses of their friends. Thus, isolation and depression are common among HIV-positive youth. The eventual development of AIDS symptoms in the adolescent can have overwhelming psychological sequelae. When their fantasy of invulnerability is broken, severe depression and suicidal thoughts are often evident.

Future planning. Adults often report that an HIV diagnosis has forced them to alter their career goals and reprioritize their future plans. Adolescents, many of whom have a fatalistic approach to life, may delay formulating goals or may decide not to plan for the future. Healthy adolescents with HIV should be encouraged to pursue goals, including job training or college. Physically stressful careers might be inadvisable for those with symptomatic illness, but if the adolescent is healthy he or she has no reason to avoid exercise and hard work. Such decisions, however, should be made in light of information about the adolescent's long-term prognosis.

Service-Provider Expectations

Sometimes service providers expect HIV-positive adolescents to exhibit adult behavior with regard to compliance with appointments, medical regimens, and treatment plans. Human service professionals need to recognize that HIV infection, by inhibiting adolescents' ability to complete the tasks of adolescence, may make these adult behaviors particularly difficult. Understanding the potential impact of HIV on the individual adolescent can help the professional develop a realistic care plan. Specifically, service providers must lower their expectations for consistent and responsible behavior, be flexible with times and places for appointments, and avoid punitive, sarcastic, or parental responses to aggravating adolescent behaviors.

Although the impact of HIV on adolescent psychosocial development varies among individuals, clearly HIV makes successful completion of adolescent tasks much more difficult. It is important to recognize, however, that the primary crisis for HIV-positive adolescents is their adolescent development, not their HIV infection.

FAMILIAL ISSUES

For many families, an HIV-positive diagnosis presents the first evidence of a teenager's sexual activity or sexual orientation, which can complicate the adolescent's struggle to separate and individuate. Some families respond by infantilizing and overprotecting the adolescent. Other families disown and reject their child, particularly if members cannot accept the risk behavior that led to infection. Although this scenario forces emancipation from the family, the adolescent is denied the opportunity to separate in a healthy way. Yet other families deny the infection and are unavailable to help the adolescent cope with the diagnosis. In such cases, the adolescent suffers extreme isolation.

SOCIETAL FACTORS

The legal and ethical issues confronted by professionals serving HIV-positive youth are extremely complicated. Although legislative solutions vary from state to state, all states have had to struggle with these issues. Positions on consent and confidentiality have been uniformly difficult to define and to resolve (English, 1987). Can adolescents consent to HIV testing? Can parents or guardians force adolescents to be tested for HIV against their will? Can adolescents receive treatment for HIV without parental consent? What about experimental treatments? Must parents be notified about positive HIV test results? The issues are complex, and all service providers must be educated about their legal responsibilities as delineated by their community and state governments.

In the United States, few services are available to identify and treat HIV-positive adolescents and to provide information about the progression of the disease in this population. Programs created for adults often are not appropriate for adolescents. Most of our testing and treatment sites do not provide specialized care for youth.

SIMILARITIES BETWEEN HIV-INFECTED ADOLESCENTS AND ADULTS

Although HIV-positive adolescents have a distinct epidemiological profile, special developmental characteristics, complex legal and ethical issues, and singular service-delivery problems, several similarities between HIV-positive adolescents and adults exist. Clinically, adolescents with AIDS are more similar to adults than to children (Gayle & D'Angelo, 1991). They develop the same opportunistic diseases, conditions, and cancers. The disease progresses a little more slowly in adolescents with hemophilia, but it is not known whether this is significant. Geographically, high seroprevalence rates among adolescents follow that of adults, primarily because adolescents are frequently infected by older individuals.

Currently, the pattern of HIV infection among adolescents is more similar to HIV patterns among minority populations than it is among gay white males (U.S. Department of Health and Human Services, 1989). Infected adolescents tend to be poor, urban, minority youth. Because they are poor and disenfranchised, services must provide basic necessities such as food, shelter, free condoms, sterile needles, and medications as well as counseling. Among both adult and adolescent populations, the mentally ill require a broad range of sensitively delivered services.

INTERVENTIONS

The philosophy underlying a particular program may be clearly articulated or may simply be stated as "the way we do things here." When working with HIV-positive adolescents, a clearly articulated intervention philosophy is needed. At Childrens Hospital Los Angeles, the intervention philosophy comprises two basic beliefs: (1) the adolescent requires and must receive services designed for his or her life phase and (2) these services must be comprehensive. Because adolescence is a complex physiological, psychological, and social developmental stage, physicians cannot simply focus on the disease, but must be cognizant of and sensitive to the context of adolescent development.

Such interventions require a multidisciplinary team that includes physicians, psychologists, health educators, and social workers. If such a team approach is not practical, service providers still must understand that adolescents require a broad range of services, from multiple pre- and posttest counseling sessions to inpatient medical care and treatment. With a team approach, adolescents hear the same message repeatedly and have a number of people with whom they might "connect." Relationships need to be open, accepting, and trusting. Having various adults providing services maximizes the possibility that the adolescent will remain in the service system. To this end, service providers need to maintain close professional ties with one another to ensure the best possible care for the HIV-infected adolescent.

Providing care for adolescents is quite complex because as a group they are so diverse. Developmentally, adolescents may think in childlike, concrete ways or they may be capable of more abstract thought. They may live at home, within the child-protective-service system, or on the streets. Psychologically, they may manifest severe mental illness, including suicidal ideation and psychoses. Socially, they present with different sexual orientations and with different degrees of dependency on various substances. Medically, they present problems from venereal warts to *Pneumocystis carinii* pneumonia.

The first wave of adolescents with HIV were those with hemophilia or who had received blood transfusions. The second wave, by all indications, will be those who exhibit high-risk activity and therefore have complex histories and behavioral profiles: polydrug users, substance abusers, homeless youth, and those involved in prostitution. Regardless of how ordinary or complex their profile, however, all adolescents need to be provided care and support in an empathetic, nonjudgmental manner. In addition to receiving a medical assessment, HIV-positive adolescents should be assessed for their social, psychological, and risk-reduction counseling needs.

Psychosocial Needs Assessment

Service providers to adolescents should be trained to conduct an in-depth psychosocial needs assessment. At Childrens Hospital Los Angeles, we use an interview called HEADSS, which stands for home, education/employment, activities/affect, drugs, sex, and suicide, to structure our assessment. This format allows the service provider to work from the least to most intrusive subject. A good psychosocial assessment will provide important information about the young person's family history, risk behavior, support system, and psychological health (see Goldenring & Cohen, 1988). Regardless of the psychosocial assessment format, special attention must be focused on drug history, sexual history, and depression/suicidal ideation.

Questions about drug use must be asked directly, and service providers need to be well versed in the predominant drugs in their community. How questions are asked is important. If the professional merely asks, "Do you use drugs?" teens are likely to provide a socially acceptable response by denying or diminishing their drug use. If the question is phrased, "Some of the young people we see use drugs; do you?" the young person is given a context for his or her own drug use and understands that the professional wants honest information. Specific information about the types and quantities of drugs used (including alcohol and cigarettes) and the dates of most recent use must also be ascertained. If injection drug use is identified, service providers should determine whether sterile needles are being used.

Similarly, a detailed sexual history must be obtained by using direct questions and explicit language. Questions about survival sex (sex for drugs, money, a place to sleep) and recreational sex may need to be asked. The sexual orientation of the adolescent may be inconsistent with his or her sexual behavior. The professional might ask, "Do you have sex with men, women, or both?" This question is effective because it focuses only on behavior.

Service providers need to feel comfortable using sexual language familiar to the adolescent. Often, professionals use sexual jargon that is meaningless to the young person. It may be necessary to discuss butt fucking instead of anal sex, blow jobs instead of oral sex, and so forth. Information about the frequency of condom use and possible drug use associated with sexual activity are important parts of the assessment process and can indicate how difficult safer sex behaviors are likely to be for the young person.

Depression and anxiety are common among adolescents in general. Such problems are often indicated by sleep disturbances, appetite changes, changes in libido, feelings of sadness and hopelessness, and dysphoric mood. In HIV-positive adolescents, depression or anxiety may not have originated over HIV issues but over social conditions (isolation, homelessness, drug abuse) that led to the high-risk activities associated with HIV transmission. The social conditions and their antecedents (such as a dysfunctional family, child abuse, family substance abuse) have considerable repercussions on the kinds of interventions that will be effective.

Suicidal history and assessment are also essential. After a measure of rapport has been established, most young people are willing to discuss ideas and plans they may have or have had for killing themselves. In that suicidal thoughts and ideation are common and recurrent in some teens, service providers working with HIV-positive adolescents must be especially sensitive to this issue and skilled at conducting suicidal assessments. Adolescents should be provided with a list of emergency phone numbers or hotlines through which they can access suicide prevention services.

Although these subject areas should be discussed during the first and second encounters with the adolescent, a psychosocial assessment is an ongoing process. Often, adolescents do not reveal important information until they begin to trust their service provider. Thus reassessment and clarification of drug-use behaviors, sexual activity, and depression/suicide are critical for establishing an effective therapeutic relationship.

INITIAL INTERVENTION

Basic needs. Initial interventions should focus on the needs and desires of the adolescent. If the professional tells adolescents what they need, rather than responding to the needs they identify, it is difficult to establish a trusting relationship. For homeless youth, initial needs usually comprise basic necessities such as food, shelter, and clothing. Service providers must have a complete list of and good working relationships with emergency shelters in their community. They must also know the names and locations of agencies that provide free food and clothing. Providing practical information such as the times and routes of buses to these locations or distributing bus tokens increases the likelihood that the adolescent will return for additional services.

Professionals need to help adolescents living at home to decide if, when, and how to tell their family that they are HIV positive. Often, families of HIV-positive adolescents are not involved in their child's care. Adolescents should be encouraged to confide in parents or guardians if these adults are supportive. In our experience, teens are usually the best judge of whether their parents will be supportive when informed of their HIV infection. For adolescents who do not want to inform their parents, at least one reliable, supportive adult in whom the adolescent can confide should be identified.

Suicidal ideation. Suicidal adolescents need immediate attention and evaluation. The assessment must determine whether the young person has a suicide plan, how detailed that plan is, and whether the adolescent will contract not to hurt him- or herself. Psychiatric help and hospitalization may be required. In such cases, it is critical that the service provider remain in contact with the adolescent in an effort to develop a sense of trust and to diminish the adolescent's feelings of isolation and abandonment.

A 19-year-old male who became suicidal after receiving his HIV-positive diagnosis visited the clinic two weeks after receiving his diagnosis from a testing center. During his first visit, he said that he did not plan to tell his family. He had no local social support system and was thinking about killing himself. Initial interventions included several different components. The service providers developed a written contract with him in which he agreed not to hurt himself and to telephone if he felt he was going to hurt himself. Weekly appointments with a physician and social worker were scheduled for the next several weeks and an appointment for psychological assessment and counseling was made. His acute depression and suicidal ideation receded over the ensuing weeks, although his problems with depression continued.

Medical care. For service providers who are not part of a medical program, making appropriate medical referrals is an essential part of the initial intervention. Although the primary care physician should be familiar with HIV infection, expertise is not mandatory. It is better that the adolescent be connected with a physician experienced in treating adolescents and who is familiar with adolescent issues. Pediatricians, family practitioners, or internists can provide appropriate care because complex HIV-related medical problems rarely occur during the initial stages of HIV infection. When more complex medical issues do occur, the primary care physician can arrange for consultation with specialists.

LONG-TERM INTERVENTIONS

Emotional support. Obviously, HIV-positive adolescents need long-term emotional support. Frequently, HIV-infected adolescents have no support networks. Offering support through extensive case management helps bond the youth to the caregiver and increases compliance in taking medications and reducing high-risk behaviors. Case managers must attempt to expand adolescents' support systems by connecting them to other agencies and getting them involved in support groups. Often, it is difficult to maintain consistent group participation, primarily because of the diversity of needs and transience of this population. Although support groups can be helpful to the receptive adolescent, service providers should also focus on individualized plans for developing support systems.

Generally, older youth are better able to find and develop support systems than are younger adolescents. This is particularly true for older-adolescent gay males, for whom community support systems already exist. Younger males and females remain more isolated because existing support systems are neither appropriate for nor acceptable to them. In addition, developmental issues—the need to separate from parents and the importance of peer acceptance—make it even more difficult for those in middle adolescence to establish support systems. Young female adolescents need considerable help in locating services that deal specifically with their issues. The HIV-positive female experiences considerable stigma. One young woman who had not disclosed her status to family or friends became transformed when she met another HIV-positive female in a support group. The cultivation of support systems for these young people is a slow and challenging process.

Substance abuse. Although injection drug use and smoking crack cocaine are risk factors for contracting HIV (Fullilove, 1989), adolescents also commonly abuse alcohol, marijuana, and other drugs. Use of these other drugs may impair judgment and thus increase the likelihood of high-risk behaviors. Drug-abuse counseling is imperative if other social problems are to be addressed. These social problems include reducing involvement in prostitution, increasing condom use, and maximizing the use of support services. Extended inpatient detoxification and treatment may be necessary but often are not available to adolescents without health insurance. This is particularly frustrating for service providers who know that without such programs these young people will remain in high-risk social situations.

Many substance-abusing youth use drugs to self-medicate. Drugs ameliorate, in the short term, depression, anxiety, and emotional pain. Drugs also enable many young people to engage more easily in survival sex. Service providers should realize that drugs will not be abandoned until the underlying problems are addressed.

In some cases, regardless of service-provider effort, young people will not give up drugs until they are ready. For example, a 17-year-old substance-abusing male resisted subtle and overt attempts to provide psychosocial help or drug treatment and would accept only medical care. Quite unexpectedly, during a medical visit two years later, this young man asked his doctor if he would give him a referral to a substance-abuse treatment program. Having decided he wanted this treatment, this young man sees his drug-abuse counselor regularly. Thus, although service providers must encourage drug treatment, they should understand that excessive pressure can alienate the adolescent.

Psychological needs. The psychological state of the adolescent must be monitored constantly. The primary caregiver—social worker or physician—should be trained in crisis-intervention techniques and have experience with dysfunctional families. Professionals must be watchful for the need for additional psychological counseling or psychiatric medication and make referrals when necessary. Depression in HIV-positive adolescents may be manifested in various behaviors: withdrawal, acting out, increased drug use, increased sexual activity, or noncompliance with treatment. Service providers must be alert to the possibility that complaints of headaches, abdominal pain, fatigue, and weight loss may be somatic manifestations of depression.

Sexual orientation. Younger adolescents often have difficulty with sexual identification and can struggle with homosexual issues. Homosexual support groups sponsored by community organizations can be helpful. Positive role models for homosexual adolescents can help youth establish healthier life-styles.

Issues surrounding sexual orientation can be even more difficult for minority youth. One 19-year-old Asian male was suicidal, depressed, and isolated for almost two years. During this time, he enrolled in many self-help groups but never invested himself in any of them. Eventually, he told his social worker that if he wanted to feel better, he knew that he had to come to terms with being both Asian and gay.

Risk-reduction counseling. All HIV-positive adolescents need education and counseling on reducing the risk of HIV transmission to others. Service providers must educate the adolescents, their families, and caregivers that HIV cannot be transmitted through casual contact. Information about how HIV is transmitted should be repeated. Fallacies that oral sex is safe and that men cannot get HIV from women must be dispelled. Adolescents should be shown how to use a condom on an imitation erect penis and shown how to clean their drug paraphernalia with bleach and water.

Numerous studies have shown that HIV education for uninfected adolescents does little to change their high-risk behaviors. Studies of the impact of education on behavior change in HIV-infected adults have also been disappointing (Becker & Joseph, 1988). Although no formal studies of high-risk behavior in HIV-infected adolescents have been conducted, our experience suggests that many of these youth continue to engage in unprotected intercourse despite the knowledge that doing so could transmit the virus. Adolescents report that they do not use condoms because they are afraid that their partners will know they are infected with HIV and thus abandon them. Role playing situations can help adolescents develop safer-sex practices. Although it is hoped that young people will change their behaviors to protect others, they are more likely to change their behaviors to protect themselves. Consequently, adolescents can be told that some researchers think that STDs are both more painful and more difficult to treat in people who are HIV infected. They should also be warned that repeated infection with HIV or STDs may hasten the progression of their illness.

Pregnancy. Many adolescent women with HIV express considerable concern about their ability to become pregnant and to have healthy babies. Current statistics in the United States indicate that 25%–30% of the babies born to HIV-positive mothers will themselves be HIV positive (Oxtoby, 1990). European studies indicate that the transmission rate may be closer to 13% (European Collaborative Study, 1991). Despite the risk of having an HIV-infected infant or of that child becoming an orphan, many female adolescents have a strong desire to experience motherhood. Although such attitudes may frustrate caregivers, the decision to become pregnant lies ultimately with the individual. Judgmental counseling will only alienate the young woman from services for herself and her child.

Confidentiality and disclosure. Confidentiality and disclosure issues permeate intervention with all HIV-infected individuals. Like adults, adolescents are extremely concerned about the confidentiality of their HIV status. Service providers must understand the laws of the state in which they work. In California, competent teens between 12 and 17 years of age may consent for their own HIV testing and treatment. The law guarantees them confidentiality with respect to their HIV status, which may be shared with persons outside the medical team only with the individual's written permission. Thus, an adolescent's HIV status cannot be given to parents, legal guardians, child protective service workers, or other social service providers without the adolescent's permission. Physicians can inform the adolescent's sexual and needle-sharing partners that they have been exposed to HIV, but this disclosure must not include the infected adolescent's name. These are California laws. Human service professionals must familiarize themselves with the laws in their states.

Disclosure is an extremely difficult issue for HIV-positive adolescents. Adolescents should be encouraged to identify at least one adult in whom they can confide. Such efforts help the young person identify people whom he or she trusts and from whom he or she can obtain support. The costs and benefits of disclosing to each of these individuals should be explored. For example, the service provider might ask: Does this person need to know your serostatus? Do you think this person will maintain confidentiality? Will this person be there for you when you need him or her? Although help with disclosure can be offered, in our experience youth typically make the disclosure on their own.

Disclosure to sexual partners or potential partners is an extremely difficult task for adolescents. They expect total rejection, and often their worst fears are realized. Service providers can offer to be present during the disclosure discussions. This helps some adolescents, especially when they must disclose to partners who are themselves at risk for having HIV and who thus need testing. Although youth typically disclose on their own, they often bring their partners to the clinic for education and/or testing.

One of the most stressful issues for a care provider is knowing that a client is endangering another person's life through unprotected sexual intercourse or needle sharing. Again, the care provider must be aware of his or her state's partner-notification laws. The adolescent's physician or the local public health department may be able to help the care provider find information about the appropriate state laws or assist him or her in notifying partners.

Service providers must constantly be aware of inadvertently disclosing the HIV status of infected young people. One teenager who did not want his parents to know that he was HIV positive was confronted by them after they received medical bills from the hospital. After discussions with the hospital's accounting department, the billing procedures for patients in the hospital's HIV risk-reduction clinic were changed.

Another disclosure problem occurs with adolescents who want to tell everyone their HIV status. Several teenagers have met with prejudice, ridicule, or isolation as a result of excessive disclosure. They have been extremely hurt at a time when they were least able to cope. Consequently, potential problems of disclosure to employers, casual friends, or new people in their lives should be discussed at length. In this way, adolescents are able to make more measured and rational decisions about whom they should confide in and when they should do it.

CONCLUSIONS

Service providers tend to focus on HIV issues in infected adolescents, while adolescents are most concerned about the stresses of growing up. Parents frequently have difficulty dealing with their child's homosexuality, sexuality, or drug use. Family problems regarding individuation are especially difficult when parents become overprotective upon learning about their child's diagnosis. Educational and employment choices are difficult when adolescents are unsure about how long they may live.

The HIV-positive adolescent, like all adolescents and people in general, needs love, affection, and good relationships with his or her peers. An HIV diagnosis can damage an adolescent's already fragile self-esteem. Service providers must supply frank and appropriate information, provide supportive counseling, and encourage healthy and responsible relationships and behaviors. It is only within the context of responsible relationships that these young people can resolve the tasks and issues of adolescence and competently and sensibly confront their lives as HIV-positive adults.

REFERENCES

Becker, M. H., & Joseph, J. G. (1988). Aids and behavioral change to reduce risk: A review. *American Journal of Public Health, 78,* 394–410.

Burke, D. S., Brundage, J. F., Goldenbaum, M., Gardner, L. I., Peterson, M., Visintine, R., & Redfield, R. (1990). Human immunodeficiency virus infections in teenagers: Seroprevalence among applicants of U.S. military service. The Walter Reed Retrovirus Research Group. *Journal of the American Medical Association, 263,* 2074–2077.

English, A. (1987). Adolescents and AIDS: Legal and ethical questions multiply. *Youth Law News, 7*(6), 1–6.

European Collaborative Study. (1991). Children born to women with HIV infection: Natural history and risk transmission. *Lancet, 333,* 253–260.

Fullilove, R. (1989, July 3). Crack cocaine use and risk for AIDS among black adolescents. *CDC AIDS Weekly,* p. 7.

Gayle, H. D., & D'Angelo, L. J. (1991). Epidemiology of acquired immodeficiency syndrome and human immunodeficiency virus infection in adolescents. *Pediatric Infectious Disease Journal, 10,* 322–328.

Goldenring, J. M., & Cohen, E. (1988, July). Getting into adolescent heads. *Contemporary Pediatrics,* 75–90.

Hernandez, J. T., & Smith, F. J. (1990). Inconsistencies and misperceptions putting college students at risk of HIV infection. *Journal of Adolescent Health Care, 11,* 295–297.

Hingson, R. W., Strunin, L., Berlin, B. M., & Heeren, T. (1990). Beliefs about AIDS, use of alcohol and drugs, and unprotected sex among Massachusetts adolescents. *American Journal of Public Health, 80,* 295–299.

Hofferth, S. L., Kahn, J. R., & Baldwin, W. (1987). Premarital sexual activity among U.S. teenage women over the past three decades. *Family Planning Perspectives, 19,* 46–53.

Johnston, L., (1991, January 23). University of Michigan News Release. Ann Arbor, MI.

Keller, S. E., Bartlett, J. A., Schleifer, S. T., Johnson, R. L., Pinner, E., & Delaney, B. (1991). HIV-related sexual behaviors among a healthy inner-city adolescent population in an endemic area of HIV. *Journal of Adolescent Health, 12,* 44–48.

Kelley, P. W., Miller, R. N., Pomerantz, R., Wann, R., Brundage, J. F., & Burke, D. S. (1990). Human immunodeficiency virus seropositivity among members of the active duty U.S. Army 1985–1989. *American Journal of Public Health, 80,* 405–410.

McCleary, K. (1988, February). Students believe they won't get AIDS. *National College Newspaper,* p. 4U.

Mehr, M. (1981). The psychosocial and psychosexual unfolding of adolescents. *Seminars in Family Medicine, 2*(3), 155–161.

Neinstein, L. A. (1990). *Adolescent health care: A practical guide* (2nd ed.). Baltimore, MD: Urban and Schwarzenberg.

Novello, A. (1988, November 18). *Final report: Secretary's work group on pediatric HIV infection and disease.* Department of Health and Human Services (pp. 17–20). Washington, DC: U.S. Government Printing Office.

Oxtoby, M. (1990). Perinatally acquired human immunodeficiency virus infection. *Pediatrics Infectious Disease Journal, 9,* 609–619.

Rotheram-Borus, M., Meyer-Bahlburg, H. F. L., Koopman, C., Rosaio, M., Exner, T. M., Henderson, R., Matthieu, M., & Gruen, R. S. (in press). Lifetime sexual behaviors among runaway males and females. *Journal of Sex Research.*

Rutherford, G. W., Lifson, A. R., Hessor, M. A., Darrow, W. M., O'Mally, P. M., Buchbinder, S. P., Barnhart, J. L., Budecker, T. W., Cannon, L., Doll, L. S., Holmberg, S. D., Harrison, J. S., Rogers, M. F., Werdegar, D., & Jaffe, H. W. (1990). Course of HIV-1 infection in a cohort of homosexual and bisexual men: An 11-year follow-up study. *British Medical Journal, 100,* 1183–1188.

Shafer, M. A., Irwin C. E., & Sweet, R. C. (1982). Acute salpingitis in the adolescent female. *Journal of Pediatrics, 100,* 339–350.

Shalwitz, J., Goulart, M., Dunnigan, K., & Flannery, D. (1990, June 20–23). *Prevalence of sexually transmitted disease (STD) and HIV in a homeless youth medical clinic in San Francisco.* Paper presented at the Sixth International Conference on AIDS, San Francisco.

Sonenstein, F. L., Pleck, J. H., & Ku, L. C. (1989). Sexual activity, condom use and AIDS awareness among adolescent males. *Family Planning Perspectives, 21,* 152–157.

St. Louis, M. E., Conway, G. A., Haymen, C. R., Miller, C., Peterson, L. R., & Dondero, T. J. (1991). Human immunodeficiency virus infection in disadvantaged adolescents: Findings from the U.S. Job Corps. *Journal of the American Medical Association, 266,* 2387–2391.

Stricof, R. L., Kennedy, J. T., Nattell, T. C., Weisfuse, I. B., & Novick, L. F. (1991). HIV seroprevalence in a facility for runaway and homeless adolescents. *American Journal of Public Health, 81*(Supplement), 50–53.

Stricof, R. L., Novick, L. F., & Kennedy, J. T. (1990, June 20–23). *HIV-1 seroprevalence in facilities for runaways and homeless adolescents in four states (FL, TX, LA, NY).* Paper presented at the Sixth International Conference on AIDS, San Francisco.

U.S. Department of Health and Human Services. (1986). *Surgeon General's report on Acquired Immune Deficiency Syndrome* (mailed to every household in the USA).

U.S. Department of Health and Human Services. (1988). *National survey of family growth.* Hyattsville, MD: National Center for Health Statistics.

U.S. Department of Health and Human Services, Centers for Disease Control. (1989). AIDS and human immunodeficiency virus infection in the United States: 1988 Update. *Morbidity and Mortality Weekly Report, 38*(supplement 4), 1–38.

Wendall, D., Onorato, I., Allen, D., McCray, E., & Sweeney, P. (1990, June). *HIV seroprevalence among adolescents and young adults in selected clinical settings, U.S. 1988–90* (abstract). Sixth International Conference on AIDS, San Francisco.

Zelnik, M., & Kantner, J. F. (1980). Sexual activity, contraceptive use and pregnancy among metropolitan-area teenagers: 1971–1979. *Family Planning Perspectives, 12,* 230–237.

13

AIDS AND THE HOMELESS: HIV PREVENTION AND CARE

VALERIE HARRAGIN

Aids and homelessness are two of the gravest problems of our day. This chapter discusses how these two issues relate to each other, the populations affected by these problems, and the services they are and are not receiving. The role of human service workers, both in direct service and administration, is discussed.

AIDS and homelessness—as separate issues—have been treated with greater depth and comprehensiveness than they are here. The material presented in this chapter is not intended to serve as a comprehensive discussion of either issue, but rather as a discussion of issues at the point where these two major social problems intersect. First, the population affected by AIDS and homelessness will be discussed. Second, AIDS prevention and care for this population will be dealt with from the perspective of the human service provider. Finally, the future treatment needs of this population, together with the goals of the human service professions, will be discussed.

An inherent difficulty in writing on this subject is that the homeless population is not a single identifiable entity. As housing becomes more expensive and public benefit programs provide less, more people, who fall into poverty for widely varying reasons, become homeless. Therefore, HIV-infected homeless persons include minority women and children, drug addicts, undocumented immigrants, and many others who have fallen through the holes of the so-called "safety net." This population also includes persons who have become homeless subsequent to and as a result of their illness.

SCOPE OF THE PROBLEM

Van Souder, Smith, and Altman (1986) found that one year after diagnosis, 50% of injection drug users and 31% of gay men who were not injection drug users were homeless. Froner (1988) discusses the "complex of factors leading to homelessness for people with AIDS," stating that AIDS is a "chronic illness that can decimate a person's savings as surely as it does their immune system" (p. 198). Complicating the housing issue further, many housing programs for people with AIDS are reluctant to take people with substance abuse or psychiatric problems, thus eliminating many homeless persons from these programs.

AIDS has also become a serious problem among runaway and throwaway youth (Hersch, 1988). These young people, lacking other means of support, may engage in sex in exchange for food, money, drugs, or shelter. In addition, children who have histories of sexual and physical abuse may lack the self-esteem to insist on safer sex even when they are aware of the risks.

Many homeless women who test positive for HIV trade sex for money or drugs. Despite widespread fear of HIV transmission by prostitutes, women who have sex with men for drugs or money are unlikely to infect them. In fact, these women are much more likely to become infected themselves (King, 1990).

It is widely believed that blacks and Hispanics, who make up a disproportionate number of the homeless, will be increasingly affected by AIDS in the future. For example, the ethnic breakdown of patients who visit the Weingart Clinic, located in a poverty-stricken area of Los Angeles, is approximately 60% black, 20% Hispanic, 15% white, and 5% "other," including Asian, American Indian, and others (John Wesley Community Health Institute, 1989).

One way to analyze HIV-infected homeless persons is to consider them as two distinct populations according to which condition—HIV or homelessness—came first. Several years ago, an article in *Newsweek* (Baker, Joseph, Harrison, Cerio, Gordon, & Hutchinson, 1988) presented two profiles, each typical of one of these populations. The first profile provided a portrait of a long-time heroin addict who lived in abandoned buildings and discovered that he had contracted HIV after entering a drug rehabilitation program. The second profile showed a man who had worked for a large corporation in Houston and was fired after telling his boss he had been diagnosed with AIDS. He subsequently lost his apartment. Social work services, beginning with prevention efforts, need to deal with these two groups differently.

Getting people with HIV infection off the streets is a difficult task. Attention must be focused on providing appropriate housing for this population. Sanders (1990) writes movingly about living with AIDS on the south side of London, where the unsuitability of the housing further complicates an untenable situation.

TASKS AND ROLES OF THE SERVICE PROVIDER

AIDS-PREVENTION EDUCATION

A major problem in providing AIDS education to homeless persons is that it is difficult to find them. For example, when the Surgeon General released the pamphlet "America Responds to AIDS," it was distributed through the mail system. Those without an address were unlikely to receive one. The homeless are also unlikely to see public service announcements on television. Most of the AIDS-prevention education for the homeless occurs through outreach efforts on the street.

Although such efforts can be effective, it takes a long time to establish credibility on the street and only a few people are reached. It is a slow and costly method for dealing with a crisis issue for which funding is tight.

Sprawling cities such as Los Angeles make street outreach very difficult. Fortunately, this geographical factor has slowed the spread of the disease among injection drug users. In fact, researchers estimate that more than one-half of New York City's injection drug users are HIV positive, whereas in Los Angeles County the rate among injection drug users is believed to be less than 5% (Scott, 1990). In 1988 the Centers for Disease Control reported that 19% of adult AIDS cases in the United States were heterosexual injection drug users; in Los Angeles County this same group made up only 3% of the AIDS cases (Smith, 1988). Although any number of variables may explain these differences, dispersion of injection drug users over a wide geographic area may be a central factor.

At the Weingart Center in Los Angeles, the HIV seroprevalence rate for the homeless is 5%. Although this percentage is significantly higher than that for the general population in Los Angeles or in other American cities, it is far lower than that for the homeless populations of Eastern cities, where injection drug use is more widespread and where large shooting galleries are more common, thus increasing the likelihood of needle sharing. In Los Angeles, even with the high rate of substance abuse among the homeless, sexual activity remains the most common form of transmission.

A study of AIDS patients living in shelters and on the street in Boston identified injection drug use as a major risk factor in 95% of cases (Avery & O'Connell, 1989). Researchers systematically collected used syringes from shooting galleries in Miami, Florida, and found that 10% of the needles contained HIV antibodies (Des Jarlais & Friedman, 1990). Hence, HIV transmission among the homeless varies considerably across the nation.

Bureaucratic and political posturing can sometimes create obstacles for AIDS prevention. For example, before 1991 Los Angeles County banned the distribution of bleach (to sterilize contaminated needles) and condoms. The Homeless Outreach Project, which conducts AIDS education with homeless injection drug users in the Los Angeles skid row area, was able to maneuver around this ban because the project is funded by the City of Los Angeles rather than the county. Thus programs are sometimes faced with the additional burden of finding ways to deliver services despite political and bureaucratic barriers.

The complex relationship between sexual identity and sexual behavior presents an additional difficulty in getting the prevention message out to the homeless. Many black and Latino men do not consider themselves to be gay or bisexual, despite having had sexual experiences with other men. Such encounters may have occurred in prison or as a result of drug use or survival on the streets. Some men believe that the partner who is penetrated anally is gay, whereas the other partner is straight. Because these men do not perceive themselves as gay, they may feel that they are not at risk of contracting HIV and thus ignore the literature, posters, classes,

189

or other educational material aimed at gay and bisexual men. Thus, it is important that prevention materials use wording such as "men who have sex with other men" as opposed to "gay" and "bisexual men." Many men, when offered the HIV antibody test, protest that they aren't gay, despite admitting to having had sex with other men.

To be effective, prevention efforts must take into account the literacy skills of those to whom educational materials are directed. Many of the homeless have little formal education, learning disabilities, a long history of drug and alcohol abuse, which in turn has affected their cognitive processes, or other barriers to their ability to assimilate written information. Obviously, materials need to be made available in languages other than English.

SECONDARY PREVENTION

Testing. Testing, commonly thought to be an important tool in secondary prevention, presents complex issues for the homeless, as it does with many other groups. According to Avery and O'Connell (1989),

> HIV testing has failed to be an effective tool in changing behavior patterns in this particular population. Persons without homes, suffering from powerful addictions to heroin or cocaine, find little reason to give up drugs when told of an imminently fatal disease. . . . Many have continued to share needles despite thorough knowledge of the virus and its transmission. [Thus] testing must be accompanied by the availability of a stable living situation such as an apartment or a long-term therapeutic community (p. 2).

This rather negative view of the efficacy of testing as a secondary tool of prevention may not be quite so applicable to populations for whom sexual transmission is the primary risk factor, even when drug addiction may be a secondary risk. At the Weingart Center, many patients who test positive for HIV are willing to learn about and practice safer sex techniques to avoid infecting others. It seems reasonable to assume that addictive behaviors are far more difficult to extinguish or modify, whereas sexual behaviors, such as use of condoms, appear to be more easily altered. Behavioral change is difficult to assess because patients may not be honest about their sexual activity. However, many homeless persons do return to request additional condoms, which suggests that they use them when they are made readily available.

Street and shelter outreach. Having a health educator provide prevention education in shelters and missions in the evenings can be effective. A health educator in the skid row area of Los Angeles presents a one-hour class at several missions and single-room occupancy hotels. He gives out condoms as well as written and oral information and provides snacks to help boost attendance. Pre- and posttesting at these classes indicate that participants are learning about the modes of transmission, but it is difficult to assess whether changes in behavior follow. The distressingly weak link between knowledge and behavioral change, however, is certainly not unique to the homeless. Smith (1988) points out that the "mini-epidemic of syphilis in Los Angeles indicates that 'safer sex' advice is not being taken" (p. 3).

190

HIV PREVENTION AMONG THE HOMELESS

Often, when we think of HIV prevention in this context, we think of preventing the spread of HIV among the homeless. Equally important, however, is the prevention of homelessness among those who have HIV. Delays in public benefits, ostracism by family and friends, and workplace and rental discrimination put individuals and families affected by HIV at risk of homelessness. As with the disease itself, prevention is far more effective than is dealing with the problem after homelessness has occurred.

Froner (1988) cites loss of employment capability, loss of savings, and inability to gain access to public assistance as major factors leading to homelessness for people infected with HIV. The legal issues of employment discrimination, even if resolved, will not prevent all AIDS-related job loss. As AIDS affects more and more low-income minority persons, the problem often becomes one of jobs that do not carry health and disability insurance. Sometimes employees may not be aware of their rights and may voluntarily quit their jobs, believing that they are eligible for Supplemental Security Income (SSI) because of seropositivity, when, in fact, an AIDS diagnosis is usually required before benefits are made available.

Traditional case management is not the most sensible approach with homeless clients, primarily because this population is so difficult to reach. In a program sponsored by the John Wesley Community Health Institute, we are developing a case-management style of service coordination. In some ways, this approach is a concession to the difficulties inherent in providing comprehensive services to the homeless. The approach involves providing short-term, narrowly focused attention with the goal of connecting the individual to medical care and public benefits. It is the casework equivalent of triage.

In successful cases, clients are out of our purview in a few months or even weeks. However, in some cases, lack of continuity keeps clients from moving through the program's first few steps. For example, a client may initiate services, then not show up for the next appointment. Or the client may have to reapply for SSI because the forms were sent to an address where the client no longer goes for mail and are returned to Social Security, prompting them to close the case.

Ironically, those clients who are perhaps least able to follow through for themselves are those who most often have to. Because we cannot reach them, we must depend on them returning to the agency without benefit of a reminder by mail or telephone. This dilemma, coupled with preexisting conditions such as AIDS dementia, mental illness, or drug addiction, makes it extremely difficult to provide advocacy and follow-up services to the homeless.

In cases in which the person has no symptoms of HIV or only mild symptoms, services are generally the same as for the general homeless population, with the exception of support groups provided for HIV-positive asymptomatic persons. However, homeless clients often do not perceive great value in these support groups because they are more concerned about immediate survival needs such as obtaining food and shelter. Scheduling and transportation difficulties may outweigh the perceived worth of participating in a group. The services that this population is most interested in and most in need of are instrumental services such as food and money. However, often these are not available to them without an AIDS or ARC diagnosis.

In Los Angeles, a person without health insurance or funds to pay for medical care may wait four to five months before being seen at a county clinic. Even though this person may be highly symptomatic of HIV disease and very ill, without an official diagnosis the person cannot begin to receive or even apply for SSI, obtain special housing for people with AIDS, or receive other benefits. The connection between tuberculosis and HIV infection is of particular concern for the homeless, in that they are much more likely to be exposed to tuberculosis and in fact have a much higher rate of tuberculosis than does the general population (Fackelmann, 1990). The Centers for Disease Control's (1987) Division of Tuberculosis Control estimates the tuberculosis rate to be from 1.6% to 6.8% among homeless populations living in shelters, a rate 150 to 300 times higher than that of the general population.

Interestingly, the service-dependent population on skid row in Los Angeles is often frightened of sharing shelter services with HIV-infected persons. They are unaware that their risk of contracting tuberculosis is much greater. Because HIV destroys the immune system, HIV-infected persons are at a much greater risk for contracting tuberculosis through transient exposure. The large warehouse-type structures used to provide emergency shelter in many cities contribute to the spread of tuberculosis.

Diarrhea, a problem for many people with HIV infection, is particularly distressing in a shelter setting that has few bathrooms and where one may have to climb over other people in the dark in an effort to get to the bathroom in a hurry. To make matters worse, many illnesses that cause diarrhea are prevalent in shelters (Gross & Rosenberg, 1987). Froner (1988) points out that, because of their frailty, people with AIDS may be especially vulnerable to the theft of money and medications while staying in shelters.

Because the number of HIV-infected people in need of housing so vastly exceeds the housing reserved for them, appropriate (or at least tolerable) living situations must be found in existing resources. Social workers who try to find housing for individual clients are likely to utilize whatever housing is available, although it may be far from ideal for people with HIV. Some inadequacies can be addressed by agency services.

For example, in Los Angeles's skid row, some HIV-infected clients reside in single-room-occupancy hotels. They are able to obtain rides to medical appointments and to agencies through a service sponsored by AIDS Project Los Angeles. Many clients walk to the Weingart Clinic, a small county clinic providing primary health care, and the Chest Clinic, a satellite tuberculosis clinic that is also part of the Los Angeles County Health Department. In some instances, people with AIDS receive home-delivered meals, visiting nurse services, and help with household chores.

Stigmatization is one of many problems faced by homeless persons with AIDS. These persons may not feel welcome in programs that are set up to deal with the homeless population in general. People may express fear of casual transmission and become hostile toward persons with the disease. In addition, HIV-infected homeless persons may not feel accepted at AIDS service agencies, where the majority of clients as well as much of the staff are white gay males who may not be prepared for work with this population. Many of these agencies, however, are working hard to improve their responsiveness to poor and minority clients.

ISSUES FOR SOCIAL WORKERS

QUALIFICATIONS OF STAFF

As with many areas of social work, debate over the most desirable qualification for professionals who work with HIV-infected homeless populations is heated and controversial. Some feel that in order to establish trust and rapport with clients, treatment personnel should be drawn from the same population, that is, recovering drug addicts working in drug-treatment programs or gay staff to work with gay clientele. Others feel that it is crucial to look at the educational and professional backgrounds of the staff and hire on the basis of credentials rather than personal background. It seems reasonable to conclude that both professional qualifications and cultural group membership are important factors for professionals who serve these clients and that this conflict may never and perhaps need never be completely resolved.

COUNTERTRANSFERENCE

Countertransference is one of the largest, if not the largest, issues confronting persons who provide services to AIDS patients and to the terminally ill in general (Dunkel & Hatfield, 1986). This is particularly true in work with the homeless, who are often a difficult group with which to empathize and an easy group to blame for their own plight.

The homeless are multiply stigmatized by society, and social workers and other helping professionals are by no means immune from these societal judgments. Social workers who have dealt with their own homophobia may still find themselves blaming drug abusers or prostitutes or persons who have been in the penal system. Few, if any, of us, can approach this population in an entirely accepting and open way. With HIV-infected homeless persons, the fact that they are dying makes it even easier to reject them emotionally in order to avoid one's own fear of loss. Individual supervision and/or support groups need to address these countertransference issues and provide insight into the "parallel nature of the client and worker processes" (Martin & Henry-Feeney, 1989, p. 337). In addition, direct service practitioners should be involved in decisions regarding policies and allocation of resources. Such efforts will reduce feelings of powerlessness and hopelessness among practitioners.

LOCATION OF PROGRAMS

As discussed above, HIV-positive homeless persons can be divided roughly according to which condition came first, HIV infection or homelessness. The location of the program providing services is critical in this regard. Members of the "traditional" HIV-affected population, that is, white gay males, are clearly not best served by having to utilize skid-row missions and shelters before they become eligible for housing assistance. Unfortunately, in some cases, this is exactly what happens.

For example, AIDS Project Los Angeles has a contract that allows them to place persons with AIDS who are homeless in HUD-subsidized housing. The person must be homeless at the time of placement. He or she cannot merely be in danger of losing housing due to discrimination or two months behind on the rent as a result of being denied disability benefits or illegally fired from a job—the person must be homeless. Thus, these persons cannot receive urgently needed assistance until a very serious situation becomes even worse.

In contrast, "traditional" homeless populations who *become* HIV-infected may be unable or unwilling to utilize resources in areas of a city that are located far away from the missions and shelters on which they depend. They may also assume that they are unwelcome in these areas and agencies, which they perceive as predominantly white and gay.

RECOMMENDATIONS

Adequate health care can be provided and complied with only when the need for housing is met (Brickner, 1985). Without housing, it is difficult to keep wounds clean and medicines refrigerated as well as to obtain enough rest to make convalescence possible. Nearby bathrooms, elevators for the upper floors, and facilities to provide for personal hygiene are essential for persons with HIV. Because weight loss and malabsorption are problems for person with HIV, nutritional needs must be addressed.

Persons on fixed incomes, who may lack adequate cooking facilities or are too weak to cook for themselves, do not have enough money to eat all their meals in restaurants. It may also be difficult for them to get out every day. Programs such as Open Hand in San Francisco and Project Angel Food in Los Angeles deliver hot meals to homebound people with AIDS, thus serving as valuable adjunct services. People with AIDS may not always be able or inclined to cook for themselves.

Housing persons with HIV infection is very costly. What is needed is a continuum of housing available for persons who have mild or no symptoms, those who are disabled by their disease, and those who are in the late stages of illness and need extensive care.

In considering types of housing beneficial to this population, it is important to realize that HIV is a progressive disease and the needs of a newly diagnosed person will be different a few years later. Is it best to develop housing that can accommodate an individual through the progression of illness or is it preferable to provide a variety of settings based on a client's needs at a particular time?

Both options have merits as well as flaws. If a continuum of care is provided in a single facility, the patient does not have to worry about being forced to leave when he or she becomes sicker. The individual can develop more durable and perhaps trusting relationships with staff and other residents. Also, a single-facility model eliminates the worry of a person falling through cracks in the system when, for example, a person is too sick for one program and not sick enough for another. On the other hand, providing care at different levels in different facilities might be less costly, because staffing levels and medical-training needs would be reduced at agencies that serve persons who are less symptomatic. It is also much easier to set up licensing and quality-assurance requirements for more narrowly focused programs. In addition, newly diagnosed clients would have an easier time adjusting to a program that is not reminiscent of a hospital or convalescent home. It may be difficult for patients who are in the earlier stages of the disease to live with people who are dying.

Although a housing shortage for this population remains, the picture is not uniformly bleak. A few existing programs may serve as models for persons with HIV.

AIDS Project Los Angeles and the Minority AIDS Project each have a house in which a person who is symptomatic but not in need of nursing care can live for up to a year. The Shanti Foundation in San Francisco maintains several apartments for people with AIDS. These programs and others like them across the nation have waiting lists and are unable to serve anywhere near the number of people requesting services.

Catholic Charities, through the Serra Corporation, operates several houses in the greater Los Angeles area that are open to people with ARC. Persons accepted into this program are eligible to stay for the remainder of their lives so that, in effect, it becomes a hospice.

Hospices have very long waiting lists. Often, hospice care is provided in the patient's home, which means the homeless die in public hospitals.

In addition to lack of funds, those developing housing for people with AIDS face the additional problem of community fear and resistance. AIDS-oriented services that attempt to place clients in housing often confront stiff neighborhood resistance, especially in residential areas. Despite educational efforts, the fear of casual transmission is so great among some people that even the residential real estate profession is arguing about whether a seller's (or previous occupant's) HIV status should be disclosed. Realtors face the dilemma that prospective buyers may not want to purchase a home if the previous owner had AIDS, yet they must consider the right to confidentiality of the seller. They face possible lawsuits either way (Baen, 1989).

CONCLUSION

A significant gap in services exists for homeless people who are HIV positive but do not have an AIDS diagnosis. The majority of AIDS-oriented services require a diagnosis of AIDS or ARC before they will accept a client. This leaves clients who are symptomatic but not yet diagnosed having to compete with the "healthy homeless" for shelter beds, meals, and other services in agencies that may not be sensitive to their needs.

Supplemental Security Income is the mainstay of people who are unable to support themselves due to permanent disability. Understandably, these funds are not available to an individual who is HIV positive but still considered able bodied. However, a person with no resources to begin with can end up without sufficient documentation to have his or her SSI application approved, even though his or her health is severely compromised.

Many of the services targeted to the general homeless are set up to increase their independence and self-sufficiency. These are laudable goals and, in some cases, may even be appropriate for someone who is HIV positive and asymptomatic. But an individual who has not finished high school, has never had a regular job, is addicted to crack cocaine, and recently tested positive for HIV is not likely to be receptive to a program that requires him or her to do a job search.

Given the existing funding constraints, in most cases, appropriate housing for HIV-infected persons will have to be created by piecing together services from various agencies. Meals, home health care, and transportation to medical appointments are the most critical needs of HIV-infected persons who are living in housing that is not designed specifically for their needs. Persons who are in a position to develop housing for people with HIV infection need to take the clients' special needs into account, that is, working elevators, adequate restroom facilities, and sanitary living conditions.

People with AIDS who need housing far outnumber available units. Thus even those who qualify for AIDS-specific benefits and services may be unable to obtain services. These persons may find themselves on the streets or in the missions, even in the late stages of the disease. Providing quality care for homeless persons with AIDS is not simple. We must use existing resources creatively and collaboratively, while working hard to develop new alternatives.

REFERENCES

Avery, R. K., & O'Connell, J. J. (1989). *HIV and homeless persons*. Boston: Boston Health Care for the Homeless Program.

Baen, J. S. (1989, Winter). AIDS and real estate: Facing the issues. *Focus, 39*, 17–30.

Baker, J. N., Joseph, N., Harrison, J., Cerio, G., Gordon, J., & Hutchinson, S. (1988, April 4). Needing a place to die. *Newsweek*, pp. 24–25.

Brickner, P. W. (1985). *Health care of homeless people*. New York: Spring Publishing.

Des Jarlais, D. C., & Friedman, S. R. (1990). Shooting galleries and AIDS: Infection probabilities and "tough" policies. *American Journal of Public Health, 80*, 142–144.

Centers for Disease Control. (1987). Tuberculosis control among homeless populations. *Morbidity and Mortality Weekly Report, 36*, 257–260.

Dunkel, J., & Hatfield, S. (1986). Countertransference issues in working with persons with AIDS. *Social Work, 31*, 114–117.

Fackelmann, K. (1990). The double whammy of TB and AIDS. *Science News, 137*, 348.

Froner, G. (1988). AIDS and homelessness. *Journal of Psychoactive Drugs, 20*, 197–202.

Gross, T. P., & Rosenberg, M. L. (1987). Shelters for battered women and children: An underrecognized source of communicable disease transmission. *American Journal of Public Health, 77*, 1198–1201.

Hersch, P. (1988, January). Coming of age on city streets. *Psychology Today*, pp. 28–36.

John Wesley Community Health Institute. (1989). *Who are the homeless?* (Skid Row Medical Outreach Project, August 1989). Los Angeles: Author.

King, D. (1990). Prostitutes as pariah in the age of AIDS: A content analysis of women prostitutes in the New York Times and the Washington Post, September 1985–April 1988. *Women and Health, 16*(3–4), 155–176.

Martin, M. L., & Henry-Feeney, J. (1989). Clinical services to persons with AIDS: The parallel nature of the client and worker processes. *Clinical Social Work Journal, 17,* 337–349.

Sanders, C. (1990, February 16). Homesick. *New Statesman and Society,* pp. 10–11.

Scott, J. (1990, January 1). Diverse L.A. drug culture threatens AIDS outreach. *Los Angeles Times,* pp. A1, A30–31.

Smith, K. (1988). *AIDS and the homeless.* Los Angeles: The Los Angeles Homeless Health Care Project.

Van Souder, P., Smith, J. T., & Altman, S. (1986). *AIDS shelter project: Final report.* New York: Institute of Public Services Performance.

14

STRESS AND COPING IN AIDS CAREGIVERS: PARTNERS, FRIENDS, AND FAMILY MEMBERS

HELEN LAND

"When your son is dying, a part of you is dying, and you keep asking yourself, 'Where did I go wrong as a parent? Why can't I put this thing right?'"

"Sometimes I forget where he stops and I begin. I see previews of the nightmare ahead for me and no one will be there to take care of me when I need it."

"A lot was going on that I didn't want to see. As his wife, how could I have been so naive? Now both me and the children are at risk."

"I've had 15 friends die in the past few months, but other than that, everything's OK."

These are the voices of lovers and spouses, parents and siblings, the loyal friends of persons with AIDS, the diverse and highly vulnerable group of AIDS caregivers. Because the needs of those with AIDS are so profound and the illness is so unrelenting, until recently little attention has been focused on the needs of AIDS caregivers. Yet various factors demand that the needs of this group be considered. Persons with AIDS often receive care from partners, friends, and family members for extended periods, due to the prohibitive costs of institutional care. Equally important, the needs of those with AIDS are better met in community-based care than in highly bureaucratized systems of institutionalized care (Pearlin, Semple, & Turner, 1988). And most important, our attention should be directed toward AIDS caregivers for moral and ethical reasons, out of concern for their well-being.

Friends, partners, and family members substantially influence the quality of life experienced by persons with AIDS. Caregivers are involved in virtually every aspect of the illness, from providing prediagnosis care to making postmortem plans. They influence medical decision making and discharge dispositions, run the household, provide nursing care or arrange for its provision, negotiate financial and legal matters, expedite the attainment of compensatory benefits such as Supplemental Security Income (SSI), counsel the dying, and serve as liaison between the person with AIDS and his or her family, friends, and service providers. In addition to managing these tasks, caregivers must maintain their own work and family life as well as manage an often intense and emotional relationship with the person with AIDS.

Several years ago, the amount of time that caregivers devoted to care of a person with AIDS was substantially less than it is today. In the early 1980s, the average life expectancy of someone diagnosed with AIDS was counted in months. Few resources were available for in-home care; hence, the patient spent more time in the hospital. As a result of these factors, the time available to terminate the relationship between the caregiver and person with AIDS was brief. If caregivers were not biological relatives, they confronted legal obstacles when they tried to manage certain tasks for the person with AIDS. They were unable to make medical and financial decisions. After the death of the person with AIDS and concomitant with the grieving process, caregivers found themselves without the right to determine burial plans or property arrangements, even when property or personal effects were jointly owned (Levine, 1990). Many felt invalidated and violated while simultaneously dealing with their grief.

Today, although the situation is far from ideal, much has changed with respect to caregiving. Hospital legal professionals, as well as persons with AIDS and their caregivers, are often able to make legal arrangements in advance of the terminal stages of the illness. Caregivers who are not blood relatives are more frequently given power of attorney by the patient, thus protecting the caregiver's rights of access to the patient and to the decision-making process. Because of advances in medical and support treatment, a diagnosis of AIDS, although always terminal, may mean that death is still years away. In addition, home health care and home hospice care are more prevalent today. However, with these advances come prolonged stresses on caregivers, and hence the increasing demand to consider their needs.

Those who have worked with caregivers know that members of this group, frequently mislabeled as the "worried well," continue to suffer from considerable stigmatization, mental conflict, life disruption, alienation, and physical and emotional exhaustion. These symptoms do not abate easily (Maloney, 1988; Trice, 1988). But despite the difficulties faced by caregivers, many professional service providers remain relatively uninformed about this highly vulnerable group.

Working with AIDS caregivers requires that professionals understand complex problems and needs involved in the caregiving response. AIDS takes many disease forms, requiring different methods and skills of caregivers. The progression of illness requires caregivers to follow the course of disease through its various physical, emotional, and mental changes and eventually to confront the patient's death. The response to the caregiving role varies according to the type of relationship the caregiver has with the person with AIDS. The age, gender, and ethnic/racial makeup of the caregiver all affect helping behaviors. The coping skills and personality of the caregiver affect his or her ability to serve as a buffer to the chronic stress engendered in both the patient and caregiver over the course of the illness.

The following sections examine the various stressors resulting from AIDS caregiving. Beginning, middle, and ending phases of caregiving are addressed. In addition, interventions designed to increase coping and limit caregiver distress are discussed.

THE BEGINNING PHASE

The type of intervention initially selected for caregivers may vary in relation to agency parameters and the role of the service provider. Despite these variant factors, service providers must be aware that primary caregivers, regardless of their relationship with the person with AIDS, are negotiating a crisis state. Thus, caregivers, too, have legitimate and separate needs that should be met to help them manage the demanding role that they have assumed.

The assessment should take into consideration the relationship of the caregiver to the patient, current and potential difficulties in the relationship, the types of caregiver stresses that are likely to be experienced during the course of the illness, the length of time of duress, the coping patterns and defenses used to alleviate stress, the strength of the support system available to the caregiver, and the caregiver's general level of functioning. While assessing the caregiver's needs, the service provider begins to establish a relationship with the caregiver and validates the difficulty of the caregiver's role. Following assessment, a plan of supportive intervention may be established that makes use of the caregiver's coping strengths.

A confirmed diagnosis of AIDS often represents the resolution of a prolonged but undefined series of illnesses and the beginning of a new set of struggles for patient and caregiver. When caregivers are partners or close friends of the patient, the traumatic news may confirm the long-suspected existence of HIV-related illness. However, in many situations, for example, the wife of a bisexual man or injection drug user or parents who did not know about their child's sexual orientation or health risks, a diagnosis of AIDS presents trauma and shock of a different nature. Each caregiving role carries with it a different set of questions, fear-based responses, and emotional needs. Although groups vary considerably in response to an AIDs diagnosis, some common response patterns may be evident.

GAY PARTNER

The gay partner caregiver may initially experience extreme separation anxiety, fear about the future of the relationship, and fear of contagion and stigma with regard to his own health status (Macklin, 1988). He may be unable to share the news of the diagnosis with his own family, thus increasing his sense of isolation in the midst of crisis. He may be grief worn from seeing a number of close friends die a slow and agonizing death. He may want to flee from the relationship, especially if it is in the beginning phases and long-term commitment has not yet been established. If the relationship has been long term and perhaps isolated from the gay community, the partner may visualize a lonely single life for himself. Under these circumstances, suicidal ideation is relatively common (Geis & Fuller, 1986; Robinson, Skeen, & Walters, 1987) and should be evaluated.

In such situations, practitioners should validate the crisis state and the many feelings the partner may be experiencing: numbness, helplessness, fear, anger, avoidance, fatigue, loneliness. It is equally important to validate the effects of the crisis on the relationship, because, by doing so, the partner's sense of control over life is heightened and anxiety is decreased. Once these goals are accomplished, the practitioner may suggest an intervention plan that includes both medical support and sociopsychological support services such as individual counseling, conjoint couple support groups, or groups for significant others.

CLOSE FRIENDS

Similar scenarios unfold for close friends who become caregivers. In some cases, the caregiver may have formerly been the partner of the person diagnosed with AIDS. Thus, the relationship may be well established, and relationship issues, although not "couple-centered," may be quite complex. Caregiver friends of both men and women with AIDS typically voice considerable commitment to the patient: "If he didn't have me, he would have no one else to take care of him," or "There but for the grace of God go I." Their sense of loyalty to the relationship is often quite profound and should be recognized and commended. Caregivers who are friends of the patient should be routinely questioned about the degree of support they receive from others and whether they have experienced multiple losses and bereavements as a result of AIDS. This group is often worn down by grief and caregiving responsibilities and may require intervention on a number of levels: acknowledgment of and praise for their caregiving, help in the bereavement process, and supportive services for their ongoing caregiver role.

SPOUSE OF A BISEXUAL MAN OR INJECTION DRUG USER

If the caregiver is the wife of a bisexual man or injection drug user, the caregiver may learn of the AIDS diagnosis at the same time she learns about her spouse's bisexual involvement or drug use. In such situations, shock (Rowe, Plum, & Crossman, 1988) and fear of loss of the relationship are accompanied by anger. Anger may first be directed at the husband for the deceit: "How dare he lie to me all this time?" Next, anger may be directed at the person with AIDS for placing the spouse's health at risk: "How could he do this to me?" Finally, the anger may be directed at herself for being blind to the situation: "I'm a fool for not seeing this coming; I guess you don't see what you don't want to see."

In some situations, the wife may have been cognizant of her husband's high-risk behaviors and she may have tried to maintain a peaceful coexistence within the marital relationship. Or she may define her husband's drug use as something that she was unable to curtail. Few family supports may be available (Greif & Porembski, 1987). Under such circumstances, the resulting dynamics upon receiving the news of an AIDS diagnosis may differ widely. Although elements of shock and disbelief are present, such feelings may be accompanied by grief and anger at having failed to make the relationship work. Finally, the spouse may experience anger and fear about her own health status. Sometimes the wife may withdraw and try to deny her anger, thus inhibiting emotional intimacy in the relationship (Maloney, 1988).

Under these circumstances, the practitioner should attempt to help the person sort out her contradictory feelings. This process may include working through or managing her anger; beginning to understand her grief, of which anger may be a part; and alleviating her sense of failure, shame, and self-blame. Because secrecy and self-isolation often occur in this population (Kelly & Sykes, 1989), joining a support group with other female caregivers in it may prove helpful. Groups often provide a sense of universality, cohesion, and a lifeline to better functioning.

PARENTS

The experience of parents who learn that their adult child has AIDS is different from those of the caregivers discussed above. In the flood of emotions expressed, parents may blame the child for contracting the illness: "I told him to take better care of himself, but he wouldn't listen." Or they may assume responsibility for their adult child's condition by blaming themselves for faulty parenting (Robinson et al., 1987). In their attempt to control an uncontrollable situation, they may blame hospital personnel for poor medical care. Alternatively, they may fear contagion and refuse to let their adult child or his or her partner visit with other family members (Frierson, Lippmann, & Johnson, 1987; Geis & Fuller, 1986).

Research indicates that ethnic-minority parents may experience particular distress because, despite their strong commitment to their child, they receive fewer supports in their communities and their children are more likely to be blamed for engaging in high-risk behaviors (Levine, 1990; Morales, 1990). Parents may blame partners and friends of their children for transmitting the disease or may condemn whole communities, such as the gay population, or ethnic groups, such as Haitians or Africans. They may rage at the federal government for inadequate funding of AIDS services and medical research. In their unbridled anxiety, parents may obsess about what to tell family members, friends, and neighbors about their child, fearing isolation and rejection (Rowe et al., 1988). Many parents become "hidden grievers" (Murphy & Perry, 1988). Because their anxiety and anger are so extreme and diffuse (Kelly & Sykes, 1989; Macklin, 1988), some parents may be unable to deal with the reality of their child's terminal illness.

The degree to which parents are able to accept their child and the diagnosis of AIDS varies enormously. Some parents may have a close and intimate relationship with their adult child and be capable of supportive care, both emotionally and physically (Cleveland, Walters, Skeen, & Robinson, 1988). However, other parents may have been unaware of their adult child's sexual orientation or high-risk behavioral patterns (Haller, 1985). In such situations, parents must confront the loss of the old identity of their adult child as well as of their child's health and future (Frierson et al., 1987). Carl (1986) has referred to this experience as the "double-death syndrome." Often, it is quite difficult to reintegrate the ill adult child into the aging family system. Physically, such care can be draining for parents who may not be in prime physical health themselves. Moreover, the psychological devastation of nursing a dying child can often result in high-risk status for aging parents (Allers, 1990).

Practitioners can help parent caregivers, whose responses are framed within a developmental, life-cycle perspective, gain insights into their situation and responses. Children are not supposed to die before their parents (Turner & Pearlin, 1989);

under the stress of caregiving, it is not unusual for parents to infantilize their adult children and for adult children to regress (Frierson et al., 1987). The parent may view the child as an extension of the parental self that will now be lost. Because the parent sees the extreme vulnerability of the dying child, a blaming, angry response may be used to protect the parent and the child. Moreover, long-standing family conflicts often emerge (Allers & Katrin, 1988).

In such situations, practitioners should slowly share these psychodevelopmental insights with parents in a manner that initially frames the parental responses as a normal part of the grieving process. If hostile responses do not subside, but rather interfere with the physical and emotional well-being of the adult child and his or her other support systems, practitioners should help the parent caregiver to examine the function of his or her responses and to refocus on more productive coping methods. For example, the clinician might suggest that feelings of anger may be easier to deal with than is pain of grief, loss of self associated with the impending loss of a child, or shock that an adult child has an identity that deviates from the family norm. The clinician might later suggest that new priorities may need to be set in the parent-child relationship, given the pressing needs of the crisis. Such work helps parents recast the conflict and to understand the vital supportive role they can play in the months ahead.

SIBLINGS

Siblings who are caregivers face dilemmas common to those faced by friends and parents. These caregivers, frequently the sisters of persons with AIDS, may assume a parental role in caregiving, yet find themselves placed in the role of friend and confidant. For older patients with elderly parents, siblings may serve as replacements for parents who are unable to assume care (Shanas, 1979). Siblings may have been geographically and emotionally separated from each other, which makes it difficult to heal emotional wounds that occurred during youth and that may resurface at this time (Turner & Pearlin, 1989). In addition, several siblings may have to coordinate caregiving among themselves, resulting in caregiving that is more difficult to manage and less stable over time (Johnson & Catalano, 1983). Service providers can provide siblings with emotional support and help them solve practical problems regarding the care situation. For example, home-based hospice care may provide some respite from a complex caregiving schedule. In addition, brief, problem-focused family therapy may help resolve family conflicts. Although some problems and/or conflicts may be impossible to ameliorate, given the level of family conflict and the complexity of the health crisis, clarifying how family conflicts interact with health crises helps siblings to gain insight into their own and the patient's behavior and to feel more in control over a seemingly chaotic situation.

CARING FOR WOMEN WITH AIDS

Caregiving for women with AIDS presents a very different scenario. First, a woman may have children who are seropositive or symptomatic who require the care of the patient herself. Thus, the woman is both caregiver and patient (Macklin,

1988). Second, few potential caregivers may be available, or response from them may be minimal, especially if the patient is unmarried. Caregivers may be unavailable for various reasons. Women with AIDS experience a different kind of stigma: they may be judged by potential family caregivers as being sexually promiscuous and/or as being irresponsible mothers and wives. They may be rejected because of their IV drug use. Many women with AIDS feel as though they are an invisible minority. Although considerable stigma exists for anyone with AIDS, women with AIDS are especially vulnerable to prejudice. Many women say, "My parents just don't and won't understand what I'm going through." Although some women may turn to their families, many turn to other women friends or to institutionalized care such as home health or hospice care.

CAREGIVER–PATIENT RELATIONSHIP

In summary, although each caregiver's individual situation and relationship with the person with AIDS in the beginning phase affect the response of the caregiver, many caregiver responses are universal. Diagnosis of a terminal illness in a young person is always traumatic, and anticipatory grieving patterns are seen throughout the course of the illness, beginning with disabling shock (Rowe et al., 1988). Following the shock and fear associated with the initial diagnosis, denial often occurs, helping the caregiver maintain sufficient strength to invest in the caregiving role (Lovejoy, 1990). In the beginning phase, service providers should identify, support, and encourage anticipatory grieving and coping methods of the caregiver.

How the caregiver manages his or her life following the initial stage of diagnosis depends on his or her combination of personality resources and patterns of health behavior, factors often rooted in family patterns and ethnic traditions. For example, some caregivers may use active cognitive coping methods to reduce stress. They may consider alternatives for handling problem situations, telling themselves that others have it worse or that they need to take life one day at a time. Or they may intellectualize, a mechanism they use to alleviate their anxiety (Lovejoy, 1990). Others may take active steps by seeking informational and educational materials about AIDS, speaking publicly on AIDS, or joining support groups (Cleveland et al., 1988; Lovejoy, 1990). Some may seek out a new philosophy that emphasizes optimistic thinking (Geis & Fuller, 1986), meditation, or other religious rituals. Because active cognitive and behavioral methods are associated with a greater sense of well-being (Moos & Billings, 1982; Lazarus & Folkman, 1984), such coping methods should be supported.

Some caregivers may attempt to cope by avoiding the situation and responsibilities, but such coping methods are usually associated with poorer outcomes. The caregiver may begin overdrinking or overeating in an effort to reduce tension or perhaps isolate him- or herself or regress into earlier patterns of relating to the person with AIDS. Emotional discharge is another common form of coping and may include projecting anger onto the persons with AIDS or onto the self (Lovejoy, 1990). Emotional responses, especially expressions of anger, are quite predictable in the process of anticipatory grieving and should be identified and validated by service providers. However, because these methods of coping tend to exacerbate an already highly stressful situation, practitioners should attempt to direct caregivers toward more productive expressions of anger and more productive strategies for coping. For example, caregivers should be helped to identify their anger as being directed at the disease rather than at the person with the disease. Some have verbalized, "Yes, I'm angry, but I'm not angry at you. I'm angry at the illness and what it's done to you, me, and us. I'm angry at society and the world."

Many caregivers seek out alternative medical treatments for the person with AIDS, such as megavitamin therapy or folk medicines such as herbs, antler powder, or teas. Some look for help from culturally indigenous healers such as *curanderos*, shamans, faith healers, priests, favored saints, or new-age philosophers. Such efforts are a sign of active coping strategies, and unless these efforts impinge on patient well-being, practitioners should avoid discouraging caregivers from seeking them out. Such efforts represent an attempt to control a situation perceived to be grossly out of control.

THE MIDDLE PHASE

The middle phase in AIDS caregiving may be short or lengthy; it may involve multiple hospitalizations and medical procedures or only a few. However, several things can be expected to occur during the middle phase: caregiving demands increase as the disease progresses; the responsibility of caregiving depletes the physical and emotional resources of even the most dedicated caregiver; social supports become fewer as the disease progresses, and, in the end, the disease wins (Geis & Fuller, 1986; Pearlin et al., 1988).

CAREGIVER ROLE STRAIN

The central experiences in the lives of AIDS caregivers during the middle phase are the daily conflicts and strains associated with the role they have assumed. Caregivers are forced to function in various capacities in relation to the person with AIDS and to the outside world. As one caregiver stated, "I'm not prepared to be a psychotherapist, priest, caseworker, mother, nurse, and lover. I'm lost in this role of providing care. I have needs, too." Eventually, the stress caused by attempting to fulfill the multiple demands of various roles depletes the caregiver's physical and emotional resources (Kelly & Sykes, 1989).

Regardless of whether service is provided for caregivers through instrumental and material support or through emotionally supportive groups, couple work, or individual counseling, practitioners should encourage caregivers to set aside time for themselves (Land & Harangody, 1990). Often, however, caregivers are reluctant to limit their time with the person with AIDS, even when their exhaustion and emotional depletion result in poorer caregiving performance. Many feel guilty about spending time away from the person with AIDS. Thus the practitioner needs to be persistent in his or her efforts to encourage the caregiver to find free time outside caregiving responsibilities.

Couples. In addition to the overload of assuming multiple roles, the caregiver also experiences role change (Pearlin, 1983). For example, during the middle phases of the illness, the romantic and sexual dimensions of a couple's relationship may change. Loss is a reverberating theme that occurs throughout the illness; each time a new loss occurs, old losses are remembered: loss of physical vitality, employment, control over life, financial security, friends, life as it was once known.

As some roles are lost, new roles, for example, increased nursing functions, are gained. The caregiving partner, as a result of assuming responsibility for negotiating services and decisions, may out of necessity assume a superior position in the relationship, perhaps upsetting established patterns and creating further stress.

Role theory suggests that the degree of stress associated with role changes is greater when the changes are out of sequence with the expected life course (Pearlin, 1983). Thus, although partners may have anticipated some role changes during later life, it is difficult for them to integrate such role changes during their young-adult years.

In addition to role change, caregivers also experience a sense of "role captivity" (Pearlin, 1983), that is, the feeling of being bound to one role or set of roles (nurse, caregiver) while wishing to play another role (spouse). To complicate the picture, the personality traits, values, and beliefs of some caregivers may not fit comfortably with the demands of the caregiving role. Such self–role incongruence can cause mental strain and diminished well-being (Smelser, 1961). Caregivers often expect themselves to have unilaterally positive feelings toward caregiving for their beloved partner. However, how they behave may not be congruent with how they feel and their self-esteem may suffer. Caregivers may project their frustrations and anger onto the person with AIDS, or they may internalize their anger and become depressed. Caregivers who struggle with role conflicts should be helped to understand and accept their limitations and feelings. Intervention may include helping caregivers locate outside help such as shopping, housekeeping, or attendant-care services. As one therapist told her client, "It would be nice if each of us played the mythic role of the all-caring Florence Nightingale, but we can't."

As the illness progresses, dependency increases while autonomy decreases in the person with AIDS. In many situations, for example, in cases of AIDS-related dementia, the caregiver is unable to relate to the patient–partner as a co-equal. The couple may be better equipped to respond to external societal pressures such as stigma than to internal relationship pressures such as dependency (Levine, 1990). When couples have contradictory expectations of roles, conflicts occur, as the following case demonstrates.

> Pedro and Jim had been a couple for four years. Soon after they celebrated their fourth anniversary, Pedro suffered an opportunistic infection and was hospitalized. As the illness progressed, Pedro began to suffer from memory loss related to neuropathy and was unable to remember if and when he had taken medication; at times he became lost in familiar surroundings, such as his own neighborhood. Jim felt that Pedro's physical safety was endangered and began to assume a more directive role in the relationship. Pedro often became angry with Jim, feeling that Jim was treating him as a child. Jim was torn between Pedro's verbal demands that Jim maintain a co-

equal partner relationship and Pedro's physical and emotional need for a more dependent relationship. In his support group, Jim often stated, "I'm unable to satisfy the conflicting expectations he has of me." In addition, Pedro expected Jim to be physically and emotionally available
at all times, whereas Jim was dealing with his anxiety about the impending loss by distancing
himself emotionally from Pedro.

In such instances, couples should be seen conjointly by the practitioner. Couples may be confused about the effects of multiple role conflicts and unaware of the
complex factors behind their overwhelming feelings of depression, depletion, and
despair. They may be unaware of the effects of their subtle messages and unspoken
demands. The practitioner should help the couple make communications explicit.
When communication is made more clear, couples can be helped to cope with their
conflicting feelings about the changing circumstances of their relationship. The practitioner can help couples work through the changes in their relationship and to contract for new behaviors. Changes may include adjusting to new roles and hierarchical
patterns, recognizing and accepting different responses to illness, accepting the partner's manner of coping with the illness, and realigning emotional boundaries.

Psychodevelopmentally rooted symptoms, such as abandonment anxiety, and
defenses, such as emotional distancing, commonly occur in couples coping with AIDS
(Macklin, 1988). However, behaviors may also be affected by family-of-origin patterns and ethnic background. When the person with AIDS and the caregiver are at
variance with regard to methods of coping with the illness, stress escalates and couple
conflict ensues (Tiblier, Walker, & Rolland, 1989). Caregivers should be encouraged
to grieve over what is lost and what has changed and to validate and value themselves
for their caregiving efforts. Despite the turmoil, some partners are able to establish a
new dimension within their relationship characterized by renewed intimacy.

Parents and siblings. When family members such as parents or siblings are
caregivers, other types of role strain are present during the middle phase. Not only
do family caregivers experience repeated losses and role overload, often they must
renegotiate family boundaries. Early research on roles demonstrated that ill-defined
role expectations resulted in lower levels of role performance (Bible & McComas,
1963) and higher levels of tension, dissatisfaction, and feelings of inadequacy
(Mason & Gross, 1955; Kahn, 1964). Families may struggle when it is unclear who
should assume the caregiving role and what responsibilities are inherent within that
role. Family power struggles may occur over decision-making, legal, and personal
obligation issues (Greif & Porembski, 1988). When the person with AIDS is gay
and has a partner, the family may find it difficult to acknowledge and accept the
couple subsystem. Research on the ambiguity of family boundaries notes the disruptive effects of ambiguous family status on family and individual functioning (Boss,
Pearce-McCall, & Greenberg, 1987; Minuchin, 1974). Such disruptions may occur
when the gay couple have not revealed their homosexual relationship to their families or when the couple are not fully accepted into the family system. Similar conflicts
occur when the caregiver is a friend of the person with AIDS. In such situations, the
boundaries of the family system become muddled, and the extended-family system

may attempt to loosen or tighten its boundaries in order to maintain integrity. Caregiver role strain and inadequate care for the person with AIDS may result from such conflicts. Strain results when family members, partners, or friends feel excluded from decision making regarding the person with AIDS (Greif & Porembski, 1988). Moreover, strain may also occur when family members are included in family subsystems in which they feel uncomfortable. For example, although the mother, sibling, partner, or friend of the person with AIDS may assume major caregiving responsibilities, the father may feel fearful or uncomfortable when he is expected to assume an active role in the caregiving process (Robinson et al., 1987). His discomfort may derive from feelings of inadequacy in performing the role in that he has not been socialized as a caregiver, or may be the result of having to acknowledge the gay-couple relationship, homosexual identity, or injection drug use of his child. As one father said,

> I felt like I could never say or do the right thing. I felt uncomfortable, so I guess even though I knew he was sick, I preferred to act like he didn't really need my help. His stepmother and sisters were there more, and his partner, Pete. But I didn't appreciate how much help he was getting from Pete, and I blamed Pete for a lot. Pete didn't speak Spanish, and we're from Ecuador, so I had a hard time with Pete, I guess. I was ashamed, for my son and for me. So I stayed away, even though he was my son, and I knew I should have been there more. Now that he's gone, I'm beginning to understand how much he meant to all of us.

CAREGIVER–PRACTITIONER RELATIONSHIP

Caring for a person with AIDS disrupts even well-functioning families (Greif & Porembski, 1988). And in less stable family systems, intervention plans designed to ease family–caregiver stress may be difficult to implement because the family system may be closed or family members may be unwilling to accept help from outside sources. However, practitioners should attempt to work with the family as a unit of care, especially with those directly involved in the caregiving role (Macklin, 1988). Boundary issues are often alleviated if family members are helped to understand how their inclusive or exclusive behavior affects the person with AIDS. When the practitioner validates and supports family caregivers, family members may become more open to changing their interactional patterns. Reframing negative interactions as deriving from good intentions but having undesirable outcomes often serves as the first step in the process of change. Other potentially successful interventions include championing the importance of all family members, identifying family triangles, seeing family subsystems (such as sister and partner) separately in order to build alliances and expand family boundaries, or using the family's expressed values regarding the importance of caregiving as a springboard to cooperative caregiving behaviors.

During the middle phase, caregivers must juggle many conflicting roles while maintaining flexibility as the patient's health changes. This scenario has great potential for inducing debilitating stress because the roles caregivers play are usually important sources of self-definition and self-esteem. Caregivers confront existential issues as well as moral and ethical decisions that affect their self-concept. Thus, the outcome of role conflicts has enduring effects on the self-image of the caregiver (Pearlin, 1989).

ENDING PHASE

By the terminal phase of the illness, both the caregiver and person with AIDS are exhausted from the strain of going though multiple relapses and remissions (Land & Harangody, 1990; Stulberg & Buckingham, 1988). At this point, the many demands on the caregiver far outweigh his or her capacity to meet the ill person's needs. Friends and visitors may disrupt the fragile hospital patterns or household routines. The care-giver often serves as consoler to friends and extended-family members (Cleveland et al., 1988), a role reversal that may engender hostility (Pearlin et al., 1988).

As death nears, the caregiver may simultaneously wish the nightmare to end while fearing his or her loneliness in the future. Dealing with these emotional conflicts results in extreme fatigue and survivor guilt, which are made worse when the caregiver is closely identified with the person with AIDS (Pearlin et al., 1988). The caregiver may verbalize his or her wish that death would come, then feel that such wishes are narcissistic and selfish. Caregivers often deny the legitimacy of their feelings, and practitioners should be gentle when confronting such issues.

As a result of emotional turmoil, caregivers may be in such a depleted, fragmented state that they are unable to think rationally or function adequately. They may wander semiconsciously through their days and nights, administering medications, hoping for remission, waiting for death. If remission occurs, the cycle is played out again and again until death finally occurs.

During the final days, caregivers need to terminate their relationship with the patient and say good-bye. Often, the person with AIDS hangs on to life for the benefit of the caregiver. Some caregivers cleave to the relationship, refusing to accept the terminal nature of the illness, bargaining and hoping that yet another medication will revive the person for a few more weeks or months. Some are not able to say good-bye, and death comes before emotional closure. Most caregivers, however, are able to say the things that need to be said, to express their love, loyalty, admiration, and pride in the person with AIDS, then give permission to their loved one to let go. The final days of life become vivid scenes that will be played repeatedly in the minds of care-givers during the bereavement process. Questions and self-doubt are prevalent: Could I have done more? Did I make the right decisions? Why did I say what I did? Should I have called in more people to say good-bye? How can I keep his memory alive?

Because these final days are so important, service providers can have an enormously positive impact if they are able to ease the transition from life into death. How caregivers respond to these final days and the supportive services available vary depending on the personality and background of the individual. Some prefer privacy, treasuring their last moments alone with their loved one, others call in many family members and friends, and still others deny that the end is imminent. Some contain their grief or express it in privacy; others express grief openly. For some, religious ritual is a comfort; for others, it is an affront.

COUNTERTRANSFERENCE ISSUES

Caregiver responses can elicit countertransference feelings on the part of the professional service provider. The approaching death of a loved one weakens the coping defenses of service providers as well as caregivers. Practitioners may feel guilty about their own health or become angry over the hopelessness of the situation (Maloney, 1988). Others may reject the anticipatory grieving process or feel the need to rescue family and friends of the person with AIDS from the grieving process. Sometimes, service providers experience contradictory or seemingly incompatible feelings in response to the imminent death of a person with AIDS, for example, feelings of closeness alternating with the need to find emotional distance. Such feelings are part of the human condition. However, countertransference feelings need to be questioned and monitored. They may be initial signs of burnout.

Service providers sometimes develop a very close therapeutic alliance with caregivers over the course of the illness. They may share a community and/or ethnic/cultural heritage and they may have similar family backgrounds or ways of coping. Regardless of the relationship between the caregiver and service provider, however, the service provider's role must be defined by the goal of empowering and enabling the caregiver and the person with AIDS. The professional's role is that of conduit, not savior.

CONCLUSION

Stress is inherent in the caregiver role. Despite this, many caregivers provide good care for persons with AIDS, even at the expense of depleted personal functioning for themselves.

To maintain an optimum level of functioning in the face of caring for a person with AIDS, caregivers need instrumental and emotional support from human service professionals. Support systems alleviate caregiver stress by helping caregivers to develop methods of coping with the debilitating course of AIDS. Some coping efforts, called problem-focused coping, serve to change or manage a stressful situation (Pearlin et al., 1988). For example, caregivers may cope with the illness by obtaining information and education about the disease and its course as well as optimum medical care. Unfortunately, AIDS caregivers are limited in their ability to change the course of the disease, which affects their ability to cope with the situation.

However, practitioners can help caregivers cope by assisting them to discover new meanings and perceptions regarding the situation (Lazarus & Folkman, 1984). Caregivers can be helped to draw on long-held beliefs and values, strengths that allow them to reappraise their situation and thus reduce the stress inherent in caregiving. Helping caregivers adopt a more positive view of life can help caregivers and patients reduce stress in the early stages of the illness. Coping methods may include denial of the terminal nature of AIDS. Such denial enables caregivers to experience some sense of control over life (Pearlin et al., 1988). In addition, the disease can have a strong impact on family relationships, sometimes drawing family members closer together or engendering greater intimacy in the couple relationship. Service providers can help caregivers define their actions as an expression of loyalty to the person with AIDS or as an act of altruism or moral allegiance to a larger social cause (Orona, 1989). "The caregiver may be bloodied but he can stand unbowed" (Pearlin et al., 1988, p. 515).

Emotion-focused coping allows caregivers to manage or control their emotions (Pearlin et al., 1988) by getting away from the situation, ventilating, and so forth. In situations that are perceived as unchangeable, emotion-focused coping strategies are relied upon heavily (Lazarus & Folkman, 1984). To the extent that emotion-focused coping helps release the caregiver from the relentless pressures of stress, such coping methods may be extraordinarily helpful both prior to and following the death of the person with AIDS. The effects of stress are not necessarily attenuated after death (Macklin, 1988), because caregivers often experience post-traumatic stress disorder (Trice, 1988). Caregivers should be encouraged to accept emotional support from others and to take the time to nurture themselves. Caregivers need to revitalize their inner strengths and resources during the middle and ending phases of the disease, when their attempts to change the situation and reframe its meaning fail to reduce tension and despair.

Providing services to caregivers may be experienced as a formidable task by some and as a privilege by others. Regardless, the needs of this population are extensive and must be met. In order to accomplish this goal, service providers must develop a package of interventions designed to vary with the course of the illness and the needs of caregivers.

Service efforts must be based on theory and research rather than on *ad hoc* experiences. Practice interventions based on stress, role, and coping theory; on developmental psychodynamic theory; and on cognitive behavioral theory have demonstrated track records of reducing stress in similar populations (Moos & Billings, 1982). Interventions are most likely to be successful if they include both direct and indirect efforts, both instrumental/ecological and emotional supports, and both individual and systemic attention such as group support and family treatment. Interventions are more likely to succeed if they incorporate the cultural values inherent in the client group, wherein culture is defined as the union of ethnicity, race, class, generation, sexual orientation, and family patterns. Service plans should always be built on a strengths/needs approach, in which the functional coping styles of client groups are validated and strengthened and needs are mutually assessed by both the client and service provider.

AIDS caregivers are a vulnerable population with special needs. If their needs remain unmet, so too will the needs of those diagnosed with AIDS, and the human service community will have lost a powerful resource in combating the war against AIDS.

REFERENCES

Allers, C. (1990). AIDS and the older adult. *Gerontologist*, *30*, 405–407.

Allers, C. T., & Katrin, S. (1988). AIDS counseling: A psychosocial model. *Journal of Mental Health Counseling*, *10*, 235–244.

Bible, B. L., & McComas, J. D. (1963). Role consensus and teacher effectiveness. *Social Forces*, *42*, 225–233.

Boss, P., Pearce-McCall, D., & Greenberg, J. (1987). Normative loss in mid-life families: Rural, urban and gender differences. *Family Relations*, *36*, 437–443.

Carl, D. (1986). Acquired immune deficiency syndrome: A preliminary examination of the effects on gay couples and coupling. *Journal of Marital and Family Therapy*, *12*, 241–247.

Cleveland, P. H., Walters, L. H., Skeen, P., & Robinson, B. E. (1988). *Family Relations*, *37*, 150–153.

Frierson. R. L., Lippmann, S. B., & Johnson, J. (1987). AIDS: Psychological stresses on the family. *Psychosomatics*, *28*, 65–68.

Geis, S. B., & Fuller, R. L. (1986). Lovers of AIDS victims: Psychological stresses and counseling needs. *Death Studies*, *10*, 43–53.

Greif, G. L., & Porembski, E. (1987). Significant others of I.V. drug abusers with AIDS: New challenges for drug treatment programs. *Journal of Substance Abuse and Treatment*, *4*, 151–155.

Greif, G. L., & Porembski, E. (1988). Implications for therapy with significant others of persons with AIDS. *Journal of Gay and Lesbian Psychotherapy*, *1*(1), 60–66.

Haller, S. (1985). AIDS and the family: Case of L. Nassaney. *People Weekly*, *24*, 135–138.

Johnson, C., & Catalano, D. (1983). A longitudinal study of family supports to impaired elderly. *Gerontologist*, *23*, 612–618.

Kahn, R. K. (1964). *Organizational stress: Studies in role conflict and ambiguity*. New York: John Wiley.

Kelly, J., & Sykes, P. (1989). Helping the helpers: A support group for family members of persons with AIDS. *Social Work*, *34*, 239–242.

Land, H. M., & Harangody, G. (1990). A support group for partners of persons with AIDS. *Families in Society*, *71*, 471–481.

Lazarus, R. S., & Folkman, S. (1984). *Stress, appraisal, and the coping process*. New York: Springer.

Levine, C. (1990). AIDS and changing concepts of family. *Milbank Quarterly*, *68*(1), 33–59.

Lovejoy, N. C. (1990). AIDS: Impact on the gay man's homosexual and heterosexual families. *Marriage and Family Relations Review*, *14*, 285–316.

Macklin, E. D. (1988). AIDS: Implications for families. *Family Relations*, *37*, 141–149.

Maloney, B. D. (1988). The legacy of AIDS: Challenge for the next century. *Journal of Marital and Family Therapy*, *14*, 143–150.

Mason, W., & Gross, N. (1955). Intra-occupational prestige differential: The school superintendent. *American Sociological Review*, *20*, 326–331.

Minuchin, S. (1974). *Families and family therapy*. Cambridge, MA: Harvard University Press.

Moos, R. H., & Billings, A. G. (1982). Conceptualizing and measuring coping resources and processes. In L. Goldberger & S. Berznitz (Eds.), *Handbook of stress*. New York: Free Press.

Morales, E. S. (1990). Ethnic minority families and minority gays and lesbians. *Homosexuality and Family Relations*, *14*(3–4), 217–239.

Murphy, P., & Perry, K. (1988). Hidden grievers. *Death Studies*, *12*, 451–462.

Orona, C. J. (1989). Moral aspects of caregiving. *Generations*, *13*(4), 60–62.

Pearlin, L. I. (1983). Role strains and personal stress. In H. B. Kaplan (Ed.), *Psychosocial stress: Trends in theory and research*. New York: Academic Press.

Pearlin, L. I. (1989). The sociological study of stress. *Health and Social Behavior*, *30*, 241–256.

Pearlin, L. I., Semple, S., & Turner, H. (1988). Stress of AIDS caregiving: A preliminary overview. *Death Studies*, *12*, 501–517.

213

Robinson, B., Skeen, P., & Walters, L. (1987, April). The AIDS epidemic hits home. *Psychology Today, 21,* 48–52.

Rowe, W., Plum, G., & Crossman, D. (1988). Issues and problems confronting lovers, families and communities associated with persons with AIDS. *Journal of Social Work and Human Sexuality, 6*(2), 71–88.

Shanas, E. (1979). Social myths as hypothesis: The case of the family relations of old people. *Gerontologist, 19*(2), 3–9.

Smelser, W. T. (1961). Dominance as a factor in achievement and perception in cooperative problem-solving. *Journal of Abnormal Psychology, 62,* 535–542.

Stulberg, I., & Buckingham, S. (1988). Parallel issues for AIDS patients, families, and others. *Social Casework, 69,* 355–359.

Tiblier, K., Walker, G., & Rolland, J. (1989). Therapeutic issues when working with families or persons with AIDS. *Marriage and Family Review, 13,* 81–127.

Trice, A. (1988). Posttraumatic stress syndrome-like symptoms among AIDS caregivers. *Psychological Reports, 63,* 656–658.

Turner, H. A., & Pearlin, L. I. (1989). Informal support and people with AIDS: Issues of age, stress, and caregiving. *Generations, 13*(4), Fall, 56–59.

15

SUSTAINING PROFESSIONAL AIDS CAREGIVERS AND THEIR ORGANIZATIONS: A PERSONAL AND ORGANIZATIONAL APPROACH TO MINIMIZING BURNOUT

JUDY MACKS

At the outset of the 12th year of the AIDS epidemic, the number of people in the United States who have been personally affected by this disease continues to increase. The epidemic has claimed the lives of more than 128,000 adults, adolescents, and children in the United States in its first 11 years. During this time, more than 200,000 people have been diagnosed with AIDS, and an additional 1.5 million are living with HIV disease (Centers for Disease Control, 1991). Simultaneously, the number of professional caregivers who have been working on the front lines and in organizations to serve people with HIV/AIDS and their families as well as individuals and communities at risk for the disease has been increasing. The AIDS epidemic has taken an enormous toll on individuals and communities and the emotional and psychological demands of working in the field have begun to diminish the effectiveness of many professional caregivers and their organizations. Faced by the daily pain and stress of caring for individuals who may experience profound physical and mental deterioration, lack of treatments and cure, inadequate resources, a deteriorating health care system, complex ethical and legal issues, and feelings of hopelessness, helplessness, anger, and inadequacy, many caregivers are finding it increasingly difficult to sustain their commitment to and energy for their work.

Research has clearly documented that practitioners working in health care and service-oriented professions are, in general, more susceptible to burnout. Professional AIDS caregivers share this vulnerability. In addition, they experience specific stressors related to the epidemic that place them at even greater risk. Burnout is costly to the individual, the organization, and the populations served. Depleted indi-

Portions of this chapter were adapted from Macks, J. A., & Abrams, D. J. (in press). Burnout among HIV/AIDS health care providers: Helping the people on the frontlines. In P. Volberding & M. A. Jacobsen (Eds.), *AIDS clinical review 1991*. New York: Marcel Dekker, Inc. I am indebted to Alan Emery for his editorial assistance and to Gary Dexter for his contribution to my thinking in the area of environmental responses to stress in the workplace.

viduals have difficulty functioning, both in the workplace and in their personal lives, and they experience increasingly poor health and psychological distress. Organizations suffer when their employees suffer. Typically, where burnout is high, organizations experience increased staff conflict, tardiness, absenteeism, higher turnover rates, and lower productivity. Most significant, clients suffer when burned-out staff withdraw from contact with them, become cynical and defensive, and fail to provide quality care.

As AIDS caregivers and organizations attempt to sustain themselves in the years to come, responding to burnout from individual, work group, and organizational perspectives will be critical to providing care to people with HIV/AIDS.

OVERVIEW OF THE POPULATION

Professional caregivers have been working with people with HIV/AIDS and their loved ones, as well as with targeted communities and the general population, since the first cases of AIDS were reported in 1981. By late 1983, 2,259 cases of AIDS had been reported to the Centers for Disease Control (CDC), with 80% of these cases concentrated in six urban areas: New York, San Francisco, Miami, Newark, Houston, and Los Angeles. The epidemic nature of this disease soon became evident; 4,569 cases were reported to the CDC in 1984, 8,406 in 1985, and more than 22,000 cumulative cases by July 1986 (Gong, 1986). This epidemiologic picture of a spiraling epidemic is the context in which AIDS providers worked during the early years of the crisis. The number of providers working in AIDS paralleled the progression of the disease.

During the early years of the epidemic, the majority of caregivers were working in metropolitan centers where HIV/AIDS was most prevalent. Initially, caregivers worked in newly founded community-based organizations or health care settings in which services were developed in response to the epidemic. Other caregivers frequently found themselves to be among only a few providers in their institutions interested in and responding to AIDS. Despite their varied professional roles and work settings, this small network of caregivers working in community-based organizations, hospitals, outpatient services, home health care, or hospice organizations shared common experiences as they pioneered new models of organizational care or new services within existing institutions in an often hostile environment. In addition, many of these providers were personally affected by HIV/AIDS: gay men, lesbians, health activists, and friends and family of people with AIDS. Demand for services increased at such a rapid pace that providers and organizations found it progressively more difficult to meet service needs. The need to respond to the crisis, the rapidly changing information about HIV/AIDS, the explosive organizational growth, the dedication and commitment of individuals, and the solidarity in fighting an unpopular disease helped keep energies focused and moving forward and served to mobilize providers' efforts.

During the early years, the HIV/AIDS epidemic had the most dramatic impact on gay men and injection drug users. Yet, it soon became clear that AIDS was disproportionately affecting people of color and posing an increasing threat to women and children. As service recipients and targets of educational efforts became progressively more diverse, the need for additional services directed to these new populations became obvious.

As the demands of the epidemic increased, the emerging picture of AIDS caregivers became one of weary providers working on the front lines. They described their experiences in terms similar to "combat fatigue." They witnessed extensive and cumulative losses, battled their own stress-inducing attitudes, combatted the stigma and moral condemnation associated with the epidemic, and faced personal limitations in regard to prevention, care, and cure. In addition, many of these providers also had to deal with their own HIV status and/or their friends', partners', and communities' illnesses and deaths. The case loads of AIDS caregivers increased commensurate with the spiraling epidemic, yet resources were not allocated to meet these demands. At the same time, AIDS organizations and services experienced the organizational stressors associated with rapid growth.

In the past six years, the network of AIDS providers has expanded dramatically. Out of both necessity and choice, existing institutions began to serve people with HIV disease and their families. These programs and services are staffed by a diverse group of providers. Some of these caregivers specifically chose to work in this arena and others incorporated it into their previous work. New organizations and services formed to respond to the specific needs of various client groups. Such programs target women, people of color, adolescents, injection drug users, children, gay and bisexual men, and lesbians. These programs have expanded across the nation in urban, suburban, and rural ares. A majority of these programs serve disenfranchised populations.

As early as 1985, a few organizations recognized the need to respond to the shared and unique stressors they were experiencing. Consequently, support groups were organized to address the severe impact of ongoing grief and loss. Support groups have been a common organizational response to the realities of a loss-saturated work environment. The recent proliferation of "care for the caregiver" workshops and related interventions attests to the growing awareness of the emotional cost of caring for people with HIV/AIDS and the necessity of responding to the stress of working as an AIDS caregiver.

STRESS AND BURNOUT

The literature on stress and burnout, particularly that which focuses on health care and social service providers, offers critical information for understanding and responding to the needs of AIDS caregivers in their work settings. Stress is an integral part of life, creating a dynamic tension between the individual and environment. Individuals respond differently to stress and potential stressors. Some people thrive on it, whereas others become debilitated. One person's stressor may be another's excitement or challenge. People respond differently to similar stressors because they have different personalities, coping styles, and access to external resources. Yet, in today's fast-paced technological world, demands on individuals often far outweigh their resources.

DEFINING STRESS AND BURNOUT

Stress has been defined in terms of demands (stressors) and resources (Selye, 1974; Rabkin & Struening, 1976). When an individual lacks adequate internal or external resources to meet a demand, he or she experiences stress. Overlying this definition of stress is the larger sociocultural perspective influencing both internal and external demands and resources (Antonovsky, 1979). External resources, which include economic, social, or tangible activities and behaviors, are more easily identifiable. However, internal resources are equally important in responding to demands and helping to decrease stress. More specifically, external resources can include support from colleagues, family, and friends; exercising regularly; or engaging in relaxing activities. Internal resources refer to an individual's abilities, skills, knowledge, attitudes, and values, which can help to ameliorate stress. A provider may need to develop a new professional skill or alter certain beliefs and attitudes that create stress by adopting new ones. One new belief might be: "I feel successful and good about my work even when I cannot meet many of my clients' pressing needs."

Demands, or stressors, can be both internally or externally based. External demands, such as changes, events, or others' needs or expectations, are more obvious. These might include diminished funding, an increased case load, a client's onset of dementia, or the death of a client. Internal demands, although less obvious, can create enormous amounts of stress for the practitioner. These stressors are based upon personal needs, expectations, standards, beliefs, attitudes, and history. For example, people who believe that they should be able to meet all of their clients' needs or who need to be liked by all of their clients may behave in ways that are stress inducing by not setting limits. As a result of these internal beliefs and demands, they are more likely to experience stress.

The person–environment fit model (French, Rodgers, & Cobb, 1974) focuses on the dynamic interplay between the skills and abilities of the individual and the supplies and demands of the environment (workplace). Occupational stress is defined as a poor fit between the individual and the job role and/or work environment.

Burnout has been defined as "the progressive loss of idealism, energy and purpose experienced by people in the helping professions as the result of the conditions of their work" (Edelwich, 1980); "a transactional process consisting of job stress, worker strain and defensive coping" (Cherniss, 1981); and "the end-stage result of the inability to manage work stress" (Scott & Jaffe, 1989). Burnout has also been described as "a state of physical, emotional and mental exhaustion caused by long-term involvement in situations that are emotionally demanding. The emotional demands are most often caused by a combination of very high expectations and chronic situational stresses" (Pines & Aronson, 1989). Thus, burnout is the individual's response to work-related stressors that have not been successfully managed or resolved.

A person's vulnerability to burnout is based upon a combination of factors, including profession of choice, personal characteristics and skills, specific stressors in the workplace, and institutional factors. Although researchers do not agree about

TABLE 1. BURNOUT SYMPTOMS.

PHYSICAL	PSYCHOLOGICAL	BEHAVIORAL
Chronic fatigue	Depression	Increased alcohol or drug
Significant changes in appetite	Anxiety	use
Muscular tension	Feelings of helplessness,	Interpersonal conflict
Somatic complaints	hopelessness, being	Withdrawal and isolation
Vulnerability to illness	trapped	Decreased contact with
Sleep disturbance	Repression of feeling	clients
Gastrointestinal problems	Anger and resentment	Criticism of co-workers
Headaches	Obsessions, phobias	Overreaction
Ulcers	Suicidal ideation and	Irritability, resentment,
	attempts	antagonism
	Negative feelings about	Overeating
	self, work, life, others	Avoiding responsibilities
	Apathy	Decreased productivity
	Alienation	Missed appointments
	Disillusionment	Chronic tardiness at work
	Unrealistic expectations	Lethargy
	Sense of omnipotence	Distractability
	Paranoia	Disorganization
	Cynicism	
	Loss of meaning	

Sources: Cherniss, 1981; Friel & Tehan, 1980; Lavendero, 1981; Maslach, 1982; McConnell, 1982; Pines & Maslach, 1978.

the weight of each of these factors, a significant interplay among personal and organizational variables undoubtedly influences the incidence of burnout.

BURNOUT SYMPTOMS

Physical, psychological, and behavioral symptoms can indicate burnout (Table 1). Many of these symptoms are also associated with stress, both personal and work-related. However, burnout is indicated when the stressors are work related and the number, duration, severity, and chronicity of symptoms are more extreme.

Burnout can also be manifested as a group and organizational phenomenon. Symptoms at these levels typically include low staff morale, communication breakdown, increased staff conflict, decreased productivity, organizational stagnation, inflexibility and rigidity, resistance to change, increased absenteeism, high turnover, scapegoating, and displaced anger.

PERSONAL AND PROFESSIONAL SUSCEPTIBILITY TO BURNOUT

Individuals who work in the human services and helping professions are vulnerable to burnout. Researchers have documented a high incidence of burnout among health care professionals (Maslach, 1976; Pines, Aronson, & Kafry, 1981; Cherniss, 1981; Vachon, 1987), particularly among practitioners who work with the terminally ill (Pines & Maslach, 1978; Shubin, 1979; Storlie, 1982).

Personal variables and characteristics indicative of increased vulnerability to burnout include the desire to make a difference and the inability to achieve real results, working close to pain and suffering, and negative relationships with colleagues (Maslach, 1976). In addition to the external demands and stresses of the HIV epidemic, researchers have identified commonly shared beliefs and personal characteristics of providers that contribute to burnout.

Individuals who are highly motivated, idealistic, and energetic and who expect their work to give their life a sense of meaning, especially those who view their work as a "calling," are most vulnerable to burnout: "We have found, over and over again, that in order to burn out a person needs to have been on fire at one time" (Pines & Aronson, 1989). Some people with altruistic, often unattainable, goals become disillusioned and question the meaning of life and their work. Unfortunately, burnout often strikes individuals with the highest level of commitment to their work.

Health care professionals share a number of internalized attitudes and beliefs that contribute to unresolved stress on the job. Three key internalized attitudes and expectations are counterproductive and stress-producing: (1) health professionals should have no personal needs or feelings, (2) providers should always be immediately available to patients, and (3) practitioners should be able to make the patient healthy or at least make a significant difference (Jaffe, 1986). Health care providers working with catastrophic illness reported the following qualities: high self-expectations, low tolerance for disappointment, need for excellence and perfection, low self-esteem when not achieving, omnipotence, need for control, and the need to save (Eisendrach & Dunkel, 1979).

Personal and Interpersonal Variables That Mediate Stress

Research indicates that personal variables mediate an individual's response to environmental and occupational stressors. Certain personality styles and coping abilities leave some individuals more susceptible to stress and burnout. Individuals with a "hardy" personality style are better equipped to respond to stressors in a positive manner. Three significant characteristics of the "hardy" personality are commitment, control, and challenge (Kobasa, Maddi, & Couvington, 1981). Commitment makes individuals feel engaged and involved in their work. Individuals who feel a sense of control in their lives believe that they can influence and affect that which occurs in their lives. They are also able to discriminate between events that they do and do not have control over and do not attempt to control those events or stressors that cannot be controlled. Certain people view change as a positive, challenging experience. These individuals are flexible and able to tolerate uncertainty.

Individual qualities influence a person's resistance or vulnerability to stress. Similarly, environmental contexts intensify stress or help buffer the individual from stress (Elliot & Eisdorfer, 1982). Such mediators include personality and coping styles; cultural, religious, and personal values; previous experience; family life and social support; health behaviors; ability to balance work and home life; and economic status.

Social support provides caregivers with the opportunity to discuss their feelings about their job and themselves and has been documented in the literature as helping to ameliorate stress and burnout. Research suggests that providers can find this type of social support either in the workplace or in their personal lives (House, 1981; McLean, 1985; Pines & Kafry, 1978; Ray, 1987).

ORGANIZATIONAL, ENVIRONMENTAL, AND ROLE-RELATED STRESSORS AND MEDIATORS

The vast majority of research on stress and burnout has focused on the individual, both in terms of causality and coping. Recent literature, however, has begun to consider organizational, environmental, social, and role-related factors (Carroll & White, 1982; Cherniss, 1981; Karger, 1981; Paine, 1982). Research in the area of occupational stress in the care of the critically ill, the dying, and the bereaved indicates that caregiver stress is more likely to be caused by the work environment and professional role issues than by actual care of dying patients and their families. Significant organizational variables identified by caregivers as stressors included team communication problems, nature of the work system and/or unit, inadequate resources and staffing, communication problems with others in the organization or outside the system, unrealistic expectations of the organization, communication problems with administration, professional role ambiguity, role conflict, lack of control, role overload, and proximity to stressors (Vachon, 1987).

A survey of burnout patterns in organizations suggested that burnout is a group rather than individual phenomenon. These researchers observed that burnout resulted from patterns of relationship and supervision of the team and was especially tied to the norms, expectations, and behavior of the supervisor. The survey suggested that an individual's personality and work style are less significant in burnout than are organizational factors. When one employee was suffering from burnout, it was likely that others in the group were also experiencing burnout (Golembiewski, Munzenrider, & Stevenson, 1986). Corroborating this finding, a primary cause of stress and burnout can be attributed to the management style within a work group. Stress and burnout tend to be clustered within work groups rather than randomly distributed throughout an organization (Maslach, 1991).

More specifically, providers working for democratic managers who promote autonomy, flexibility, and a team approach to client care experience less stress than do those working for autocratic managers (Arches, 1991; Mather & Frakes, 1983; Taylor & Gideon, 1981). In addition to a lack of perceived autonomy, the inability to participate in decision making, demands from funding sources, and increased bureaucratization have been identified as key contributors to burnout and job dissatisfaction among social workers (Arches, 1991). Researchers have further documented that supportive relationships with superiors and co-workers buffer stress and burnout (Albrecht, Irey, & Mundy, 1982; Cherniss, 1981; House, 1981; McLean, 1985). The effectiveness of supervision as a mediator of stress is linked to how, when, and why supervisory support is offered (Maslach, 1982).

221

The role of managers in buffering or increasing stress in their workplaces and the concomitant stress associated with a managerial role have also been studied. Managers' success at assisting employees to cope with workplace stressors is significantly related to whether supervisees feel satisfied with their jobs (Kadushin, 1976; Orsolits, 1984; Waxman, Carner, & Berkenstock, 1984). Stress has also been associated with managers' occupational roles and responsibilities. Inadequate training, lack of management experience and skill, and placement in middle-management positions can all heighten stress. The most common stressors experienced by managers result from frustrated hopes and expectations about their ability to have an impact upon the work environment (Pines & Aronson, 1989). Furthermore, because managers act as role models, their response to stress is an important predictor of staff stress (Soos, 1991).

Rapid organizational growth can result in decreased staff participation in decision making as well as the erosion of employee autonomy, flexibility, and creativity. Such organizational growth has also been identified as a factor in increased stress and burnout. Paradoxically, an organization's growth is one marker of success, yet staff often feel disillusioned with the accompanying bureaucratization. Staff working in organizations founded to promote social ideologies or respond to a cause are particularly vulnerable to burnout during organizational growth. This occurs because emphasis shifts from philosophy and ideology to bureaucratic controls in the growth process (Messinger, 1955).

The following variables have been correlated with burnout in organizations: (1) lack of participation in decision making, (2) organizational conflict arising from roles or expectations of co-workers' roles, (3) lack of role clarity, (4) lack of job satisfaction, and (5) lack of emphasis on staff development. The only personal variable found to be statistically significant is an active, rather than passive and defensive, coping style (Joseph et al., 1989).

Health care professionals share some common role-related and institutional stressors. These include making decisions under pressure, working in a technical environment where mistakes can have deadly consequences, enduring long hours, working with life-and-death issues, witnessing pain and suffering, and facing limits in their ability to help (Scott & Jaffe, 1989).

CRITICAL ISSUES FOR AIDS CAREGIVERS AND THEIR ORGANIZATIONS

The sociocultural, political, medical, and psychological contexts of HIV disease and the AIDS epidemic create unique challenges and stressors for AIDS caregivers and their organizations. Although AIDS caregivers share common experiences, stressors, vulnerabilities, and characteristics with other providers, as described in the literature, the complex dynamics resulting from their particular circumstances contribute to AIDS caregivers' sense of combat fatigue and high risk for burnout.

THE CONTEXT

The AIDS epidemic has emerged during a period in the history of the United States in which particular social, cultural, political, medical, and economic conditions frame the context for the experiences of AIDS caregivers and their organizations. Many of the conflicts and problems faced by AIDS caregivers and their organizations are not unique to people working in health care, social services, and advocacy, and in fact represent larger societal problems. Still, the AIDS epidemic has served as a focal point for many of these issues because of its nature and timing.

The AIDS epidemic, in its early years, predominantly affected gay and bisexual men. Because of the sexual transmissibility of the disease and societal abhorrence of homosexuality, the epidemic quickly became viewed as one associated with immorality and sin. As a result, early programs and interventions were pioneered largely by gay men, lesbians, health activists, and others who were not homophobic. The stigma associated with AIDS and with how the disease is transmitted set it apart from other life-threatening illnesses. The division between the general public's response to the epidemic and that of those who initially addressed the crisis magnified preexisting divisions and prejudices in the culture, which in turn led to the politicization of HIV disease.

As the epidemic unfolded and it became clear that people of color were being disproportionately affected, as were women, adolescents, and injection drug users, preexisting social inequities, deficiencies, and inadequacies were further intensified. Again, not surprisingly, services to these populations were slow in coming. Building alliances among these diverse affected populations has been difficult. The obstacles AIDS providers have experienced in building coalitions and alliances reflect deeply rooted societal inadequacies and prejudices that pit disenfranchised groups against one another to compete for very limited resources. Similarly, conflict has increased between programs serving people with HIV and those serving persons with other health care needs and life-threatening illnesses.

The HIV epidemic has focused serious attention on the inadequacies of the health care system in the United States. It has further highlighted the inaccessibility of health care services for people of color, women, the poor, and, increasingly, the middle class. The HIV epidemic also emerged at a time when the general population and the medical profession believed and expected that a cure existed or could be found for any illness. Lulled by the illusion and expectation that answers to any medical problem could be found through science and technology, professionals and consumers of health care have come to feel impotent and angry that HIV is an ongoing reality.

The second decade of the epidemic has brought soaring health care costs as a majority of the individuals infected in the 1980s develop symptoms and require increased medical intervention in the 1990s. These needs are juxtaposed against a depressed economy, shrinking resources, increased competition for resources, and the matter of survival for many individuals and organizations.

CUMULATIVE LOSS

All AIDS providers, programs, and organizations experience losses associated with their young clients' severe physical and mental deterioration and inevitable death. Care providers contend with fluctuating feelings of sadness, anger, helplessness, despair, rage, uncertainty, and fear. The number and severity of the losses and the degree to which they affect individual providers and organizations differ according to several variables.

One variable is the degree to which a community of individuals, such as the gay community, has suffered losses as a result of the epidemic. The "gay community" is not homogeneous. It includes diverse individuals of various ethnic and racial backgrounds, ages, and physical abilities. Even if all of its members do not identify with a gay community as part of their primary identity, every gay person, in some way, shares the commonality of a sexual orientation that is relegated to second-class status in the United States. The connection to a gay community offers individuals a positive context and alternatives to counter societal hostility toward them. It also offers validation for relationships, love, and sexual orientation as well as collective and personal grief and mourning. Although the degree to which gay and bisexual men have lost members of their community varies, most everyone in the community has been touched by HIV/AIDS. In fact, gay communities have been devastated by the epidemic. The sense of loss is deeply felt at a community as well as personal level.

A second variable is the degree to which the client population suffers other losses in addition to those associated with HIV. The AIDS epidemic has disproportionately affected people of color and is increasingly affecting women. These populations frequently experience significant economic deprivation. HIV/AIDS adds to their disenfranchised status, and their cumulative losses are associated both with their illness and the conditions of their lives.

"Bereavement overload" is a term that was first used to describe the experience of the elderly dealing with multiple deaths among their peers in a relatively short period (Kastenbaum, 1977). In a vastly different context, AIDS caregivers suffer from a similar phenomenon when they must deal with the repeated diagnoses, illnesses, and deaths of their clients, co-workers, and loved ones as well as the very difficult economic circumstances of many of their clients. Because of the number and rapidity of the losses, caregivers are unable to complete grieving one loss before confronting the next. This unresolved grief exacerbates the grief process, resulting in difficulties in coping and managing one's life and work, increased staff conflict, resistance to change, loss of personal and organizational vitality, and other problems in the workplace.

Many AIDS caregivers chose their work because they had some affiliation with the populations most affected by the epidemic. As a result, a disproportionate number of providers are infected with HIV, have friends and loved ones with HIV disease, and have suffered the illnesses and deaths of co-workers and volunteers.

Over time, these conditions have taken their toll on providers and their organizations, a situation that parallels experiences documented in the literature regarding survivors of traumatic and catastrophic losses.

The pioneering work on survivors of catastrophic loss appeared in a study of survivors of the Coconut Grove fire in Boston (Lindemann, 1944). The literature was greatly expanded by researchers who documented the long-term deleterious psychological effects of surviving trauma in interviews with Holocaust survivors and World War II prisoners of war (Krystal, 1968; Kluznik, Speed, van Valkenburg, & Magrow, 1986; Niederland, 1968). This research, as well as the burgeoning literature on Vietnam war veterans (Foy, Carroll, & Donahue, 1987; Foy, Resnick, Sipprelle, & Carroll, 1987; Laufer, Gallops, & Frey-Wouters, 1984; Wilson, 1980) and other survivors of trauma, such as the Buffalo Creek disaster (Erikson, 1976), documents the symptomatology associated with post-traumatic stress disorder and delayed grief as described in the *Diagnostic and Statistical Manual of Mental Disorders* (American Psychiatric Association, 1987). Some of these symptoms include reexperiencing the trauma, numbing of responsiveness to or involvement with the external world, and guilt about surviving. Evidence suggests that the severity of symptoms is correlated with the length of exposure to the stress or trauma and that symptoms can present years after the trauma occurred.

Although the AIDS epidemic is a trauma of a different magnitude from combat and Holocaust survival, similar symptoms are beginning to emerge among some AIDS caregivers, albeit to a less severe degree. Caregivers who have experienced the most loss, either as a function of their professional role and/or personal life situations, have experienced the most trauma. Many of these people are not only professional caregivers but are caregivers to friends, partners, and family members as well.

It is not uncommon for AIDS caregivers to experience survival guilt for being HIV negative. Such guilt leads caregivers to question themselves about issues of meaning, fairness, responsibility, and fate. For some, survivor guilt has led to increased isolation, decreased coping, and ultimately burnout.

PERSONAL, PROFESSIONAL, AND ORGANIZATIONAL STRESSORS

Personal, professional, and organizational stressors further distinguish AIDS from other life-threatening illnesses and pose greater risk of burnout for AIDS caregivers. These providers, especially those who began working early in the HIV epidemic, share many of the characteristics and beliefs that have been correlated with susceptibility to burnout. They were unusually committed, energetic, and altruistic. They worked long hours and were determined to make a difference. In the short run, these qualities led to creativity, hard work, initiation of new services, and programmatic and organizational growth. However, over time, these same qualities and the underlying attitudes and beliefs that they reflect have contributed to increased burnout among AIDS caregivers.

Typical attitudes and beliefs include "I'm not doing enough," "I should be able to meet all immediate needs and crises," "I can do more," "I can't say no," "There's no time to focus on myself," "There's no time to grieve," "I can't make mistakes." Such beliefs can result in behavioral and emotional manifestations, for instance, poor limit setting, lack of planning, low self-esteem, addictive relationship to work, increased substance use, interpersonal problems, low tolerance for disappointment and mistakes, and rigidity.

The medical complexities of HIV and its treatment have challenged AIDS caregivers to keep up with a rapidly changing and expanding knowledge base while maintaining overflowing case loads. Not only is the level of care demanding, but adequate resources are not available to meet the medical and psychosocial needs of people with HIV. As a result, AIDS caregivers are expected to fulfill multiple roles for which they frequently have not been trained, such as patient advocate, hospice counselor, educator, academician, grant writer, financial manager, or administrator. AIDS providers find themselves caught in the middle between patients' physical and psychosocial needs and the little care they can offer because of shrinking resources and an inadequate health care system.

Societal prejudices toward people with HIV influence the level of support AIDS caregivers receive from family, friends, and society at large. One survey noted that parents of young physicians working with people with HIV once were proud of their son's or daughter's work, but were now ashamed to discuss their child's work with others because of the association with HIV. This was particularly true for gay physicians whose parents had not discussed their child's sexual orientation within their social milieu (Vachon & Dennis, 1989). Similarly, many caregivers working in medical settings have reported not only a lack of support from their families and friends but hostility and conflict arising as a result of their working with people with AIDS.

The fact that many AIDS providers are members of the affected communities presents unique problems for client care and service organizations. Caregivers often experience additional strains posed by their own health status or that of their loved ones. Because working with people with HIV disease triggers caregivers' concerns about their own health status and that of those for whom they are caring in their personal lives, caregivers may find it difficult to empathize with their clients or may overidentify with them. The lack of separation between AIDS-related stressors at work and at home adds to these caregivers' susceptibility to burnout.

These difficulties are also experienced at the organizational level. The issues and dynamics associated with the mixed health status of staff are difficult to address directly, yet are felt by all. The staff member with HIV is concerned about personal health, confidentiality, interpersonal interactions related to his or her health status, accommodation, flexibility, respect, and cumulative loss. For the HIV-negative staff person who is a member of an affected community, cumulative loss, survivor issues, and caregiver functions outside work are of paramount significance. AIDS caregivers who are not members of affected communities express other concerns. A key issue has been a desire to support their HIV-infected and -affected colleagues. Because of the lack of professional role separation and increased identification, these staff members often feel uncertain about how to respond to or approach their HIV-infected peers in the context of daily work. Another concern has been the anger about, and concomitant guilt associated with, the lack of validation for the non–AIDS-related illnesses, deaths, and other crises experienced by these providers. These concerns are difficult to discuss openly and may be manifested in covert ways. Their existence can contribute to increased staff conflict, poor team communication, low morale, and a diminishing appreciation and celebration of positive events.

Cumulative loss and grief among staff, when left unattended, can seriously impair organizational functioning. There are few precedents and even fewer models for responding to the effect of grief and loss in the workplace. The organizational symptoms that manifest when such issues are not addressed parallel those of burnout: poor staff morale, communication breakdown, increased staff conflict, decreased productivity, entire work groups feeling overwhelmed or stagnant, inflexibility and rigidity, resistance to change, increased absenteeism, high turnover, scapegoating, and displaced anger.

AIDS services and organizations have grown extremely rapidly over a relatively short period. They were founded in response to a health crisis and grew in response to immediate rather than planned needs. They were crisis oriented and managed, and they relied on the dedication of hard-working and committed staff. As a result, the cultures that have developed within these organizations and services frequently promote and reinforce stress-inducing attitudes, beliefs, and behaviors through messages, norms, and systems of reward.

With rapid growth, the founding philosophies and expectations of AIDS services and organizations have shifted. Participatory decision-making processes have evolved into more bureaucratic and hierarchical ones. As the literature suggests, organizations face developmental crises as they mature and grow. Each stage requires a different response, leadership style, and organizational structure.

Paradoxically, the solutions to one phase lay the foundation for problems in the next (Lippitt & Schmidt, 1967). These phases include creativity, direction, delegation, and consolidation (Management Assistance Group, 1984). Most AIDS organizations have experienced the shift from the first phase—creativity—which is driven by the cause and characterized by commitment, informal structure and communications, and rewards related to mission and meaning. Many organizations are now in the second phase—direction—which is characterized by a focus on efficiency, centralization, and formalization of structure and communication systems. A small number of the older AIDS organizations and programs have moved into the third and fourth phases of their life cycle. The delegation phase is characterized by expansion of services, decentralization, and delegation. The consolidation phase involves more formal planning, consolidation, and team orientation. In the world of medical and social services, AIDS organizations are by definition very young and have had to mature rapidly to respond to and keep up with what has become a world-wide health crisis. During this process, many people moved into management positions without adequate managerial training, skills, or experience. The degree to which rapid growth is associated with stress and burnout is largely dependent upon the organizations' abilities to resolve the corresponding crises. This extremely rapid growth has challenged AIDS organizations and programs to respond effectively to developmental crises while maintaining quality service provision.

INDIVIDUAL AND ORGANIZATIONAL STRATEGIES TO MINIMIZE STRESS AND BURNOUT

The relevance of the literature on stress and burnout to the AIDS caregiver as well as the impact of cumulative losses and the societal context within which AIDS emerged clearly show the significant challenges faced by AIDS providers and their organizations as they attempt to manage stress and minimize burnout. Most solutions to managing stress and preventing burnout described in the literature focus on the individual and are based on cognitive, behavioral, and social-support theoretical frameworks. These strategies are useful in helping the individual to cope with occupational stressors. However, research indicates that key environmental and role-related stressors must also be addressed to decrease occupational stress and minimize burnout. Thus, managing stress and minimizing AIDS-related burnout require a collaborative effort between the individual and the organization, whereby stress is managed through a comprehensive organizational strategy.

Managers identify financial and time constraints as key barriers to designing and implementing comprehensive organizational strategies to minimize burnout. In a recent study of the economic impact of burnout on a large AIDS organization of 61 employees, Soos (1991) documented the annual cost as ranging from $39,234 to $157,357. This calculation was based on the following four indices: excess absenteeism, increased worker's compensation premiums, excess job turnover, and productivity losses. The costs were considered a conservative estimate because they did not include additional cost sources that were not easily quantifiable, such as increased property, casualty, and medical insurance premiums; increased costs of employee retention and termination; increased drug and alcohol use; low employee morale; interpersonal antagonisms; and decreased quality of services. The annual cost of implementing the comprehensive "Staff Care Plan" developed by this organization in response to staff burnout ranged from $27,354 to $180,045. The estimated mid-range cost of $73,026 was thought to reflect most accurately the actual costs by calculating that only half of the employees would utilize the optional benefits. Although this range is wide, data indicate that intervention can be far less costly than is burnout.

AIDS organizations and programs have implemented various strategies to assist their staff members in coping with stress. Seven of the larger AIDS service organizations in the United States attribute their success in responding to burnout to liberal benefit packages and generous time-off policies, manageable case loads, management training and coaching, support groups, and training to enhance multicultural awareness and sensitivity (Soos, 1991).

INDIVIDUAL STRATEGIES

Individual stress-management strategies can include relaxation activities, cognitive restructuring, goal setting, behavioral change, developing and maintaining healthy habits, counseling, support groups, conflict resolution, managing grief and loss, time management, and other stress-management skills. Most of these strategies require caregivers to learn new ways of thinking and behaving that can be used both inside and outside the workplace.

Many of these intervention approaches focus on minimizing stress-inducing internal demands by helping caregivers develop new attitudes, beliefs, and expectations. As evidenced by the literature describing the personal and professional characteristics that leave an individual susceptible to burnout, strategies that focus on cognitive restructuring and behavioral change can be particularly useful. These strategies include setting realistic expectations and goals, setting appropriate limits, and finding different kinds of meaning in one's work. Additionally, these strategies can help caregivers develop the qualities described by Kobasa, Maddi, and Couvington (1981) as the "hardy personality." Caregivers can buffer their stress by recommitting to and reengaging in their work, developing a greater sense of control and influence over what occurs in their lives, accepting what they cannot control, and viewing change as a challenging and positive experience.

Social support helps ameliorate stress and burnout. Support groups focus on the prevention of individual burnout through social support and skills development. In group settings, caregivers can explore and ventilate feelings associated with their work, decrease isolation, give and receive feedback, share insights with their peers, develop and express their sense of humor, and enhance mutual support in a structured setting. Support groups are most effective when they are facilitated by a trained professional from outside the organization, are offered during work hours or with compensatory time, and do not turn into "gripe sessions."

Professional training and development can help diminish stress and burnout by offering staff opportunities for new challenges, growth, and skills development. Formal training and educational opportunities, career counseling, skills development, and "job swapping" can have positive results.

ORGANIZATIONAL STRATEGIES FOR PREVENTING BURNOUT

Organizational interventions are essential not only to support the individual's attempts at effectively managing stress and self-care but to alter the institutional causes of burnout. In response to individual and organizational stressors and the high risk of burnout associated with working in the field of HIV, JKRAssociates developed a model to work with loss-saturated work environments.[1] The goal of this model is to help organizations and their employees identify and implement organizational and individual strategies to respond to ongoing and cumulative stress and grief. It is based on the assumption that stress and grief in the workplace are experienced and expressed, overtly and subtly, at the personal, interpersonal/work group, and organizational levels. The model involves several steps: (1) organizational assessment and problem definition, (2) identification of a planning task force representative of the diversity in the organization, (3) task-force planning, (4) education and training, (5) problem-solving and strategy design, (6) implementation and intervention, (7) follow-up and evaluation, and (8) second-stage implementation. This model has been adapted to work with a wide variety of health care institutions, social service agencies, community-based organizations, and groups of private practitioners working in the same discipline.

Several key factors are necessary to ensure the success of this model. First, all staff in the organization must be included in the assessment, problem-solving, and implementation phases to ensure that employees are heard, have a voice in the outcome, and help create the solution. Soliciting input from staff and providing a process that offers staff a role in shaping policy can be even more important than the specific interventions (Maslach, 1991). Second, management must actively support and participate in this process. Third, strategies must target the individual, work groups, and the organization as a whole. Fourth, strategies should address all of the following: policies and benefits; ongoing acknowledgment of losses; the role of management; enhancing communication systems; formal support; informal communication; appreciation mechanisms; ways to acknowledge and honor cultural diversity; issues among staff who are HIV infected, personally affected, and professionally affected; job structure and workload; and staff development.

An initial assessment of the problem is essential to developing intervention. At a minimum, assessment must focus on the impact of stress and burnout on the organization. Optimally, an organizational assessment should be conducted from a much broader perspective to identify problems in various aspects of the organization that ultimately contribute to burnout. The assessment involves a two-step process. First, discussions are held with the management team to assess the timeliness of the project, given other major changes or events occurring within the organization. Second, and most important, staff are surveyed via a written questionnaire. They are asked about the impact of grief and loss on themselves, their work group, and their organization; the most significant stressors associated with their job tasks; the degree to which they feel supported and appreciated at work; their expectations of the organization's role in responding to grief, loss, stress, and burnout; and other related dimensions. Questionnaires are anonymous and are correlated based upon demographic and work group or departmental dimensions.

After the assessment has been completed and the task force assembled, planning of the all-staff retreat takes place. This meeting includes three components. First, staff read and respond to a report that summarizes the data collected in the assessment and confirm that it accurately reflects their perceptions and concerns. Second, training is conducted on grief, cumulative loss, stress, and burnout, and the impact of these factors on the workplace. Third, staff engage in a group problem-solving session to generate potential strategies to respond to identified stressors and problems.

The next step in this process is carried out by the task force. They compile the ideas generated at the all-staff meeting and, on the basis of this information, make recommendations for an implementation plan, including a phased timeline. After the organization's executive director approves a plan, implementation begins. At the six-month point, the implementation plan is evaluated by means of a written, all-staff survey. A follow-up meeting is scheduled with the staff to review the evaluation data, identify gaps in the implementation plan or adaptations that need to be made, and discuss strategies to respond to these gaps and adaptations. This, then, provides the basis upon which the task force coordinates the second-stage implementation plan.

It is critical for organizations to design strategies that address a wide range of areas, including policies and benefits, workload, communication systems, supervision and managerial role, honoring of cultural diversity, issues related to the health status of staff and volunteers, ongoing acknowledgment of losses, celebrations, appreciation mechanisms, and formal support. Implementing policies and benefits that help mitigate stress and burnout directly also gives clear messages to staff that self-care is encouraged. Policies should be consistent yet allow for flexibility regarding vacation and sick leave, compensatory time, bereavement leave, educational leave, mental health days, part-time options, leave without pay, and other related benefits. Organizations also need to design an effective system to orient new staff members to policies and procedures and periodically to bring current staff members up to date on any new policy or procedure.

Because workload and scarce resources are frequently cited as primary stressors in AIDS organizations and other work settings, interventions to address AIDS-related burnout may need to focus on job structure, role-related tasks and responsibilities, work distribution, and time schedules. Some organizations have found it helpful to reorganize jobs to avoid repetition, vary tasks and case loads, share jobs or tasks, and develop more flexible time schedules. A redivision of work can help by adding variety to a job and by reducing the intensity, duration, and frequency of stressors (Maslach, 1979).

Poor communication is frequently cited as a key organizational stressor. Creating support mechanisms and fostering open communication through formal and informal communication systems are important strategies in a comprehensive response to stress and burnout. Ameliorating this problem by addressing communication among individuals, work groups, teams, management, and staff will help decrease the likelihood of staff burnout. In addition, informal communication needs to be encouraged by scheduling opportunities for staff to be together in fun, relaxing, and informal ways.

Managers must provide consistent supervision and become sensitive to employee stressors and symptoms of burnout. Effective, consistent supervision encourages each staff person to recognize his or her signs and symptoms of burnout and helps the individual to strengthen coping skills and to manage stress. Depending upon the needs of the individual, supervisors can help employees to ask for help, set reasonable limits, manage their time, recognize their strengths and weaknesses, accept their own and others' limitations, take time off, and set long- and short-term goals. In order to be most effective, managers may need additional training in supervisory and leadership skills and in how to assist others in managing their grief, loss, stress, and burnout. Managers also find that peer support from other managers helps them better cope with the stress associated with their occupational role.

AIDS organizations and programs need to develop systems to acknowledge losses on an ongoing basis. Although they can take various forms, systems should be implemented to inform colleagues about the deaths of co-workers and clients, acknowledge losses, and develop group rituals for remembering those who have died. Cultural diversity must be recognized and interventions designed to accommodate individual and cultural responses to grief and loss. The organization also needs to address openly the dynamics and issues resulting from the differing degrees to which HIV affects staff members personally. By opening a discussion on this vital subject on a regular basis, in a safe and structured environment, covert issues and dynamics can be brought into the open, responded to, and worked through in a thoughtful manner.

Organizations must also implement mechanisms to appreciate staff for their hard work and commitment and to recognize contributions. Celebrations need to be organized to acknowledge significant life events such as birthdays and achievements.

Strategies for improving organizational and job design (Dexter, 1984) are also fundamental underpinnings to guide organizations in any comprehensive effort to minimize stress and burnout. These include (1) allowing the individual worker to influence his or her own work situation, working methods, and pace; (2) allowing for an overview and understanding of the work process as a whole (the individual should see where his or her contribution "fits" in a broader scheme); (3) allowing the individual worker to use and develop all of his or her skills; (4) creating opportunities for human contacts and cooperation in the course of work; and (5) making it possible for the individual worker to satisfy time claims from roles and obligations outside work (e.g., family, social, and community commitments). In addition to the strategies described in this section, effective and stress-reducing interventions might require larger-scale organization-development interventions, including organizational redesign, restructuring, and strategic planning.

CONCLUSION

The cumulative toll of stress on AIDS caregivers and their organizations demands increasing attention. Individual stress-management strategies must be encouraged and expanded so that caregivers can remain productive and healthy. At the same time, greater focus must be placed on organizational strategies for preventing burnout. An integrated part of an organization's planning must include organizational efforts to minimize stress and prevent burnout. These strategies must be longitudinal and adequately funded.

The AIDS epidemic will become increasingly demanding of the best efforts of AIDS caregivers and their organizations throughout the 1990s. Planned, budgeted, and ongoing organizational strategies to address and minimize AIDS-related stress and burnout will help ensure that AIDS caregivers and organizations will meet the demands of this epidemic.

NOTE

1. JKRAssociates is a consulting firm in San Francisco, California, providing assistance to organizations in managing grief, loss, stress, and burnout in the workplace.

REFERENCES

Albrecht, T. L., Irey, K. V., & Mundy, A. K. (1982). Integration in a communication network as a mediator of stress. *Social Work, 27,* 229–234.

American Psychiatric Association. (1987). *Diagnostic and statistical manual of mental disorders* (3rd ed., rev.). Washington, DC: Author.

Antonovsky, A. (1979). *Health, stress and coping.* San Francisco: Jossey-Bass.

Arches, J. (1991). Social structure, burnout, and job satisfaction. *Social Work, 36,* 202–206.

Carroll, J., & White, W. (1982). Theory building: Integrating individual and environmental factors within an ecological framework. In W. S. Paine (Ed.), *Job stress and burnout.* Beverly Hills, CA: Sage Publications.

Centers for Disease Control. (1991, December). *HIV/AIDS surveillance.* Atlanta, GA: Author.

Cherniss, C. (1981). *Professional burnout in human service organizations.* New York: Praeger.

Dexter, G. (1984). *Altering stress in the workplace: A comparison of individual vs. environmental interventions* (diss.). Ann Arbor, MI: University Microfilms International.

Edelwich, J. (1980). *Burnout: Stages of disillusionment in the helping professions.* New York: Human Sciences Press.

Eisendrach, S. J., & Dunkel, J. (1979). Psychological issues in intensive care unit staff. *Heart and Lung, 8,* 751–758.

Elliott, G. R., & Eisdorfer, C. (Eds). (1982). *Stress and human health: Analysis and implications of research.* New York: Springer.

Erikson, K. (1976). Loss of community at Buffalo Creek. *American Journal of Psychiatry, 133,* 302–305.

Foy, D., Carroll, E., & Donahue, C. P. Jr. (1987). Etiological factors in the development of PTSD in clinical samples of Vietnam combat veterans. *Journal of Clinical Psychology, 43*(1), 17–27.

Foy, D., Resnick, H., Sipprelle, C., & Carroll, E. (1987). Premilitary, military and post-military factors in the development of combat-related posttraumatic stress disorder. *Behavior Therapist, 10,* 3–9.

French, J. R. P., Rodgers, W., & Cobb, S. (1974). Adjustment as person–environment fit. In G. Coelho, D. Hamburg, & J. Adams (Eds.), *Coping and adaptation* (pp. 316–333). New York: Basic Books.

Friel, M., & Tehan, C. B. (1980). Counteracting burnout for the hospice caregiver. *Cancer Nursing, 3,* 285–293.

Golembiewski, R. T., Munzenrider, R. F., & Stevenson, G. (1986). *Stress in organizations: Toward a phase model of burnout.* New York: Praeger.

Gong, V. **(1986).** *AIDS: Facts and issues.* New Brunswick: Rutgers University Press.

House, J. S. (1981). *Work, stress and social support.* Reading, MA: Addison-Wesley.

Jaffe, D. T. (1986). The inner strains of healing work: Therapy and self-renewal for health professionals. In C. Scott & J. Hawk (Eds), *Heal thyself: The health of health care professionals.* New York: Brunner-Mazel.

Joseph, V., et al. (1989). *The impact of organization on staff and agency burnout.* Paper presented at the NASW Annual Conference, October 12, 1989, San Francisco, CA.

Kadushin, A. (1976). *Supervision of social work.* New York: Columbia University Press.

Karger, H. (1981). Burnout as alienation. *Social Service Review, 55,* 271–283.

Kastenbaum, R. J. (1977). Death and development through the life span. In H. Feigel (Ed.), *New meanings of life.* New York: McGraw-Hill.

Kobasa, S. C., Maddi, S. R., & Couvington, S. (1981). Personality and constitution as mediators

233

in the stress-illness relationship. *Journal of Health and Social Behavior, 22*, 368–378.

Kluznik, J. C., Speed, N., van Valkenburg, C., & Magrow, R. (1986). Forty-year follow-up of United States prisoners of war. *American Journal of Psychiatry, 143*, 1443–1446.

Krystal, H. (1968). *Massive psychic trauma.* New York: International Universities Press.

Laufer, R. S., Gallops, M., & Frey-Wouters, E. (1984). War stress and trauma: The Vietnam veteran experience. *Journal of Health and Social Behavior, 25*, 65–85.

Lavendero, R. (1981). Burnout phenomenon: A descriptive study among nurses. *American Journal of Nursing, 11*(11–12), 17–23.

Lindemann, E. (1944). Symptomatology and management of acute grief. *American Journal of Psychiatry, 101*, 141–148.

Lippitt, G. L., & Schmidt, W. H. (1967, November–December). Crises in a developing organization. *Harvard Business Review, 45*, 102–112.

Management Assistance Group. (1984, February). Passages: Changing organizations and boards. *Conserve Neighborhoods, 35*, 334–335.

Maslach, C. (1976). Burned out. *Human Behavior, 5*(9), 16–22.

Maslach, C. (1979). The burn-out syndrome and patient care. In C. Garfield (Ed.), *Stress and survival.* St. Louis, MO: C. V. Mosby.

Maslach, C. (1982). *The cost of caring.* Englewood Cliffs, NJ: Prentice-Hall.

Maslach, C. (1991). Personal interview as reported by Soos, J., in *Caring for the caregiver: An evaluation of staff burnout at Shanti Project and a benefit–cost analysis of the "staff care plan."* Unpublished manuscript, Graduate School of Public Policy, University of California, Berkeley, Berkeley, CA.

Mather, C. D., & Frakes, K. (1983, November–December). The hospice philosophy: They bring out the best in you. *Nursing Life, 3*, 50–51.

McConnell, E. A. (1982). The burnout syndrome. In E. A. McConnell, (Ed.), *Burnout in the nursing profession: Coping strategies, causes, and costs* (pp. 70–74). St. Louis, MO: C. V. Mosby.

McLean, A. A. (1985). *Work stress.* Reading, MA: Addison-Wesley.

Messinger, S. L. (1955). Organizational transformation: Case study of a declining social movement. *American Sociological Review, 20*(1), 3–10.

Niederland, W. G. (1968). The problem of the survivor. In H. Krystal (Ed.). *Massive psychic trauma.* New York: International Universities Press.

Orsolits, M. (1984). Effects of organizational characteristics of the turnover in cancer nursing. *Oncology Nursing Forum, 11*(1), 21–26.

Paine, W. S. (1982). *Job stress and burnout: Research, theory and intervention perspectives.* Beverly Hills, CA: Sage Publications.

Pines, A., & Aronson, E. (1989). *Career burnout.* New York: Free Press.

Pines, A., Aronson, E., & Kafry, D. (1981). *Burnout: From tedium to personal growth.* New York: Free Press.

Pines, A., & Kafry, D. (1978). Occupational tedium in social services. *Social Work, 23*, 499–507.

Pines, A., & Maslach, C. (1978). Characteristics of staff burnout in mental health settings. *Hospital and Community Psychiatry, 29*, 233–237.

Rabkin, J. G., & Struening, E. L. (1976). Life events, stress and illness. *Science, 194*, 1013–1020.

Ray, E. B. (1987). Support relationships and occupational stress in the workplace. In T. L. Albrecht & M. Adelman (Eds.), *Communicating social support: Process in context.* Beverly Hills, CA: Sage Publications.

Scott, C. D., & Jaffe, D. T. (1989). Managing occupational stress associated with HIV infection. *Occupational Medicine, 4*, 85–93.

Selye, H. (1974). *Stress without distress.* Philadelphia: Lippincott.

Shubin, S. (1979). Rx for stress—your stress. *Nursing, 9*(1), 52–55.

Soos, J. (1991). *Caring for the caregiver: An evaluation of staff burnout at Shanti Project and a benefit–cost analysis of the "staff care plan."* Unpublished manuscript, Graduate School of Public Policy, University of California, Berkeley, Berkeley, CA.

234

Storlie, F. J. (1982). Burnout: The elaboration of a concept. In E. A. McConnell (Ed.), *Burnout in the nursing profession: Coping strategies, causes, and costs* (pp. 81–85). St. Louis: C. V. Mosby.

Taylor, P. B., & Gideon, M. (1981). Day in and day out you minister to others. *Nursing, 11*(10), 58–61.

Vachon, M. (1987). *Occupational stress in the care of the critically ill, the dying and the bereaved.* New York: Hemisphere.

Vachon, L. S., & Dennis, J. (1989). HIV, stress and the health care professional. In J. W. Dilley, C. Pies, & M. Helquist (Eds.), *Face to face: A guide to AIDS counseling.* San Francisco: AIDS Health Project, University of California, San Francisco.

Waxman, H. M., Carner, E. A., & Berkenstock, G. (1984). Job turnover and job satisfaction among nursing home aides. *Gerontologist, 24,* 503–509.

Wilson, J. P. (1980). Conflict, stress, and growth. In C. R. Figley & S. Leventman (Eds.), *Strangers at home: Vietnam veterans since the war.* New York: Praeger.

PART 3

SPECIAL TOPICS IN CLINICAL WORK

16

COPING WITH THE TRAUMA OF AIDS LOSSES

RICK BIDGOOD

The AIDS pandemic has resulted in irrevocable losses, which, in turn, have led to pervasive and chronic grief for persons living with HIV/AIDS. More than 133,000 people in the United States died of AIDS between June 1981 and December 1991; worldwide, the figure is estimated to be more than half a million. In areas such as San Francisco, it is estimated that three people per day die from AIDS (*San Francisco Examiner*, 1992). As of 1991, more than 200,000 cases of AIDS have been diagnosed in the United States. The estimated 1.5 million AIDS diagnoses worldwide foreshadow the siege of loss to come.

But figures can't convey the pain and loss experienced by those affected personally by this epidemic. Those who are affected by AIDS grieve continuously. In addition, the stigma attached to HIV/AIDS and the young ages of persons who contract the disease create special bereavement issues for both persons living with the disease and practitioners.

Although loss and bereavement are universal experiences, individuals react to and cope with these experiences uniquely. Grief is a normal and natural adaptive response to loss. It affects our thoughts, feelings, behaviors, physical well-being, and spirit. It is both an interpersonal and intrapersonal process.

BEREAVEMENT THEORIES

Lindemann (1944) identified three stages of grief response among persons who experienced loss as a result of Boston's Coconut Grove nightclub fire: shock and disbelief, acute mourning and acceptance of the loss, and resolution of grief and a return to regular life activities. Bowlby (1960) described a mourning process involving similar stages of grief. Kübler-Ross (1969) suggested a five-stage model: denial,

The author acknowledges and thanks Scott A. Shipe for his support and contribution to this chapter.

anger, bargaining, depression, and acceptance. Others believe that psychosocial factors, the complexity of emotional responses, and the nature of the death affect the bereavement process. Worden (1982) proposed four tasks that must be accomplished to complete the grieving process: accepting the reality of the loss, experiencing the pain of grief, adjusting to life without the person, and reinvesting emotional energy into life. Although these tasks do not *necessarily* follow a particular order, they do have direction. For example, it is difficult to deal with the emotional impact of a loss if one has not yet accepted the reality of that loss. Staudacher (1987) discusses bereavement in terms of the types of loss—parent, spouse/partner, child, accidental death, suicide, murder—suggesting a process of retreat, acceptance, and resolution. The process varies among individuals and often is shaped by cultural values and practices (Eisenbruch, 1984).

BEREAVEMENT AND HIV/AIDS

With regard to HIV/AIDS, far less has been written about loss and grief than about other aspects of the pandemic. Shearer and McKusick (1986) discussed grief reactions of persons affected by HIV/AIDS losses. They state that the multiple losses in the gay/lesbian community are creating an atmosphere of denial. As social support networks crumble beneath the weight of so many deaths, many survivors are losing the necessary connections and resources to facilitate grieving. With less capacity to grieve, defenses such as denial are used more often. Klein and Fletcher (1986) list some of the nontraditional issues that gay survivors of HIV/AIDS losses face: the majority of deaths are among young men, members of this group come from a subculture whose life-style is often socially condemned, low self-esteem and guilt are easily exacerbated by internalized homophobia, financial benefits are not usually guaranteed to survivors, and those who survive are often treated like outsiders by the deceased person's family of origin. Such issues place HIV/AIDS survivors outside the typical bereavement process, which in turn causes survivors to have less control over the grief process. Schindelman and Schoen (1988) discussed how the stigma of AIDS makes it difficult for survivors to disclose the cause of death, thus prolonging grief and intensifying sorrow. They point out that persons living with HIV may even confuse grief reactions with AIDS symptoms: tightness in the chest, weight loss, fatigue, difficulty concentrating. Martin (1988) discussed how bereavement among gay men is complicated by multiple losses and by the high likelihood that the bereaved person also faces AIDS-related health issues. These men may find it difficult to process realities of death in that losses of significant others remind them of how vulnerable they are to the same fate.

Anderson, Gurdin, and Thomas (1989) examined the disenfranchisement of foster parents grieving for children with AIDS. Their grief may be misunderstood or discounted because they are not the biological parents. Combined with the stigma of HIV/AIDS and the consequent discrimination and lack of social support, foster parents can be at risk for bereavement complications.

Dick (1989) explored the grief of health care professionals caring for persons with AIDS. Their grief may be unrecognized and not addressed because of the stigma of AIDS and their limited inclusion in the sorrow shared among the deceased person's family of origin and family of choice. Monette (1988) provided a personal account of the long and difficult process of caring for a partner from diagnosis to death. The story illustrated the painful journey of AIDS-related grief undertaken by the author. Meyer (1991) discussed how cultural and ethnic differences influence the grieving process, suggesting that for a Latino family whose adult child dies of AIDS, the highly regarded value of interdependence, especially if the deceased was estranged, complicates resolution of the death. The AIDS stigma is more devastating because of mutuality within Latino families; an estranged child can be a shameful family issue. Together these factors can impede bereavement by making the loss more painful and difficult to accept.

This short review of the literature highlights some of the issues surrounding grief resulting from HIV/AIDS losses. However, the various populations affected by HIV/AIDS—gay and bisexual men, needle-sharing drug users, blood-product recipients, women, children, people of color—all have unique issues of loss that have not been adequately addressed in the literature. Their concerns relate to the central components of the AIDS stigma, which take on different themes for each population. These themes include homophobia; social condemnation of drug use and abuse; lack of social support, and consequent isolation, for recipients of infected blood products; inadequate resources for and limited access to health care for women; lack of nurturing family and school environments for infants and children; and social and economic oppression for people of color. These issues are difficult to address, especially in combination with the AIDS stigma, which may explain the lack of attention to these issues in the literature. It is difficult for us to understand the grief, fear of death and dying, and the multiple losses experienced by persons with AIDS.

Although traditional bereavement models offer pragmatic approaches to dealing with the grief process, they are not able to address the traumas that result from multiple losses, cumulative grief, HIV/AIDS stigma, and the daily horrors of HIV infection. Individuals and communities living with HIV/AIDS face an inordinate amount of psychological distress. Stressors include a sustained threat to life and physical integrity, threat and harm to loved ones, destruction of the community, and numerous deaths. These descriptions of trauma meet the criteria for *traumata* as defined by the *Diagnostic and Statistical Manual of Mental Disorders* (American Psychiatric Association, 1987). Martin (1988) studied the mental health effects associated with AIDS-related losses in gay men and found traumatic stress responses, such as panic attacks, nightmares, and numbing, to be prevalent. Dilley, Pies, and Helquist (1989) discussed the incredible stresses endured by those affected by HIV/AIDS and how these stresses result in psychic trauma.

Trauma and grief are distinct clinical phenomena. However, because a single event can precipitate both responses, the two are often confused (Spencer & Pynoos, 1985). When this phenomenon is overlooked, intervention and treatment planning may focus too much on bereavement issues as a means of addressing trauma (Singh & Raphael, 1981), thereby risking maladaptive trauma resolution. Coexisting trauma complicates grief work. For these reasons, approaches incorporating both bereavement models and traumatology are needed to serve populations affected by HIV/AIDS.

LOSS AND TRAUMA ISSUES FOR BEREAVED GAY MEN

In the United States, gay and bisexual men still constitute the largest group of persons living with HIV. For more than a decade, this population and its communities have sustained tremendous losses. Although their experience is unique in many ways, their loss and trauma issues may cross over to other AIDS populations and be helpful in developing responsive approaches to AIDS bereavement.

DEVELOPMENTAL ISSUES

Over the past decade, the widespread deaths of people in the prime of life have forced gays and lesbians and their communities to wrestle with issues that are not usually encountered until later in the developmental cycle.

Most people in their twenties and thirties are able to deny death; they are healthy and productive, enjoy sufficient social support, and do not identify with the issues of their elders who are dying. Those affected by HIV/AIDS, however, witness health problems, interruption of productivity, and diminishing social supports. The distance between themselves and death collapses when friends and acquaintances die. Furthermore, the social phenomena of avoiding death and cloaking it in mystery shatter when the reality of death is incorporated into daily life through attending memorial services and providing care for persons who are sick and dying. Kimmel (1980) discusses how early exposure to death can result in developmental changes geared to resolving issues such as mortality, generativity, and the meaning of one's life. Less time is spent working through issues that are normally important for young-to-middle-aged persons: career, relationships, family, life goals. The nearness of death makes time precious. The consequent anxiety can lead to feelings that one must "live fast" or "do it all now." Others may avoid situations that expose their vulnerability to the experience of death.

Denial and avoidance can be healthy coping responses for individuals who are faced with overwhelming life situations. However, if denial obscures reality so that adaptive responses are impaired or unable to develop, problems occur. Thus clinicians need to evaluate carefully the client's situation before confronting the denial and avoidance of those grieving chronic AIDS losses. Their constant adjustments to a grieving process that is continuously interrupted by new losses may require that they be given permission to engage in such defenses.

Another consequence of developmental dysynchronicity (i.e., changes in the life cycle that accelerate developmental issues not typical to a person's age) is an increased intensity of the grief response. In the grieving process, a wide range of conflicting feelings is normal. Fluctuating among feelings of sadness, despair, relief, anger, elation, loneliness, guilt, emptiness, meaninglessness, and meaningfulness may make clients feel as though they are going "crazy." Clinicians need to normalize these experiences. Because the majority of clients have not developed a context into which such devastating losses can be fit, clinicians need to help them develop such a context. Helping clients understand that their contradictory feelings are understandable and normal is a step in this direction.

SURVIVOR GUILT

Clinicians need to help clients develop adaptive responses to their life events and circumstances. Gay males face unique issues with regard to survivor guilt (Odets, 1990). They may wish they had not survived and hope they will not further survive. Guilt complicates bereavement by making it extremely difficult to think and talk about feelings related to surviving loss. It hinders internal coping resources and individuals' connections to external resources. In avoiding the thoughts, feelings, and circumstances related to surviving, gay men experience hopelessness, helplessness, and anxiety, resulting in dysfunctional behaviors and psychological disorders. Odets discusses social isolation among bereaved gay men who wish to avoid additional loss and guilt; the widespread emergence of mood, anxiety, and adjustment disorders due to multiple losses; hypochondriasis as a result of fear of HIV infection; and sexual dysfunction and risky sexual behaviors. Because unprotected sexual behavior is a transmission route for HIV, many gay men may project their survivor guilt onto the sexual act, thus finding it difficult to experience pleasure in the sexual act. Others, who feel hopeless, may engage in unsafe sexual practices. Without access to personal and social resources, gay men are at risk for many psychological and behavioral problems.

Survivor guilt complicates bereavement and trauma resolution by causing nonadaptive numbing. Such numbing can obstruct attempts to address the realities of loss and trauma, to process feelings, and to develop adaptive responses.

TRAUMATIC STRESS, COPING, AND BEREAVEMENT

Traumatic stress studies and coping theory provide explanatory frameworks with which clinicians can address the needs of bereaved gay men that are not addressed by bereavement models. Many of these studies are based on work with combat veterans, survivors of community and natural disasters, and survivors of sexual and violent traumas. Traumatic stress occurs when an individual is overwhelmed by personal and environmental circumstances and lacks adequate supports to address these stressors. Clinical themes include how the individual experiences the stressor, the range of emotional conflicts, and associated symptoms of traumatic stress. For bereaved gay men, these themes are adapted as follows: (1) the stressors are experienced as chronic, immense, extensive, and devastating; (2) the central emotional conflicts involve life and death, sickness and health, intimacy and abandonment issues; (3) symptoms include helplessness, hopelessness, shock, numbness, disbelief, feeling out of control, feeling vulnerable or unsafe, sadness, crying, despair, diffused affect, feeling abandoned, moodiness, excessive worrying, anxiety, panic, hypervigilance, difficulty concentrating, confusion, disturbing images, disturbing memories or dreams, sleep disturbances, irritability, anger, increased risk-taking behaviors, physical fatigue, exhaustion, relationship and family problems, a sense of a foreshortened future, avoidance of thoughts or situations reminiscent of the loss, and recollection of other losses or traumas.

Trauma work involves appraising the traumatic event, understanding its emotional impact, grappling with its meaning, and integrating the experience until adaptive resolution occurs. Both psychodynamic and cognitive processes (Horowitz, 1976; Janoff-Bulman, 1989) and psychosocial issues (Green, Wilson, & Lindy, 1985) are involved.

Coping with HIV/AIDS trauma is complicated by various factors. Appraisal is made difficult by the overwhelming nature of the experience and the formidable task of understanding its emotional impact. Grappling with meaning is obstructed by feelings such as "nobody's left" or "I'm next to get sick and die." Finally, working through these traumas may require deep reexamination of beliefs, which in itself is an overwhelming and disruptive task.

Sowder (1985) discusses other factors that increase the likelihood of maladaptive resolution of trauma, many of which apply to HIV/AIDS trauma: the intense horror of the disease, the length of illness before death, the lack of resources to respond to loss, the perceived loss of control, and the prolonged alteration of lifestyle and environment as a result of the trauma. Gay men often relate the difficulty of dealing with HIV/AIDS over a period of months and years. They often feel out of control as a result of having to deal constantly with sickness and death. Community resources are inadequate. They feel as if their lives have changed fundamentally and that their lives will never be the same as they once were.

In adapting to traumatic experiences, clients need help in integrating their conceptualizations of life events with their conceptualizations of themselves and their world. Persons who experience chronic trauma feel that their lives have been altered and may feel like victims. Janoff-Bulman (1985) reports that life events that make clients feel like victims challenge clients' belief in their personal invulnerability, their self-esteem, and their belief in a meaningful and rational world. Epstein (1989) describes four basic assumptions that are disrupted by trauma: the world is benign, the world is meaningful, the self is worthy, and people are trustworthy. Moreover, clients' reactions to traumatic events are often distorted by changes in their cognitive functioning. These changes may be subtle or shattering, depending on the discrepancy between their cognitive functioning pre- and post-trauma. Such dissonance often causes clients to feel that their life will never be the same as it was before the trauma occurred.

Trauma victims often cope with loss through avoidance behavior, withdrawal, immersion (e.g., into work), substance abuse, and other addictive behaviors. Initially, clients may attempt to maintain the status quo because the familiar is less stressful. (This reaction may partially explain why many gay men lapse into risky sexual behaviors.) Their identification as victims causes them to feel discouraged, immobilized, and vulnerable to other traumatic events as well as post-traumatic distress. Helping clients identify themselves as survivors may alleviate their traumatic anxiety, activate internal resources, and facilitate adaptive appraisal of their situation.

To develop a more resonant fit between self and the world, clients need to find meaning in their trauma (e.g., self-knowledge) (Lyons, 1991). Explanations of life events need not be reality based; in fact, illusory meaning may be more adaptive than having to confront an ambiguous reality (Janoff-Bulman, 1985). It may be difficult for clients to develop a sense of meaning in their lives if the trauma is too harsh or its implications too disturbing. Explanations that do not exactly fit the reality of clients' trauma may, nevertheless, help clients find some meaning for their life and consequently some resolution to their trauma. Such explanations may be useful temporarily until the client is able to withstand a more accurate appraisal of the trauma.

Berube (1989) discusses meanings that clients and the public attribute to AIDS and other disasters:

> When people respond with answers, they are likely to explain why AIDS happens at particular times to particular people and what AIDS teaches us. They can cause harm with definitive answers that keep people from finding their own meanings, blame people for their illnesses, or fill the silences in which people can face their fears and grieve. When people respond to the tragedy of AIDS without answers, they are likely to challenge moral explanations and open up the possibility of wondering, listening and being silent together (p. 1).

Thus, adaptive resolution should be the guiding criterion in helping clients search for meaning in traumatic life events.

Burgess (1975) suggests that victim-oriented thought, such as horror over the manner of death of a loved one, interferes with ego-oriented thought, such as mourning the loss of a loved one. The horrific circumstances of death command more attention than does the death itself. In other words, it is difficult to process reactions to death with coexisting trauma. Spencer and Pynoos (1985)) assert that traumatic anxiety is a priority concern for the ego, compromising the individual's ability to grieve a loss. Alleviation of traumatic anxiety helps clients grieve their loss. Lindy, Green, and Grace (1983) discuss how this approach worked with survivors of the 1977 Beverly Hills Supper Club fire:

> In cases where both . . . trauma and loss were present, working through . . . the overwhelming anxiety of death, feelings of helplessness, shame, as well as defenses protecting against these strong affects, came first. When they were sufficiently dealt with . . . a spontaneous progression seemed to ensue in which the patient was able to take on the as yet not worked through aspects of grief relating to losses in his experience (p. 608).

This approach should be considered in treatment planning for those traumatized by HIV/AIDS losses. It provides a framework from which to address the complex issues presented by this population.

TREATMENT STRATEGIES

Various treatment approaches facilitate adaptive resolution of trauma from HIV/AIDS losses. The discussion that follows is based on my clinical experience working with individuals and groups of gay men dealing with cumulative and multiple HIV-related losses.

Before planning treatment, clinicians need to consider interventions that account for the client's age, gender, culture, and ethnicity. Next, the client's traumatization from HIV/AIDS losses needs to be thoroughly assessed. In addition to standard clinical assessment issues, clinicians should focus on the following issues: (1) the degree, extent, and types of losses; (2) the client's appraisal of the loss-related events and his interpretation of their meaning; (3) the central emotional conflicts represented by the trauma of loss; (4) the impact of the loss on social support systems and client functioning; (5) the impact of the loss on cognitive schemas (cognitive manifestations of psychological needs) of self and the world; (6) defenses used to adapt to the traumatic experience; (7) patterns of symptoms associated with trauma and loss, as well as their frequency and duration; (8) previous and current coping strategies, techniques, and resources; (9) previous loss and trauma-related experiences and how these were resolved; and (10) the client's health status, especially short-term prognosis.

Following this initial assessment, specific treatment goals can be established: (1) developing a meaningful appraisal of the client's traumatic experience of loss; (2) exploring the cognitive, emotional, behavioral, physical, and spiritual/existential consequences of traumatic loss; (3) containing the ambiguities of the experience in order to help the client find meaning within himself and his community; (4) developing ways to integrate resolution of the trauma into the client's experience of self, others, and the world.

The following intervention strategies are helpful in achieving these goals: (1) providing education about the effects of trauma and loss and ways to cope with traumatic stress and the grief process; (2) identifying the traumatic stressors, central emotional conflicts, associated symptoms, and cognitive schemas altered by the trauma; (3) promoting a "common language," or context, to understand the traumatic experience by normalizing responses to trauma and loss; (4) improving existing coping skills and strategies and developing new ones; (5) providing social support and community resource referral.

Clients should be encouraged to explore issues on both the individual and community levels. Such efforts facilitate resolution of altered cognitive schemas by helping clients find ways to match their conceptualizations of self and the world. Such work also addresses psychosocial issues such as homosexuality, homophobia, AIDS phobia, and sexual behaviors. Shifting the client's identity from that of victim to survivor is made easier by developing a context of shared experience whereby clients do not overidentify with traumatic effects.

Effective treatment techniques include the following: (1) repeated storytelling about persons who have died and the circumstances of their deaths; (2) taking an inventory of losses to address the scope of the trauma; (3) working with videos, photographs, and mementos of those who have died; (4) rituals to acknowledge aspects of loss, such as writing letters expressing feelings to those who have died, then symbolically burning them; (5) creating a calendar marking important occasions in the lives of the survivor and persons who have died; (6) expressing the trauma and loss nonverbally (e.g., by drawing representations of one's grief or through music or dance); (7) creating a loss box, a visual container in which names of those lost can be placed to hold the grief so that exposure to it can be controlled by the client; (8) ceremonies whereby the names of those lost or feelings related to the loss are written on materials that can be burned or buried to symbolize "letting go"; (9) guided visualizations and relaxation training to assist clients in relieving traumatic stress symptoms and developing a sense of distance from the trauma and control over their experience; (10) affirmations that facilitate cognitive restructuring (e.g., "It's OK for me to be alive with my grief"); (11) journal writing to identify issues and focus the client on them; (12) bibliotherapy; (13) a humor box with funny quotations, jokes, stories, and cartoons to balance the pain; (14) participation in community events such as candlelight marches and memorials; (15) making a quilt panel for the Names Project; (16) holding anniversary observances of the loved one's death; (17) participation in community activities such as demonstrations and political action. Other methods can be developed, and clinicians should involve clients in creating them.

Clinicians may also ask clients to identify how they survived previously stressful life events and apply such skills and knowledge to their current situations. Some clients in substance-abuse recovery find that the 12-step method helps to contain traumatic loss by providing both a structure and support in wrestling with the meaning of life events. Involving clients in the application of problem-solving methods can help them to reframe and redefine their experience and to develop concrete coping plans. Conducting skill-building and role-playing exercises are also useful.

A skill-building model called the Five Cs—control, connection, commitment, challenge, and compassion—has been used clinically with individuals and groups. This model is based partially on the concept of a "hardy" personality style (Kobasa & Maddi, 1981) and serves as a handy reference for skills that promote adaptive resolution of trauma.

To have *control* is to have a degree of personal power or influence over one's environment. In treatment, clients are encouraged to identify that which is within their control or influence and to let go of that which they are unable to control. Because HIV/AIDS clients often have experienced multiple losses, they are encouraged to evaluate how much, who, when, where, and what they are going to grieve. A sense of control helps clients address their helplessness and vulnerability to events and life experience.

Connection involves having clients identify values that they respect in others and incorporate such values in their own relationships. Clients are encouraged to develop behaviors that generate respect in others so that they can experience common bonds with others. The primary effort here is to develop social supports that buffer the clients' isolation as a result of traumatic experiences.

Commitment addresses existential issues and changes in cognitive functioning by encouraging clients to explore new ways of thinking about the meaning or purpose of their life. Working with metaphors is helpful. For example, a client who is stuck in his or her trauma might be asked to try on new ideas and insights "for size." This effort might be facilitated through the metaphor of shopping for new clothes. The aim here is to help clients make a commitment to life by taking action that involves them with life.

Challenge speaks to the opportunity inherent in any life experience. This does not mean that clients are supposed to put on a "happy face" in the midst of devastating circumstances. Rather, it involves optimistic cognitive appraisal, for example, highlighting the self-knowledge that might be acquired from facing a traumatic experience. Such work helps clients identify themselves as survivors and to accept death as part of the life process.

Compassion focuses on the disillusionment and collapse of the heart, mind, body, and spirit from the experience of multiple, traumatic losses. Clients should be gently encouraged to evaluate how they care for themselves and to correct deficiencies. Clients might be asked to consider the amount and quality of time spent resting, relaxing, exercising, eating healthfully, and socializing. Clients should be encouraged to think about how others can help them with self-care. Such work addresses both the intrapersonal and interpersonal dimensions of grief.

The Five-Cs model helps clients organize their lives in the wake of traumatic experiences and thus clear the way for the grieving process. Certainly, more work is needed to determine the effectiveness of this approach with HIV/AIDS-affected clients.

CLINICIAN'S ROLE

Clinicians need to assume an active, sometimes directive role, while remaining empathic, focused on traumatic themes, and resourceful. Clients should be empowered to define their own situation and experience. To fully understand this role, clinicians need education and training on traumatic stress as it relates to grief and loss. Without it, they will be ill-prepared to respond conceptually and intuitively to the issues presented.

In undertaking this work, clinicians should be aware of their own reactions to clients' traumatic material. McCann and Pearlman (1990) discussed the fundamental changes that can occur in the cognitive schemas of clinicians who work therapeutically with traumatic stress. They applied constructivist self-development theory to understand the long-term psychological effect of working with trauma victims.

This process—"vicarious traumatization"—differs from clinician burnout, which the authors conceptualized as the psychological strain of working with difficult populations. Burnout results from professional isolation, the emotional drain of excessive empathy, ambiguous successes, nonreciprocal giving, and failure to live up to one's own expectations. Certainly, clinicians can experience burnout in work with HIV/AIDS populations: the stigma of AIDS isolates professionals, clients and the issues they present are emotionally demanding, the success of interventions is unclear, and the effect of clinicians' work on the larger social and community issues of HIV/AIDS is difficult to determine. However, working with trauma victims produces an effect different from burnout as a result of exposure to emotionally shocking images of horror and pain.

McCann and Pearlman (1990) also discuss countertransference, which they perceive as an inadequate construct to explain the shifts in cognitive schemas of clinicians from exposure to traumatic material. Countertransference refers to clinicians' unresolved or unconscious conflicts and concerns activated by their work with clients; the focus is on the preexisting personal issues of the clinician. Professionals who have not addressed or resolved personal issues of guilt, rage, horror, grief, loss of control, inability to contain intense emotions, uncertainty, and defenses such as numbing, denial, or avoidance will certainly find HIV/AIDS work extremely demanding. However, in work with HIV/AIDS-affected clients who have suffered multiple losses, clinicians must deal with difficult situations that result from external events as opposed to internal conflict. The interaction between the psychological needs and cognitive schemas of clinicians and the traumatic stressors inherent in external events leads to vicarious traumatization.

Trauma disrupts cognitive schemas and an individual's reaction to trauma depends largely on the significance of the disruption to the individual. Working with trauma survivors can permanently change the ways in which clinicians view themselves and the world. Clinicians need a supportive environment to work through the pain inherent in work with HIV/AIDS-affected clients. McCann and Pearlman (1990) view vicarious traumatization as a normal reaction to stressful and traumatizing work that needs to be monitored by clinicians.

CONCLUSION

Traumatic stress and bereavement models have been useful in work with the traumatic loss issues presented by gay men. Many of these issues are similar to issues presented by other HIV/AIDS groups: AIDS phobia and stigma, multiple losses, the developmental changes that result from early exposure to death, and the impact of facing death on psychological defenses such as denial and avoidance, lack of social support, the fear of progressive HIV-related illnesses, the intensity of the grief response, and survivor guilt. Although the treatment model presented here has not been thoroughly studied and evaluated, in my work with HIV/AIDS clients it has proven helpful. Clinicians need education and training in how traumatic stress relates to HIV/AIDS losses. Moreover, they should monitor their personal reactions to work with populations that have experienced multiple and traumatic losses. Clinicians should consider how differences in culture, ethnicity, age, gender, and sexual orientation shape individuals' reactions to traumatic experiences (e.g., women's cognitive schemas may differ substantially from men's).

Social support as well as the comfort, assistance, and information received formally and informally through individuals and groups can serve as a buffer to the effects of chronic trauma. For HIV/AIDS-affected clients, social support may be less available because of multiple losses in their support network, community devastation, and social stigma. Multiple strategies may be necessary to cope with multiple losses. Self-help and support groups, group therapy, individual and relationship counseling, community forums, educational workshops on grief and loss and on stress and coping, and educational materials made available by the community help alleviate HIV/AIDS-affected clients' sense of isolation and despair. Moreover, professionals need education and training on traumatic stress and loss as they apply to HIV/AIDS issues. Although funding for HIV/AIDS is woefully inadequate, services need to be provided for survivors of this catastrophe.

The Chinese poet Lu Xun (1881–1936) wrote:

> Hope can be neither affirmed nor denied. Hope is like a path in the countryside; originally there was no path. Yet, as people walk all the time in the same spot, a way appears.

Although the trail of HIV/AIDS losses may seem to go nowhere, survivors may find direction in the healing process itself.

REFERENCES

American Psychiatric Association. (1987). *Diagnostic and statistical manual of mental disorders* (3rd ed., rev.). Washington, DC: Author.

Anderson, G. R., Gurdin, P., & Thomas, A. (1989). Dual disenfranchisement: Foster parenting children with AIDS. In K. J. Doka (Ed.), *Disenfranchised grief: Recognizing hidden sorrow* (pp. 43–53). Lexington, MA: Lexington Books.

Berube, A. (1989). AIDS and the meaning of natural disaster. *Focus: A Guide to AIDS Research and Counseling, 5*(1), 1–2.

Bowlby, J. (1960). Grief and mourning in infancy and early childhood. *Psychoanalytic Study of the Child, 15,* 9–52.

Burgess, A. W. (1975). Family reaction to homocide. *American Journal of Orthopsychiatry, 45,* 391–398.

Dick, L. C. (1989). An investigation of the disenfranchised grief of two health care professionals caring for persons with AIDS. In K. J. Doka (Ed.), *Disenfranchised grief: Recognizing hidden sorrow* (pp. 55–65). Lexington, MA: Lexington Books.

Dilley, J., Pies, C., & Helquist, M. (Eds.). (1989). *Face to face: A guide to AIDS counseling.* San Francisco: AIDS Health Project, University of California, San Francisco.

Eisenbruch, I. M. (1984). Cross-cultural aspects of bereavement, I: A conceptual framework for comparative analysis. *Culture, Medicine, and Psychiatry, 8,* 283–309.

Epstein, S. (1989). The self-concept, the traumatic neurosis, and the structure of personality. In D. Ozer, J. M. Healy, Jr., & A. J. Stewart (Eds.), *Perspectives on personality* (vol. 3). Greenwich, CT: JAI Press.

Green, B. L., Wilson, J. P., & Lindy, J. D. (1985). *Conceptualizing post-traumatic stress disorder: A psychosocial framework.* In C. R. Figley (Ed.), *Trauma and its wake* (pp. 53–69). New York: Brunner/Mazel.

Horowitz, M. J. (1976). *Stress response syndromes.* New York: Jason Aronson.

Janoff-Bulman, R. (1985). The aftermath of victimization: Rebuilding shattered assumptions. In C. R. Figley (Ed.), *Trauma and its wake* (pp. 15–35). New York: Brunner/Mazel.

Janoff-Bulman, R. (1989). Assumptive worlds and the stress of traumatic events: Applications of the schema construct. *Social Cognition, 7*(2), 113–136.

Klein, S. J., & Fletcher, W., III (1986). Gay grief: An examination of its uniqueness brought to light by the AIDS crisis. *Journal of Psychosocial Oncology, 4*(3), 15–25.

Kimmel, D. C. (1980). *Adulthood and aging* (2nd ed.) New York: John Wiley.

Kobasa, S. C., & Maddi, S. R. (1981). Personality and constitution as mediators in the stress-illness relationship. *Journal of Health and Social Behavior, 22*, 368–378.

Kübler-Ross, E. (1969). *On death and dying.* New York: Macmillan.

Lindemann, E. (1944). Symptomatology and management of acute grief. *American Journal of Psychiatry, 101*(2), 141–148.

Lindy, J. D., Green, B. L., & Grace, M. (1983). Psychotherapy with survivors of the Beverly Hills Supper Club fire. *American Journal of Psychotherapy, 37*, 593–610.

Lyons, J. A. (1991). Strategies for assessing the potential for positive adjustment following trauma. *Journal of Traumatic Stress Studies, 4*(1), 93–111.

Martin, J. L. (1988). The impact of AIDS-related deaths and illnesses on gay men in New York City. *Focus: A Guide to AIDS Research, 3*(7), 1–2.

McCann, I. L., & Pearlman, L. A. (1990). Vicarious traumatization: A framework for understanding the psychological effects of working with victims. *Journal of Traumatic Stress, 3*(1), 131–149.

Meyer, P. (1991, Fall). Too much grief. *Lavender Reader: News and Review for Santa Cruz County's Gay and Lesbian Community*, pp. 26–27.

Monette, P. (1988). *Borrowed time.* New York: Harcourt Brace Jovanovich.

Odets, W. (1990). *The psychological epidemic: The impact of AIDS on uninfected gay and bisexual men.* Unpublished manuscript, Oakland, CA.

San Francisco Examiner. (1992, January 26), p. 1.

Schindelman, E., & Schoen, K. (1988). Gay and grieving: Bringing grief out of the closet. In M. Shernoff & W. Scott (Eds.), *The sourcebook on lesbian and gay healthcare* (2nd ed.). Washington, DC: National Gay and Lesbian Healthcare Foundation.

Shearer, P., & McKusick, L. (1986). Counseling survivors. In L. McKusick (Ed.), *What to do about AIDS* (pp. 163–169). Berkeley, CA: University of California Press.

Singh, B., & Raphael, B. (1981). Postdisaster morbidity of the bereaved. *Journal of Nervous and Mental Disorders, 169*, 203–212.

Sowder, B. J. (1985). *Disasters and mental health: Selected contemporary perspectives.* Rockville, MD: National Institute of Mental Health.

Spencer, E., & Pynoos, R. (1985). Interaction of trauma and grief in childhood. *Progress in Psychiatry Series 1985.* Washington, DC: American Psychiatric Press.

Staudacher, C. (1987). *Beyond grief: A guide for recovering from the death of a loved one.* Oakland, CA: New Harbinger Publications.

Worden, J. W. (1982). *Grief counseling and grief therapy: A handbook for the mental health practitioner.* New York: Springer.

17

HIV AND THE LAW:
THE EMPOWERMENT OF THE INDIVIDUAL AND THE SYSTEM
MARK S. SENAK

In any medical care setting today, the importance of legal and ethical issues surrounding medical treatment is second only to the medical treatment and procedures themselves. And the importance of legal and ethical issues has become more apparent than ever with the advent of the HIV epidemic. AIDS has brought about monumental changes in our medical system and the way we administer care. Although traditionally the legal system has supported the changes and developments in the nation's medical system, the startling changes wrought by AIDS have strained society's ability to respond adequately. Now more than ever, professionals, patients, and their families need legal and ethical guidelines that offer clear and rational support for our public health care policies. Under the circumstances of the rapidly changing AIDS epidemic, we are experiencing a crisis in the legal and ethical community as well as in the health care community.

Advances in medical science frequently pose problematic issues for the legal and ethical community. When science resolves a medical dilemma, it often opens up new ethical debate from which legislation must flow. For example, although medical researchers have discovered benefits in placing fetal tissue in the brains of persons with Parkinson's disease, serious ethical questions surround the procedure.

The pressures brought to bear on ethics due to the HIV epidemic are twofold: (1) conflicts arise from diseases associated with sex, death, and drugs and (2) conflicts arise as a consequence of advances in medical treatment and science. For example, a notable advance was the development of the HIV antibody test. Licensed in 1985 for the purpose of screening the nation's blood supply for HIV antibodies (not HIV itself) (Scherzer, 1987), the medical community perceived the test as a solution to society's helplessness in the face of the virus. However, when testing proceeds without legal restraint or ethical consideration, it can affect the insurability, job status, and housing of individuals who are tested (Senak, 1988). Thus the test can undermine rather than enhance our ability to combat the epidemic.

More recently, uses of the test and its derivations, such as home testing kits and saliva and urine testing, have caused legal and ethical concerns regarding easy testing and testing of body fluids other than blood. Such innovations also raise ethical issues of surreptitious testing or testing without counseling. These scientific advances can severely strain our ability to respond to legal and ethical dilemmas according to clear guidelines. Developments in the AIDS epidemic do not occur in a medical or scientific vacuum but have serious consequences in the legal, social, and ethical realms. Thus, it is important to distinguish what the law can do and what an ethical code can accomplish.

Ideally, with the progression of the epidemic and accompanying advances in medical science, our ethical code should evoke a legal response to each medical development. Ethics reflects the values of our society and defines societal principles of right and wrong conduct. In many instances, societal values may not be immediately clear to policymakers, as in the case of fetal tissue for treatment of Parkinson's disease mentioned above.

The law, on the other hand, embodies society's ethical values in a code of enforcement. The law reflects ethics, and ethics in turn reflects our values. Medical and scientific developments create ethical dilemmas that interact with legal precedents. Whereas the medical problems posed by the AIDS epidemic demand immediate actions and solutions, these actions and solutions can create complex problems for our legal and ethical systems.

Nevertheless, with the considerable advances in medical science, the legal system has also responded to the HIV/AIDS epidemic. In the past few years, virtually hundreds of laws have been proposed to various state legislatures of the nation that address some aspect of HIV (Senak, 1991). These proposed laws vary from Alabama's approval of Medicaid coverage for AZT treatment to sophisticated testing issues in other states (Senak, 1991). Many jurisdictions have enacted confidentiality laws that prohibit disclosure of a person's antibody status to third parties. Supported by antidiscrimination legislation, these laws protect the rights of individuals who might otherwise suffer severe social and economic consequences. Many legislatures throughout the United States have also reacted to this protective infrastructure by proposing legislation aimed at mandatory testing of health care workers and patients.

In debate over such legislation, discussion of the issues often pits the rights of the infected against the rights of the uninfected. This polemic clouds ethical issues with emotional argument. For example, in the case of the transmission of HIV from an infected Florida dentist to five of his patients, debate has centered on the question of whether health care workers should be tested (Brennan, 1991). The charged emotional context of such debate weakens our ability to make rational decisions and ultimately results in laws that fail to support our public health care policies. Discussion of HIV and the law must view the epidemic in terms of how the individual is affected by laws and how those laws in turn might affect the health care provider and public health care system. Ethical debates should not pit one sector of the population against another but seek a fair solution and support a sound public health care policy. Ideally, ethics should be the driving force in any legislative development in health care. This chapter examines ethical issues that have arisen in the wake of the HIV epidemic. Legal considerations deriving from these ethical issues are subsequently discussed.

THE DEVELOPMENT OF HIV ETHICS

Even before the discovery of HIV as a viral agent, the legal implications of the disease that came to be known as AIDS began to surface. Fear ran rampant, and during the period when the disease was called GRIDS (gay-related immune deficiency syndrome), legal and ethical crises occurred in a setting of medical ignorance. The public knew only that a communicable and deadly disease existed and that the disease was capable of achieving epidemic proportions through the sexual practices and drug use of groups of people who traditionally were disenfranchised by society. In the presence of so many taboos and prejudices, the environment was hostile to any rational decision-making process.

THE "FIRST" HIV ETHICS CRISIS

Ethical dilemmas share common themes. Perhaps the first instance of an HIV-related ethical dilemma might be traced, hypothetically, to a city hospital in New York, San Francisco, or Los Angeles in 1981. An attendant wearing gloves, gown, mask, and headcover leaves a breakfast tray on the floor of the hallway, well out of reach of an AIDS patient. The breakfast gets cold. Driven by the fear of the unknown, that simple act, or refusal to act, is the basis for every ethical dilemma that has occurred since then. Fear is a rational reaction in the presence of danger that can, however, lead to irrational acts, as indicated by the above illustration. This hypothetical situation contains all of the essential components of the ethical dilemmas presented by HIV: a patient with AIDS, knowledge of others that the patient has AIDS, fear of AIDS contagion, and a decision to act or not act based on the needs of the caregiver (or other third party) and not the patient.

To extend this hypothetical situation, perhaps the patient's family and friends were afraid to hug him when he was discharged from the hospital. His siblings refused to let him see his nieces and nephews. During a later hospitalization, he became incontinent and no one would clean him. Even in death, he was discriminated against when one funeral home would not take his body and another charged his family "extra" for burial.

The ethical issues suggested here have not yet been entirely resolved, although the law has addressed many of them. Basic fears still surround care of a person with AIDS and create ethical dilemmas for our legal and health care systems.

ANTIBODY TESTING

The HIV antibody test has probably given rise to more ethical dilemmas and has stimulated more legislation than any other issue in the AIDS epidemic (Gostin, Curran, & Clark, 1987). Questions regarding whom to test, when to test, how to test,

255

and who has the right to know the results of the test galvanized attention from all sectors of society. Legislatures, many of whom are ill informed, create policies in an emotionally charged atmosphere that are then carried into the health care setting. Arguments that advocate mandatory testing policies, although on the whole unsuccessful, have arisen in virtually all health care settings, leaving the American public confused.

Originally, the HIV antibody test was developed for the purpose of screening the nation's blood supply, not the population. But because no vaccine or new drugs were available to combat the disease, the test was quickly perceived as the only tool that health care providers could use to battle HIV in a variety of settings. Thus, the test quickly became a cornerstone of our public health care policy. That policy encourages people to come forward voluntarily for testing, learn their status, obtain medical care if they test positive, engage in safer sexual and/or needle-sharing practices, and thereby stem the flow of transmission. Testing backed up by counseling and drug treatment was the best policy we could hope for given the circumstances.

Nevertheless, with the advent of testing, abuses occurred. Many insurance companies began testing for HIV antibodies with or without the consent or knowledge of the individual (Senak, 1991). In many jurisdictions, testing without consent violates the law of informed consent, which is designed to protect patients from medical procedures that are unwarranted. Moreover, insurance companies did not always keep test results confidential. As a result, people lost their insurance, jobs, homes, and family relationships. Moreover, a new class of "uninsurables" was created through insurance companies' practice of testing potential clients for HIV.

These practices also set the dangerous precedent of testing for health conditions that may or may not develop over time. This precedent is particularly troublesome because of advances in genetic science, whereby genetic predictor tests are or will soon be available to test people for latent genetic defects that may cause disorders such as Alzheimer's disease. If insurance companies are able to require applicants to undergo such testing, fewer people will be able to obtain medical insurance and will be forced to shoulder high medical costs. Clearly, such issues present profound ethical problems.

ACCESS TO HEALTH CARE

The loss of insurability points to one of the most potent ethical debates to emerge from the HIV epidemic. The issue of access to medical treatment is much broader than the HIV crisis and affects our entire system of health care. Although testing and medical-procedures issues will continue to be debated as we attempt to set policies for HIV and health care, conflicts will continue to arise on many fronts if society fails to provide everyone with equal access to health care services. For example, placement of fetal tissue in the brain of a Parkinson's disease victim may be an ethical and desirable health care practice. If, however, only the insured or wealthy are able to afford this technique, ethical issues arise.

As more HIV-infected persons become ill and the burden of the illness shifts demographically to economically disenfranchised populations, our public health care system is experiencing severe strain. The inadequacies of the Medicaid system indicate the need for a national response to these health care problems. Moreover, our failure to develop ethical responses to these problems will result in increased financial strain on the taxpayer.

DEVELOPMENT OF AIDS LAW

EARLY LAW

Because laws are often outgrowths of ethical dilemmas, the history of AIDS law parallels that of ethical crises. In the days of GRIDS, the general public knew little about the disease. Public awareness of transmission routes was evident only in those geographic areas where AIDS was prevalent. As the number of AIDS patients increased, many lawyers volunteered time to assist patients in writing their deathbed wills.

As the epidemic spread, medical and legal issues became more complex. Legal issues affecting health care providers ranged from one's duty to diagnose and treat a patient to issues of confidentiality and breaches thereof, all of which have a significant impact on the way physicians and hospitals deliver and report on medical care (Bayer, 1991).

For persons with AIDS during the mid-1980s, it seemed that their financial and social support network was eroding faster than their immune system. Before AZT and other medical interventions, persons with AIDS lived for a shorter period and in worse health than they do today. In the mid-1980s, people were diagnosed with AIDS and became legal clients almost at the same point at which they became medical patients, whereas today many people are diagnosed as being HIV positive early in the disease process and thus have time to sort out legal and health care options.

The law is designed to respect legally sanctioned relationships. Because the first AIDS cases were primarily gay men, estranged families often appeared when a patient died, taking the belongings not only of the deceased but of the surviving lover as well. Moreover, the surviving lover often lost his job and insurance when it was discovered that he had had a relationship with someone who had died of AIDS. Thus, a circle of discrimination was drawn around gay white men. As the epidemic progressed, lawyers who attempted to write wills for clients with AIDS discovered that their clients' problems were more complicated than bar-exam questions. Clients often had little property because they had lost their jobs as a result of discrimination. They were threatened with eviction and, once they were placed on disability income, plagued by creditors. To force the law to respect same-sex relationships, the gay community had to obtain legal help. In addition, the gay community's need for legal services increased as more and more persons lost their jobs because of their disease.

Whereas a will becomes effective when a person dies, power of attorney may operate while the person is alive. Power of attorney delegates legal authority for a person's affairs to another individual. For example, if an individual is unable to handle his or her finances, he or she can delegate check-signing authority to another. Power of attorney can be drawn up broadly (I appoint John Doe to do anything I can do) or narrowly (I appoint John Doe to sign check number 101 in an amount not to exceed $100). Many persons with AIDS signed a medical power of attorney, thus appointing another individual to make medical decisions for them. This addressed the needs of many persons with AIDS, who in the early days of the epidemic had been abandoned by families and friends. These instruments were initiated on a widespread basis, and many states adopted measures to formalize the procedures.

Many power of attorneys were signed before the discovery of HIV (Senak, 1988). The discovery of HIV confirmed many of the worst fears of the gay community. Because the disease was viral in nature it was communicable. At issue was whether a communicable disease would be recognized as a disability by local, state, and federal antidiscrimination laws.

Gay white men with AIDS were not the only persons feeling the burden of discrimination; so too did the women and children who were close to them. Discrimination cases increased, many of which involved persons who, for one reason or another, were perceived to have AIDS. For example, children were forced out of schools because a family member had been diagnosed with AIDS.

As the circle of discrimination widened, so too did the net of antidiscriminatory statutes protecting persons with disabilities. Statutes at the federal level and at most state levels prohibited discrimination against persons with disabilities; such statutes were expanded to cover persons with AIDS. Moreover, such statutes were expanded to protect persons from discrimination based on the perception of a disability (Leonard, 1987). Thus, if an employer believed an employee had AIDS because of the employee's weight loss, sexual preference, or symptomatology and the employer acted in a discriminatory fashion, the employee was protected by statutes whether or not he or she had AIDS. The carryover of protection from persons who were actually symptomatic of HIV to those who were perceived to have HIV was one of the first developments in AIDS law that directly benefited women and children.

In 1984, as the demographics of the disease began to shift radically in New York City, another emerging need became apparent. Like gay men who had lost everything but still made wills in order to protect an unmarried partner, women with little or no property found themselves making wills to express their custody preferences for their children. This was the case particularly for women living in poor urban areas who had been injection drug users or the sexual partners of injection drug users. As AIDS made inroads further into society, whole families died of the disease. Children who were the subject of their mother's will with respect to custody found themselves the subject of yet a second will written by their new custodians who were also dying of AIDS.

LEGAL ISSUES FOR THE HEALTH CARE PROVIDER

The legal issues that beset individuals with AIDS spilled over to affect health care providers. As the number of uninsured people increased, fewer patients were able to pay their medical bills. Discrimination often resulted from widespread knowledge of HIV-antibody status. Due to lack of HIV/AIDS training, physicians failed to diagnose AIDS-related conditions, resulting in liability for such physicians. Public fear flared when the first cases of HIV transmission from health care worker to patient were reported, resulting in proposals for mandatory testing supported by criminal sanctions for health care workers (Altman, 1991).

THE NEED FOR CONFIDENTIALITY

With regard to issues of discrimination in the workplace, places of public accommodation, housing, and loss of insurance, confidentiality has far-reaching effects. Without confidentiality, health care policies that encourage at-risk individuals to come forward voluntarily for antibody testing are compromised. Thus, legislation has been introduced in many jurisdictions to protect the confidentiality of individuals who wish to be tested (Wood, Marks, & Dilley, 1990). Typically, such legislation makes it illegal to inform another person of a tested individual's positive status for HIV antibodies without the tested person's consent (Wood et al., 1990). The purpose of such legislation is not to protect one group's rights over another's, but rather to encourage people to be tested.

Such legislation has been difficult to draft, requiring a delicate balance between confidentiality and the occasional need to breach such confidentiality. In the purest sense, such statutes would not permit any disclosure of HIV status to another individual without the signed permission of the HIV-positive person. Because this is not practical in health care settings, exceptions that allow health care professionals to share antibody-status information in the course of treatment are generally made.

Confidentiality may also be breached, depending on the jurisdiction, when the physician or health care provider is treating a patient he or she knows to be intransigent when it comes to issues of safer sexual or safer needle-sharing practices. For example, in California, physicians *may* breach confidentiality, though they are not required to do so, when they know that the tested individual refuses to take safety precautions, thus transmitting the virus to a known third party. The California statute requires a physician to (1) counsel the client regarding safer sex and needle sharing and (2) inform the sexual or needle-sharing partner of the risk without identifying the patient or (3) inform the county health department (again without identifying information with respect to the patient), who then notifies the sexual or needle-sharing partner of the patient (Wood et al., 1990).

In California, no other exceptions to confidentiality are permitted. Sharing of test results usually requires the written permission of the patient. Issues concerning written consent and informed consent make charting of medical history difficult for health care providers. Policies regarding charting methods within a particular institution are best accomplished by multidisciplinary teams that include nurses, physicians, and legal representatives.

TESTING IN THE HEALTH CARE SETTING

Patients' interests are best served by taking an initial HIV test in an anonymous setting. Anonymous testing is much different from confidential testing, though the two are often confused. Confidential testing means that the agency performing the testing promises to keep the results secret. This type of testing, however, is subject to legislative whim; whereas one legislature may protect the results, another legislature may overturn such policies. With anonymous testing, the identity of the patient is never known.

MANDATORY TESTING OF PATIENTS

Demands for mandatory testing have come from various sectors of society. Understandably, medical societies and physician's groups sometimes call for mandatory testing or routine screening of hospital patients. In urban areas, particularly where the virus is rampant, physicians seek to know the HIV status of patients. A hospital in New Jersey recently reported that 7% of its patients were HIV positive. In hospital settings in which a significant number of patients are HIV positive, physicians often ask for routine screening, especially prior to invasive procedures.

Although such requests appear reasonable, in the long run the repercussions of routine hospital testing could be quite dangerous. Routine testing allows health care professionals to rely on test results, some of which may be false negatives, and thus employ fewer general precautions against unconfirmed infectious disease, thus increasing the risk of HIV transmission. In addition, such testing represents a departure from the way medicine has been practiced. Traditionally, tests have been performed for the benefit of the patient, not the physician. It is illegal and unethical for a physician to order an HIV test to determine whether to treat a particular patient. Moreover, a negative antibody test does not ensure the absence of infection or ensure that transmission is not possible, in that false negatives occur and HIV antibodies may have not yet formed.

TESTING OF HEALTH CARE WORKERS

Testing of health care workers has been an extremely controversial issue. From a public health standpoint, testing of health care workers does not provide the security one might assume it does. A person can test negative when he or she is in fact positive. To be truly effective, testing would have to be performed daily. Regardless of antibody status, if proper infection-control procedures are established and followed, transmission will not occur. Nevertheless, public fear of HIV/AIDS has created an outcry for testing, rather than for strict adherence to infection-control procedures, despite the fact that more health benefits flow from the latter. Infection does not occur because someone is antibody positive, but because transmission was allowed to occur. The public's perception of the antibody test is that it is an "AIDS test" as opposed to an antibody test and that testing is the only tool we have for battling AIDS.

The transmission of HIV from a Florida dentist to five of his patients, the only documented transmission of HIV by a health care worker in the past 10 years, has resulted in public discourse via the talk-show circuit rather than responsible debate by public health care professionals. Again, by focusing on extreme cases, we increase public fear and fail to confront the real problem of developing good procedures for infection control.

To put this controversy in context, more known cases of transmission of HIV 2, a deadly strain of virus similar to the HIV we know to cause AIDS, have occurred in the general population than have cases of HIV transmission from health care worker to patient. The antibody test for HIV 2 is different from that for HIV, and an "AIDS test" does not reveal the presence of HIV 2. Rather, a second test must be performed. Yet, we do not test people for HIV 2 nor do we test the nation's blood supply for HIV 2. This decision is based on cost. It makes more sense to allocate our resources for thorough testing of the nation's blood supply (Gostin et al., 1987) rather than for mandatory testing of health care workers, among whom only five cases of transmission have been documented.

CRIMINALIZATION OF HIV TRANSMISSION

Supporters of mandatory testing of health care workers have even included proposals at the federal level to make it a crime punishable by imprisonment for a health care worker to continue working after discovering his or her HIV status. In addition, various jurisdictions have proposed laws, which for the most part have been passed, that make willful transmission of HIV a crime. For example, when a person with HIV knowingly engages in unprotected sexual relations with another without revealing his or her HIV status first, he or she will be held criminally liable.

Obviously, the knowing transmission of HIV is morally reprehensible. However, when designing legislation, we must evaluate the laws that *are not* passed as well as laws that are passed. For example, legislation requiring mandatory HIV education for school children is mired in controversy, despite the fact that AIDS is the sixth leading cause of death among adolescents in the United States and by the year 2000 will be the leading cause of death. If our goal is public health, legislation that will help save the most lives should be made a priority. Although criminalization of willful transmission of HIV will punish a few people, it is not likely to save a single life. Persons who knowingly transmit HIV are not likely to be easily swayed by criminal statutes because they have little left to lose. Moreover, mental health measures already exist in many jurisdictions that allow restraint of persons who present a danger to themselves or others.

CONCLUSION

HIV/AIDS has had an incredible impact on our legal system. With the exception of the Great Depression of 1929, probably no other event of this century has evoked so much legislation, and certainly no other event has generated so much heated controversy in the public health arena. Although society is faced with an urgent need to find solutions to large and troubling problems connected with AIDS, our decisions must take into consideration competing and complex sets of values and the ethical repercussions on society. Our efforts to create good public health care policy to battle HIV are often clouded by our fear of sex, death, and drugs.

Until we become more concerned about saving lives rather than punishing them, we will continue to lose the battle against AIDS.

REFERENCES

Altman, L. (1991, July 16). AIDS tests urged for many doctors. *New York Times*.

Bayer, R. (1991). AIDS: The right to care, the right to privacy. In J. Mukand (Ed.), *Rehabilitation for patients with HIV* (pp. 425–436). New York: McGraw-Hill.

Brennan, T. A. (1991). Transmission of the human immunodeficiency virus in the health care setting—time for action. *New England Journal of Medicine, 325*, 1504–1507.

Gostin, L. O., Curran, W., & Clark, M. (1987). The case against compulsory casefinding in controlling AIDS, testing, screening and reporting. *American Journal of Law and Medicine, 12*(1), 7–53.

Leonard, A. S. (1987). AIDS in the workplace. In H. Dalton & S. Burris (Eds.), *AIDS and the law* (pp. 109–125). New Haven, CT: Yale University Press.

Scherzer, M. (1987). Insurance. In H. Dalton & S. Burris (Eds.), *AIDS and the law* (pp. 185–200). New Haven, CT: Yale University Press.

Senak, M. (1988). Legal issues facing AIDS patients. In K. Blanchet (Ed.), *AIDS: A health care management response* (pp. 99–115). Rockville, MD: Aspen Publishers.

Senak, M. (1991). The legal and ethical aspects of HIV infection. In J. Mukand (Ed.), *Rehabilitation for patients with HIV disease* (pp. 437–449). New York: McGraw-Hill.

Wood, G. J., Marks, R., & Dilley, J. W. (1990). Confidentiality. In *AIDS for mental health professionals* (pp. 15–49). The AIDS Health Project, University of California, San Francisco.

18

MEDICAL ISSUES IN HIV-RELATED ILLNESS

PAUL D. HOLTOM

Since the AIDS epidemic was first recognized in 1981, clinicians have been faced with two treatment tasks: (1) the therapy of the primary disease caused by human immunodeficiency virus (HIV) infection and (2) therapy for infections related to the immune deficiency caused by HIV infection. These infections are termed *opportunistic* because they are caused by organisms that do not usually cause disease in humans with intact immune systems but take advantage of a host with impaired immunity. Cases of AIDS were defined by these opportunistic infections before the HIV virus was discovered. The Centers for Disease Control's definition of AIDS cases focuses primarily on the development of these previously uncommon infections or tumors in people with no other known cause for immune-system suppression.

Since the first reports of *Pneumocystis carinii* pneumonia occurring in young otherwise healthy men (Gottlieb et al., 1981; Masur et al., 1981), physicians have been challenged to develop new therapies for diseases that were previously rare and for which effective therapies were unknown. Progress has been made in developing therapies for some infections, and many new drugs have been developed and introduced into practice, such as zidovudine (AZT), didanosine (ddI), fluconazole, ganciclovir, and foscarnet. Other infections have been treated with drugs that had been already released, and many investigational agents may soon be released for use (dideoxycytidine and itraconazole). Common opportunistic conditions seen in AIDS are listed in Table 1, together with the current therapies used for them. Despite the introduction of AZT and ddI, both of which may slow progression of HIV infection, truly effective therapy for the underlying immunodeficiency has not yet been found. For diseases such as the diarrhea caused by cryptosporidiosis, no effective therapy is available; for other infections, such as those caused by *Mycobacterium avium-intracellulare* and cytomegalovirus, drugs are available to ameliorate the infection but not to cure it. Much research remains to be done to develop better and more effective therapies for practically all the opportunistic infections associated with AIDS.

TABLE 1. Common opportunistic conditions of AIDS.

Causative Agent	Location of Disease	Symptoms of Condition	Methods of Diagnosis	Types of Therapy	Comments
Pneumocystis carinii	Lungs, rarely other organs	Cough, fever, shortness of breath	Chest X-ray, sputum exam, bronchoscopy with BAL	TMP-SMX (trimethoprim-sulfamethoxazole), pentamidine	Prophylactic therapy decreases rate of recurrence
Kaposi sarcoma (cause unknown)	Skin, mouth, gastrointestinal tract, lungs, other organs	Visible lesion, swelling of legs, pneumonia, abdominal pain	Biopsy of skin or other organs	Local: radiation, intralesional injection; chemotherapy	
Bacteria					
Mycobacterium tuberculosis Tuberculosis	Lungs, brain (meningitis) bone marrow, liver, spine, intestines	Cough, fever, weight loss, shortness of breath; varies with other organs	Chest X-ray, sputum exam, cultures of affected organs	Effective: isoniazid + rifampin + pyrazinamide (+ ethambutol)	Communicable to others; often confused with MAC until cultures come back
Mycobacterium avium-intracellulare (MAI or MAC)	Lungs, blood, liver, bone marrow, gastrointestinal tract	Fever, night sweats, weight loss, weakness, diarrhea, abdominal pain	Cultures from blood, stool, bone marrow, or other organs	None completely effective: rifampin, ethambutol, clofazimine ciprofloxacin, amikacin	Not contagious; may be present in more than half of patients with AIDS
Treponema pallidum Syphilis	Skin, brain (meningitis), multiple other organs	Often has no symptoms; initially with chancre (meningitis has fever, headache, stiff neck)	Blood test (serology), lumbar puncture	Penicillin; best regimen not known	
Other bacteria	Lungs, sinuses, skin	Depends on site involved	Cultures, X-rays	Standard therapy depending on organism	Chronic sinusitis is common
Viruses					
Cytomegalovirus	Retinitis (eye), lungs,	Decreased vision/blindness,	Eye examination, cultures	Ganciclovir (DHPG),	Drugs can be

	Sites affected	Symptoms	Diagnosis	Treatment	Comments
	gastrointestinal tract, brain, other organs	diarrhea, abdominal pain, confusion, fevers	of blood, urine, stool	foscarnet	given only intravenously
Varicella-zoster	Skin, other organs	Shingles: skin rash, pain, fever	Examination of rash, cultures	Acyclovir	
JC virus	Brain	PML (progressive multifocal leukoencephalopathy); confusion, paralysis	Clinical findings, brain biopsy	None known	Progressive deterioration; death in less than 3 months
FUNGI					
Candida albicans	Mouth (thrush), esophagus, skin, blood	Mouth pain, loss of taste, pain on swallowing, fevers	Clinical exam, cultures, endoscopy	Nystatin liquid, clotrimazole, fluconazole tablets	Thrush is not an AIDS-defining illness
Cryptococcus neoformans	Lungs, brain, blood, skin	Headache, fever, confusion	Lumbar puncture, blood cultures, blood antigen level	Amphotericin B, flucytosine (5-FC), fluconazole	Disease may recur after therapy; lifelong maintenance therapy with fluconazole
Histoplasma capsulatum	Lungs, bone marrow, liver/spleen, brain, other organs	Fever, weakness, abdominal pain	Blood culture, biopsy of affected organ	Amphotericin B	Lifelong maintenance therapy
PROTOZOA					
Toxoplasma gondii	Brain (encephalitis), eyes (retinitis)	Confusion, seizures, strokes, blindness	CT scan or MRI, brain biopsy, blood titers	Pyrimethamine and sulfadiazine	Lifelong maintenance therapy
Cryptosporidium	Gastrointestinal tract	Diarrhea	Stool exam	Symptomatic therapy only; no specific therapy	
Isospora belli	Gastrointestinal tract	Diarrhea	Stool exam	TMP-SMX (trimethoprim-sulfamethoxazole)	

The following sections focus on current therapies for some of the most common opportunistic conditions associated with AIDS. Treatment of these infections is constantly evolving, and new agents will be introduced in the coming years that will make many of the current therapies obsolete as well as provide therapies for conditions that are now without effective treatments.

HUMAN IMMUNODEFICIENCY VIRUS

An array of diseases result from HIV infection. Approximately six weeks after infection, a person may develop an illness that resembles infectious mononucleosis, which can last for several weeks. Most people will then go for many years without developing any symptoms from the virus, which is nonetheless present and causing subtle changes in the immune system. Eventually, more severe symptoms such as persistent swollen lymph nodes, fevers, night sweats, and thrush (a fungal infection in the mouth) occur. As immune system function further deteriorates, opportunistic infections occur. The syndrome of AIDS is defined by the occurrence of an opportunistic infection as defined by the Centers for Disease Control (CDC).

In addition to opportunistic infections, HIV causes various clinical symptoms (see Table 2), including a progressive neurological deterioration termed HIV encephalopathy or AIDS dementia. Ninety percent of patients with AIDS have cognitive, affective, and psychomotor disturbances (McArthur, 1987). Dementia can be the presenting symptom in a person with AIDS. It has a major impact on patients' ability to care for themselves as well as their ability to follow instructions, comply with therapy, and make decisions regarding their medical care.

The need for developing an effective drug to treat HIV was clear from the dismal survival rates of patients with AIDS in the early 1980s. The one-year survival rate for AIDS patients in New York City between 1981 and 1985 was less than 45% for patients initially presenting with *Pneumocystis carinii* pneumonia, less than 72% for those presenting with Kaposi sarcoma, but less than 39% for patients with other AIDS-defining illnesses (Rothenberg, Woelfel, Stoneburner, Milberb, Parker, & Trumen, 1987).

The development of AZT, the first drug approved by the Food and Drug Administration (FDA) to treat HIV, was a major advance in the management of patients with AIDS. The use of AZT in patients with AIDS or AIDS-related complex (ARC) was shown to be effective both in decreasing mortality and in decreasing the number of opportunistic infections (Fischl et al., 1987). These results led to recommendations that all patients with AIDS be started on AZT.

Unfortunately, AZT therapy has been associated with considerable toxicity. Patients often report nausea, vomiting, myalgias (muscle aches), and severe headaches while using the drug. The major toxicity is bone-marrow suppression, leading to anemia (often requiring transfusions) and leukopenia (low white-blood-cell count). Toxic effects from AZT occur frequently; in one clinical trial 45% of the patients had to have their AZT dose reduced or stopped due to side effects (Richman et al., 1987). For this reason, trials have been done with reduced doses, and a recent

TABLE 2. MANIFESTATIONS OF INFECTION WITH HIV.

Acute retroviral syndrome: an acute mononucleosis-like illness
Persistent generalized lymphadenopathy
Wasting syndrome
Anemia; low platelet count
Constitutional symptoms: fevers, night sweats, fatigue
Diarrhea
Arthralgias and arthritis
Peripheral neuropathy: pain, numbness, and occasionally weakness
Muscle pain, tenderness, weakness
Dementia or encephalopathy

study has shown that 500 mg per day (one-half the original recommended dose) was at least as effective as the higher dose and was less toxic (Fischl, Parker, Pettinelli, et al., 1990). New trials are being conducted with even lower doses.

Some newer drugs for HIV infection are being developed. Didanosine (ddI) has been released for treatment of HIV in patients who are unable to take AZT. Although it is generally better tolerated than is AZT, toxic side effects such as peripheral neuropathies and pancreatitis have been noted. Dideoxycytidine (ddC) is currently undergoing clinical trials and may soon be released by the FDA. Neither of these drugs, however, has been shown to be more effective than AZT. Clinical trials are also investigating the effectiveness of combinations of AZT and ddI or ddC to determine whether such combinations are more effective than AZT alone.

Although progress in the field of antiretroviral drugs (drugs effective against HIV) has been exciting, it has also led to frustration and uncertainty among patients. Many clinical trials are in progress; as the results become available, treatment recommendations change. Patients naturally feel frustrated that no absolute answer exists to their questions concerning the best treatments for their disease. They do not want to wait several years for trials to be completed. Some patients react to these frustrations by abandoning traditional medicine and using vitamins or herbal medications. Others obtain experimental drugs through "buyers' clubs." Such actions can lead to difficulties if patients do not inform their physicians about the drugs they are taking so that their treatment can be monitored properly. Other patients, however, often agree to participate in ongoing clinical trials, which contributes to our medical knowledge of HIV.

When it was shown that AZT was effective in treating patients with AIDS, the question arose as to whether it would be effective in early treatment of HIV patients. One measure of the severity of immune compromise is the number of CD4 lymphocytes (also known as "T cells" or T4 lymphocytes) that can be detected in the patient's blood. A recent study demonstrated that patients with a CD4 lymphocyte count of less than 500 benefit from the use of AZT (Fischl, Richman, Hansen, et al., 1990). The current recommendation is that all patients with a CD4 lymphocyte count of less than 500 be started on AZT. Studies are currently being conducted to determine whether HIV-infected people with CD4 lymphocyte counts greater than 500 would benefit from AZT.

Because of these new recommendations, many patients become fixated on the results of their T-cell counts. This concern leads to anxiety among patients when their counts fluctuate. Because of the lack of reproducibility of T-cell counts, many physicians take two counts one week apart before making any therapeutic decisions. It can be difficult to alleviate patients' anxiety when their latest T-cell count is low. Moreover, the CDC is considering redefining AIDS to include all patients with CD4 lymphocyte counts less than 200. For some patients, this will lead to an earlier diagnosis of AIDS and thus additional anxiety.

Because HIV is a virus that becomes incorporated in the genetic material of the cell, it is unlikely that any drug will be able to eradicate the virus in an infected person. For this reason, the development of a vaccine against HIV infection has been given high priority. Great strides have been made in the basic research that must precede the development of an effective vaccine, but much work is left to do. Special ethical considerations need to be taken into account when designing and conducting trials for potential HIV vaccines. Volunteers need to be counseled on ways to reduce the risk of HIV infection and thus lower the overall rate of infection and prolong the trial, on the need for strict confidentiality, and on the social and economic problems that can accompany HIV seroconversion in patients who have been immunized. It will probably be many years before an effective vaccine is commercially available.

PNEUMOCYSTIS CARINII INFECTIONS

The first cases of AIDS were described in 1981 in young homosexual men who presented with pneumonias due to an organism called *Pneumocystis carinii*. Pneumonia caused by this organism had been seen before, but only in patients whose immune systems were markedly depressed, such as cancer patients receiving chemotherapy. Since that time, *Pneumocystis carinii* pneumonia (PCP) has been recognized as a very common problem in people with HIV, occurring in more than 60% of people as the first AIDS-defining illness. Some advances in the treatment of PCP have been made, but more important has been the recognition that the incidence of PCP can be decreased by the use of prophylactic medication. Because of the tremendous rise in the number of cases of PCP in the United States, from fewer than 60 cases per year in the 1970s to a predicted 60,000 cases in 1991, and because of the fatality rate of 10% to 20% despite therapy, improved treatment strategies are critical.

Pneumocystis carinii is a protozoan (or perhaps a fungus; taxonomists are currently arguing about its classification) that occurs worldwide. Studies show that most healthy children are exposed to the organism by an early age (Meuwissen, Tauber, Leewenberg, Beckers, & Sieben, 1977). The infection is transmitted through the air, but the precise source remains unknown. In healthy people the organism does not cause disease, but in patients with impaired immune systems a pneumonia can occur approximately four to eight weeks after infection.

TABLE 3. COMMON CAUSES OF PNEUMONIA IN AIDS.

BACTERIA
Mycobacterium tuberculosis
Mycobacterium avium-intracellulare
Streptococcus pneumoniae
Hemophilus influenzae

FUNGI
Cryptococcus neoformans
Coccidioides immitis
Histoplasma capsulatum
Candida albicans

NON-SPECIFIC PNEUMONITIS

PNEUMOCYSTIS CARINII

TUMORS
Kaposi sarcoma
Lymphoma (non-Hodgkin's)

VIRUSES
Cytomegalovirus

The presenting symptoms of PCP include shortness of breath, fever, and a cough that is usually not productive of sputum. In patients with AIDS the symptoms can be subtle and persist for weeks or months. The findings on a chest X-ray or arterial blood gas examination may be suggestive of PCP, but the only way to differentiate *Pneumocystis carinii* from other forms of pneumonia is to identify the organism (see Table 3). Through the use of special staining techniques, physicians can examine a specimen of sputum that has been induced by inhalation of a saline mist to determine the presence of PCP (Kovacs et al., 1988). If the diagnosis cannot be made by sputum examination, then a bronchoscopy with a bronchoalveolar lavage (BAL) must be performed. Diagnosis of PCP can be made in more than 90% of patients with AIDS through the use of bronchoscopy and BAL.

Pneumocystis carinii pneumonia (PCP) occurs commonly in patients with AIDS. Because the initial symptoms of the disease are often subtle, all patients with AIDS who have a cough or shortness of breath should be evaluated by a physician. It is often difficult to convince a patient with only a cough and mild shortness of breath to undergo uncomfortable procedures such as an arterial blood gas examination or a bronchoscopy. Because there are so many different causes of pneumonia in patients with AIDS, a number of invasive tests (including a bronchoscopy) may need to be done to diagnose the problem. This type of medical workup is essential, however, because early treatment of PCP can decrease mortality. Persons who wait until they are severely ill with pneumonia respond less well to therapy than do those who are seen early. Patients need to be encouraged to seek medical attention early and to comply with the diagnostic testing and therapy. Patients often need counseling and reassurance during the medical procedures.

Two drugs are currently used in the United States in the treatment of PCP: trimethoprim-sulfamethoxazole (TMP-SMX) and pentamidine isethionate. Patients with PCP usually have to be hospitalized and receive one of these drugs intravenously. Treatment generally lasts 21 days. In patients with moderate to severe pneumonia, the addition of corticosteroids to the antibiotics improves survival

(Bozzette et al., 1990; Gagnon, Boota, Fischl, Baier, Kirksey, & La Voie, 1990). Unfortunately, both TMP-SMX and pentamidine commonly have adverse reactions. In patients with AIDS, TMP-SMX frequently causes a skin rash and can cause severe nausea and vomiting. Pentamidine cannot be given orally, and in patients with pneumonia, it must be given intravenously. It can cause life-threatening adverse reactions, such as low blood sugar. Nevertheless, both drugs are effective for therapy, and the survival rate for the first episode of PCP is probably better than 90% (Brenner et al., 1987; Wharton et al., 1986).

None of the therapies available can cure the infection; current therapies only suppress the infection and lead to resolution of the pneumonia. Even after successful treatment, more than 50% of patients will have recurrence of PCP. For this reason, all patients now receive some form of prophylactic therapy to prevent recurrence. The best form of prophylactic therapy appears to be oral therapy with TMP-SMX, but over half of the patients will have adverse reactions. Alternative therapies include daily oral dapsone or monthly treatment with aerosolized pentamidine. Studies currently under way are comparing these therapies. Therapy must be continued throughout life to prevent recurrence of pneumonia. Because of possible adverse reactions to all of these therapies (rash and nausea with TMP-SMX and depsone, cough with pentamidine) compliance with such long-term therapy can be a problem.

Because PCP is so common in patients with AIDS and is associated with morbidity and mortality, strategies have been developed to try to prevent development of the disease. *Pneumocystis carinii* pneumonia rarely occurs in patients who have CD4 cell counts higher than 200. The current recommendation is for all HIV-infected patients with CD4 cell counts less than 200 to begin lifelong prophylactic therapy for PCP. The therapies being used are the same ones described above for the prevention of relapse. As mentioned above, compliance can be a problem.

KAPOSI SARCOMA

Kaposi sarcoma (KS) is the most common tumor in HIV-infected patients. Before the AIDS epidemic, this tumor was rare and occurred primarily in elderly men in the United States and among people in central Africa. The tumor arises from the lining of small blood vessels. Kaposi sarcoma affects HIV-infected male homosexuals disproportionately compared with other groups (such as injection drug users). This finding suggests that KS is an infectious disease, although its cause is still unknown.

Kaposi sarcoma most frequently affects the skin. The lesions are typically violaceous to red, nodular, and vary in size from several millimeters to 10 centimeters in diameter. The lesions can be widely scattered on the body and can be associated with swelling and pain in the legs or face. Besides affecting the skin, KS lesions can involve the oral cavity, the gastrointestinal tract (sometimes causing diarrhea or intestinal obstruction), or the lungs (causing a syndrome resembling PCP).

Diagnosis of KS can be confirmed through biopsy and examination of the specimen by a pathologist. When visceral organs are involved, procedures such as bronchoscopy, endoscopy, or colonoscopy need to be performed to obtain a biopsy specimen. Factors such as the number of lesions present, the rate of appearance of new lesions, the presence of KS in visceral organs, and the degree of immunological impairment due to HIV infection all appear to influence the patient's prognosis.

Because the clinical course of KS is variable, ranging from indolent to rapidly fatal, therapy must be individualized on the basis of an estimate of the patient's prognosis. Local problems due to lesions can be treated with radiation, which can rapidly shrink individual lesions. Intralesional and topical therapy is also being tried. For patients with unfavorable prognosis, systemic interferon-alpha or combination chemotherapy can be used, with a relatively high response rate.

Kaposi sarcoma can be a disfiguring disease when it appears on the face or exposed extremities, causing patients to experience the social stigma associated with AIDS. Additionally, it can be a very painful disease, particularly when significant swelling occurs in the legs. Because the lesions act as visible reminders of AIDS to the person infected, these patients often need counseling and emotional support.

MYCOBACTERIUM AVIUM-INTRACELLULARE COMPLEX

Mycobacterium avium-intracellulare complex (MAI or MAC) is similar to the organism that causes tuberculosis. In fact, on special stains the bacteria look identical to the tuberculosis organism (*Mycobacterium tuberculosis*) and can be differentiated only on the basis of culture characteristics, which can take up to six weeks to determine. Humans are frequently exposed to these organisms, but in immunologically normal hosts they rarely cause disease. It is thought that the organism cannot be transmitted from one person to another. As many as 25% to 50% of HIV-infected patients develop infection with MAC.

Infections with MAC commonly present as a systemic illness with fevers, night sweats, weight loss, and fatigue. Patients often have diarrhea and abdominal pain and can present with pneumonia. The infection usually involves many organs, and many organisms are present in the bloodstream (Young, 1988). It typically occurs in patients with profound immunosuppression as well as other serious infections. The diagnosis is usually made by culturing the organism from the blood, stool, or bone marrow, but can also be made by analyzing a biopsy specimen from any infected organ.

Although most patients with AIDS develop infection with MAC, it is not clear how this infection contributes to AIDS mortality. Moreover, currently no therapy is effective for MAC infections. The organism is resistant to many of the standard drugs used to treat tuberculosis. Clinicians currently use a multiple-drug regimen that may include rifampin or rifabutin, ethambutol, clofazimine, a quinolone (such as ciprofloxacin), and amikacin. A new drug, clarithromycin, has shown promise, but has not yet been approved for treatment of MAC. Such therapy is not curative, but may result in improvement of symptoms.

Compliance with therapy is a major problem. Because as many as five drugs are used, patients need to take approximately eight pills a day, and amikacin can be given only intramuscularly or intravenously. Several of the drugs used can cause gastrointestinal upset, which further complicates compliance. Research is ongoing to find new and more effective (as well as less toxic) agents for therapy.

MYCOBACTERIUM TUBERCULOSIS

Tuberculosis is not truly an "opportunistic" infection. It was known to the ancient Greeks and in the 17th and 18th centuries caused one-fourth of adult deaths in Europe. With the development of effective therapy in the 1950s and 1960s the number of tuberculosis cases in the United States declined, leading some to predict that tuberculosis would be eradicated. Unfortunately, cases of tuberculosis have increased in the past decade, due in large part to AIDS (Centers for Disease Control, 1988). Between 2% and 10% of AIDS patients are estimated to have tuberculosis (Chaisson, Schecter, Theuer, Rutherford, Echenberg, & Hopewell, 1987; Centers for Disease Control, 1987).

It is believed that many people are exposed to *Mycobacterium tuberculosis* at a young age and become chronically infected. In most people this infection remains dormant and is controlled by their immune system. Years later, this infection may reactivate and cause disease in the lungs (pulmonary tuberculosis) or disseminate to other parts of the body (extrapulmonary tuberculosis) such as the brain, kidneys, spine, lymph nodes, joints, bone marrow, or other organs. During the years that the infection is clinically silent, its presence can be detected by a tuberculin skin test.

HIV infection interacts with tuberculosis in several ways. First, some of the risk factors for HIV infection (such as IV drug use) are also risk factors for infection with *Mycobacterium tuberculosis*. Second, HIV infection can change the course of tuberculosis infection. Patients who are HIV infected are more likely to reactivate their tuberculosis infection (Selwyn et al., 1989). They are also more likely to have disseminated disease (in up to 50% of HIV-infected patients, compared with 15% in patients without HIV infection). Because of patients' HIV infection, their symptoms of tuberculosis may not be typical and their diagnosis may be delayed. In addition, strains of tuberculosis that are resistant to many or all drugs have been found in HIV-infected patients.

Tuberculosis is a communicable disease that can spread from person to person via airborne respiratory secretions. For the protection of other patients as well as health care personnel, it is important to make the diagnosis of pulmonary tuberculosis quickly and to initiate therapy as soon as possible. All patients who are HIV-positive should receive skin tests for tuberculosis to find out if they have clinically silent infections. Those who are positive should receive treatment to prevent the development of the disease. Unfortunately, patients with severe immunosuppression may not react to the skin test even if they have tuberculosis.

The standard prophylactic therapy is one year of isoniazid tablets. Although isoniazid is very effective in other patients, it is not known if it is adequate therapy in HIV-infected people. Some authorities now recommend life-long therapy with isoniazid. Studies are being done to determine the optimal therapy.

Patients with active infection most often present with symptoms of lung disease such as cough and shortness of breath. As mentioned in the section under *Pneumocystis carinii*, many different conditions can cause these symptoms in patients with HIV infection. Tuberculosis must be diagnosed quickly because of the possibility of communicating the disease to others. Other patients may present with symptoms showing involvement of other organ systems (headache, stiff neck, confusion, anemia, joint swelling or pain) without any lung symptoms.

Tuberculosis is diagnosed by culturing the organism. This may be done from sputum for lung involvement or may require special procedures such as lumbar puncture (spinal tap), bone marrow biopsy, or liver biopsy. The organism can be differentiated from *Mycobacterium avium-intracellulare* only by culture, which can take up to six weeks.

Several drugs are known to be effective in the therapy of tuberculosis. AIDS patients generally respond well to standard therapy if the infecting organism is sensitive to standard drugs. The most common drug regimen uses isoniazid with rifampin and pyrazinamide for a total of six months, although many physicians now add ethambutol for HIV patients. It is not known whether therapy should continue longer in patients who are HIV infected; studies are now under way to examine this question. Other drugs such as cycloserine and ethionamide are available for therapy of resistant infection.

Because tuberculosis is communicable, it is essential that patients are diagnosed and begun on therapy as soon as possible. In general, therapy can be provided on an outpatient basis. Patients cease to be communicable one to two weeks after starting therapy. However, even though patients may respond relatively quickly to therapy, treatment needs to be continued for a full course or relapse may occur. If patients do not complete a full course of therapy, the possibility of relapse is great. Often, relapse is caused by organisms that are resistant to standard therapy.

OTHER BACTERIA

Many other bacteria cause infections more frequently in HIV-infected patients than they do in non–HIV-infected patients. These bacterial infections involve primarily the skin, lungs, and the sinuses. Chronic sinusitis is relatively common in HIV-infected patients and often presents with cough, nasal congestion, and headache. The diagnosis can often be made by X-ray. These patients usually respond well to standard antibiotic therapy.

Syphilis is another bacterial infection that has a more aggressive course in HIV-infected patients. Many reports have been published of uncommon presentations and severe infections. Because both syphilis and HIV are sexually transmitted diseases, they often occur simultaneously. We have found that more than 20% of HIV-infected patients who present at our clinic show evidence of inadequately treated syphilis (Holtom, Larsen, Leal, & Leedom, in press). Thus HIV patients should be encouraged to be tested for syphilis.

A major problem is the frequent progression of the syphilis infection to the nervous system (neurosyphilis). Diagnosis may be difficult, and the ideal type and length of therapy are currently being debated, because recommended therapies may not be effective in all cases. All HIV-positive patients with evidence of infection with syphilis should have a lumbar puncture to evaluate for neurosyphilis. Unfortunately, many patients have irrational fears of lumbar punctures and are reluctant to undergo the procedure. Because the presence of neurosyphilis will radically alter the type of therapy recommended, patients need to be reassured about the safety of the procedure and informed of the importance of the results. Untreated (or undertreated) neurosyphilis can result in meningitis, strokes, seizures, and frank psychosis.

CYTOMEGALOVIRUS

Cytomegalovirus (CMV) is a member of the herpesvirus family. Infection with CMV is common, and somewhere between 40% and 100% of adults have been infected, depending on the country surveyed (Krech, 1973). Like other herpesviruses, once infection occurs it remains latent in the patient but can reactivate and cause disease if the immune system fails. In patients with AIDS, the virus commonly causes retinitis (infection of the retina of the eye) but it can also cause pneumonia, infection of the gastrointestinal tract, hepatitis, and problems with the endocrine glands.

When CMV infection involves the eye, patients experience progressive visual impairment and blurred vision, which can be irreversible. Patients may have their infection discovered on a routine examination before they have symptoms. A fundoscopic examination by an ophthalmologist experienced in dealing with CMV is essential for the diagnosis and also for serial evaluation of the result of therapy.

Currently only two FDA-approved drug are available for the treatment of CMV disease. Both ganciclovir (DHPG) and foscarnet can arrest the progression of disease in the eyes and in other organs. However, the disease relapses in a few weeks if therapy is stopped. Both of these drugs are important additions to treatment of CMV disease. Unfortunately, both drugs have severe side effects and must be administered intravenously. Patients treated with foscarnet may live longer than patients treated with ganciclovir, but this may be due to the fact that patients taking foscarnet can continue taking AZT, whereas patients taking ganciclovir cannot because of toxicity.

Cytomegalovirus retinitis is a devastating disease for patients, because it eventually results in blindness. Patients also have a difficult time accepting the need for a permanent indwelling catheter and the need for daily intravenous injections. New research is focusing on finding alternative drugs that can be taken orally.

CANDIDA ALBICANS

Candida albicans is a fungus that can cause various syndromes in HIV-infected patients. It is a microorganism found in all people. Disease is caused by an overgrowth of the normal flora and is not transmitted from one person to another. The most common form is oral candidiasis, or thrush, an infection of the mouth cavity and throat. Patients can have white or reddish plaques in their mouth, sometimes with pain or loss of taste. Diagnosis is usually made by clinical examination, but a culture can be taken or a biopsy performed. Thrush is not an AIDS-defining illness, but the incidence of disease increases with progressive immunodeficiency.

Esophageal candidiasis is the presenting AIDS diagnosis in approximately 3% of AIDS cases in the United States. Patients commonly present with pain or difficulty swallowing, chest pain, loss of appetite, nausea, and weight loss. Since other infections of the esophagus (such as cytomegalovirus and herpes simplex virus) can mimic infection with *Candida albicans*, a definite diagnosis can be made only by an upper endoscopy with biopsies. Unlike thrush, esophageal candidiasis is an AIDS-defining illness.

Infections with *Candida albicans* can be treated with a variety of antifungal drugs. Thrush can be treated topically with a liquid form of nystatin swished in the mouth, by sucking on troches of clotrimazole, or by taking fluconazole tablets. Esophageal infection must be treated with systemic drugs. The current drug of choice is the new agent fluconazole, which can be administered by tablet once a day. Other drugs, such as oral ketoconazole or intravenous amphotericin B, can also be used. Most patients respond well to therapy, although thrush frequently recurs when treatment is stopped and therapy may need to be continued for life.

CRYPTOCOCCUS NEOFORMANS

Cryptococcus neoformans is a ubiquitous fungus present in the soil and in bird droppings. People acquire infection by inhaling the organism into the lungs. Although symptomatic infection can occur in patients with normal immune systems, an explosion in the number of cases of cryptococcal meningitis has occurred since the start of the AIDS epidemic.

Systemic infection occurs in up to 10% of people with AIDS (Dismukes, 1988). Although a number of clinical syndromes have been reported, most patients present with meningitis, an infection of the brain and its coverings. Eighty percent of patients complain only of fever, night sweats, malaise, and a dull headache (Kovacs et al., 1985), although some patients can have severe headaches, confusion, seizures, or paralysis. *Cryptococcus* is not communicable from person to person and presents no risk to caregivers.

Diagnosis of meningitis can be made only by performing a lumbar puncture and examining the fluid. A blood test is available that can indicate the presence of infection, but cultures are still needed for diagnosis. Because the symptoms of cryptococcal meningitis can be vague and the disease is invariably fatal without therapy, patients with fevers and new headaches need to be encouraged to have a prompt diagnostic workup.

Two different therapies are currently available for cryptococcal meningitis in the United States, and several new drugs are in development. The standard therapy is intravenous amphotericin B. This drug has been shown to be fairly effective, with a survival rate of approximately 80% at the end of therapy (Chuck & Sande, 1989). Unfortunately, the drug is relatively toxic, causing uncomfortable side effects during administration (such as chills, nausea, and vomiting) and long-term side effects such as kidney failure and anemia. Fluconazole can be given orally, but it is not yet known whether it is as effective as amphotericin B in the treatment of meningitis.

Even after patients have been successfully treated for meningitis, they are at a high risk for relapse of cryptococcal disease. It has been shown that long-term therapy with oral fluconazole can markedly decrease the risk of relapse. As with many other therapies in patients with AIDS, this treatment must be continued for the rest of the patient's life. Members of the health care team must reinforce the need for lifelong therapy. Patients who have a relapse of meningitis are much less likely to respond to therapy.

HISTOPLASMA CAPSULATUM

Disseminated histoplasmosis is caused by the fungus *Histoplasma capsulatum*, which occurs in the soil in many parts of the United States, especially in the Ohio and Mississippi river valleys. This infection can present as a prolonged subacute fever with weakness and weight loss or as a fulminant infection with marked blood abnormalities and respiratory failure. The diagnosis usually can be made from cultures of the blood or from biopsy specimens, especially bone marrow or liver biopsy.

Disseminated histoplasmosis is a very common AIDS-defining illness in areas where the fungus is endemic (Johnson, Khardori, Naijar, Butt, Mansell, & Sarosi, 1988). Without treatment, the disease is invariably fatal. Currently, the recommended therapy is intravenous amphotericin B, but this therapy has many side effects, as mentioned above. One investigational agent, itraconazole, has shown great promise in the therapy of histoplasmosis and has the advantage that it can be given orally.

Like cryptococcosis, histoplasmosis also is likely to recur after therapy is stopped, and lifelong treatment is indicated. The problem with the current therapy with amphotericin B is that it requires lifelong weekly IV injections with a toxic medication. Trials of maintenance therapy with itraconazole are currently under way in the United States.

TOXOPLASMA GONDII

Toxoplasmosis is caused by the protozoan *Toxoplasma gondii*, a pathogen for both humans and animals. Many adults have been infected with the organism in childhood and have latent, asymptomatic infections that can reactivate later in life, especially if the person's immune system is not functioning well. Although infection with *Toxoplasma gondii* can cause many manifestations, including pneumonia, retinitis, and heart muscle inflammation (myocarditis), the most common result of infection in patients with AIDS is encephalitis or brain inflammation. Although tox-oplasmic encephalitis was once rare, it is estimated that it occurs in 5% to 10% of patients with AIDS in the United States and approximately 25% of AIDs patients in Western Europe (Luft & Remington, 1988).

Most patients present with headaches and confusion, and approximately half have neurological signs such as seizures, difficulty walking, or focal paralysis. The diagnosis can often be suggested by findings on the head scan, although similar findings may be caused by other infections or conditions such as tumor (lymphoma). If the diagnosis is in doubt or the patient does not respond to medication, a brain biopsy may be required to make the diagnosis.

Most patients with toxoplasmosis respond to standard therapy with two drugs: pyrimethamine and sulfadiazine. Unfortunately, adverse effects are common with both drugs (such as rash, nausea, and low white-blood-cell count), and no alternative drugs are clearly effective. Clinical trials are being done with several new agents, and it is hoped that better therapies will become available. As with many other infections in AIDS patients, relapse occurs when the therapy is stopped; thus the drugs must be continued for life.

CRYPTOSPORIDIUM AND ISOSPORA BELLI

Human disease due to *Cryptosporidium*, a protozoan, was first reported in 1976. In immunologically normal individuals, infection causes watery diarrhea and abdominal cramps. Infections last for an average of 10 to 14 days, although they can be prolonged. The parasite is distributed worldwide and appears to be a relatively common cause of diarrhea in underdeveloped countries.

In patients with AIDS, the course of infection with *Cryptosporidium* is much more variable and often much more severe. Patients may experience voluminous diarrhea and abdominal pain that can last for months. Because of the massive fluid loss, they may need hospitalization for IV fluid replacement. These patients can also develop profound weight loss and severe wasting. Additionally, *Cryptosporidium* can infect the gallbladder and cause cholecystitis.

Diagnosis of diarrhea due to *Cryptosporidium* can be made by laboratory examination of a stool specimen using special stains. For any AIDS patient with diarrhea, it is important to identify the cause so that a treatment plan can be made. Possible causes include all the many viruses and bacteria that can cause diarrhea in the general population, the HIV virus itself, cytomegalovirus, *Cryptosporidium*, and *Isospora belli* . Unfortunately, infection with *Cryptosporidium* has no known effective therapy. Studies have been done with several different agents, including spiramycin, but as yet none has proven to be effective. Current management involves fluid replacement to prevent dehydration and the use of nonspecific antidiarrheal agents.

Isospora belli, another protozoan, causes watery diarrhea and abdominal pain, with a prolonged course in immunocompromised patients. It also can be identified by examination of a stool specimen using special stains. Unlike *Cryp-*

tosporidium, however, *Isospora* infection responds to therapy with oral trimetho-prim-sulfamethoxazole. Because patients with AIDS have a high frequency of relapse, they are often given a regimen of suppressive therapy indefinitely.

CONCLUSION

Looking back over the first decade of the AIDS epidemic, tremendous strides have been made in our understanding of the medical aspects of and therapeutic modalities for the disease. The HIV has been identified and two antiretroviral drugs (zidovudine, or AZT, and didanosine, or ddI) are now in wide use, while others are being developed. Many previously rare infections have been identified as oppor-tunistic infections in people with AIDS, and therapies have been identified for many of them.

Unfortunately, we have a long way to go. Although AZT can decrease oppor-tunistic infections and prolong life, it remains a toxic therapy. Newer, less toxic, and more effective medications are needed to combat the immune deficiency. Better therapies are needed to prevent or reverse the dementia that is common with AIDs. Some opportunistic infections still have no effective treatment, and many need more effective and less toxic therapies.

Because of the pain associated with many of the medical procedures, the toxic-ity of medications, and the need for lifelong therapy, medical treatment of persons with HIV and AIDS requires participation of all members of the health care team. Good patient care requires appropriate medical diagnostic tests and therapy as well as emotional support and the informational services that allow patients to make informed medical decisions. Patients need to be provided with the opportunity to ventilate their frustrations and fears before they are able to understand the therapies that are being presented. They need ongoing reinforcement regarding the need for lifelong therapy.

These areas represent some of the challenges facing the medical community in confronting the AIDS epidemic. It is hoped that the next decade will see dramatic increases in our knowledge about these diseases and new therapies will result in marked improvements in medical care and quality of life for persons with AIDS.

REFERENCES

Bozzette, S. A., Sattler, F. R., Chiu, J., Wu, A. W., Gluckstein, D., Kemper, C., Bartok, A., Niosi, J., Abramson, I., Coffman, J., Hughlett, C., Loya, R., Cassens, B., Akil, B., Meng, T. C., Boylen, C. T., Nielsen, D., Richman, D. D., Tilles, J. G., Leedom, J., McCuthchan, J. A., and the California Col-laborative Treatment Group. (1990). A controlled trial of early adjunctive treatment with corticos-teroids for *Pneumocystis carinii* pneumonia in the acquired immunodeficiency syndrome. *New Eng-land Journal of Medicine, 323,* 1456–1457.

Brenner, M., Ognibene, F. P., Lack, E. E., Simmons, J. T., Suffredini, A. F., Lane, H. C., Fauci, A. S., Parrillo, J. E., Shelhamer, J. H., & Masur, H. (1987). Prognostic factors and life expectancy of acquired immunodeficiency syndrome patients with *Pneumocystis carinii* pneumonia. *American Review of Respiratory Diseases, 136,* 1199–1206.

Centers for Disease Control. (1987). Tuberculosis and acquired immunodeficiency syndrome—

New York City. *Morbidity and Mortality Weekly Reports, 36*, 785–795.

Centers for Disease Control. (1988). Tuberculosis, final data—United States, 1986. *Morbidity and Mortality Weekly Reports, 36*, 817–820.

Chaisson, R. E., Schecter, G. F., Theuer, C. P., Rutherford, G. W., Echenberg, D. F., & Hopewell, P. C. (1987). Tuberculosis in patients with the acquired immunodeficiency syndrome: Clinical features, response to therapy, and survival. *American Review of Respiratory Diseases, 136*, 570–604.

Chuck, S. L., & Sande, M. A. (1989). Infections with *Cryptococcus neoformans* in the acquired immunodeficiency syndrome. *New England Journal of Medicine, 321*, 794–799.

Dismukes, W. E. (1988). Cryptococcal meningitis in patients with AIDS. *Journal of Infectious Diseases, 157*, 624–628.

Fischl, M. A., Parker, C. B., Pettinelli, C., Wulfsohn, M., Hirsch, M. S., Collier, A. C., Antoniskis, D., Ho, M., Richman, D. D., Fuchs, E., Merrigan, T. C., Reichman, R. C., Gold, J., Steigbigle, N., Leoung, G. S., Rasheed, S., Tsiatis, A., & the AIDS Clinical Trials Group. (1990). A randomized controlled trial of reduced daily dose of zidovudine in patients with the acquired immunodeficiency syndrome. *New England Journal of Medicine, 323*, 1009–1014.

Fischl, M. A., Richman, D. D., Grieco, M. H., Gottlieb, M. S., Volberding, P. A., Laskin, O. L., Leedom, J. M., Groopman, J. E., King, D., & the AZT Collaborative Working Group. (1987). The efficacy of azidothymidine (AZT) in the treatment of patients with AIDS and AIDS-related complex. A double-blind, placebo controlled trial. *New England Journal of Medicine, 317*, 192–197.

Fischl, M. A., Richman, D. D., Hansen, N., Collier, A. C., Carey, J. T., Para, M. F., Hardy, W. D., Dolin, R., Powderly, W. G., Allan, J. D., Wong, B., Merrigan, T. C., McAuliffe, V. J., Hyslop, N. E., Rhame, F. S., Anderson, J., & the AIDS Clinical Trials Group. (1990). The safety and efficacy of zidovudine (AZT) in the treatment of subjects with mildly symptomatic human immunodeficiency virus Type 1 (HIV) infection. A double-blind, placebo-controlled trial. *Annals of Internal Medicine, 112*, 727–737.

Gagnon, S., Boota, A. M., Fischl, M. A., Baier, H., Kirksey, O. W., & La Voie, L. (1990). Corticosteroids as adjunctive therapy for severe *Pneumocystis carinii* pneumonia in acquired immunodeficiency syndrome. *New England Journal of Medicine, 323*, 1444–1450.

Gottlieb, M. S., Schroff, R., Schanker, H. M., Weisman, J. D., Fan, P. T., Wolf, R. A., & Saxon, A. (1981). *Pneumocystis carinii* pneumonia and mucosal candidiasis in previously healthy homosexual men: Evidence of a new acquired cellular immunodeficiency. *New England Journal of Medicine, 305*, 1425–1431.

Holtom, P. D., Larsen, R. A., Leal, M. E., & Leedom, J. M. (in press). Prevalence of neurosyphilis in human immunodeficiency virus (HIV) infected patients with latent syphilis. *American Journal of Medicine.*

Johnson, P. C., Khardori, N., Naijar, A. F., Butt, F., Mansell, P. W. A., & Sarosi, G. A. (1988). Progressive disseminated histoplasmosis in patients with acquired immunodeficiency syndrome. *American Journal of Medicine, 85*, 152–158.

Kovacs, J. A., Kovacs, A. A., Polis, M., Wright, W. C., Gill, V. J., Tuazon, C. U., Gelmann, E. P., Lane, H. C., Longfield, R., Overturf, G., Macher, A. M., Fauci, A. S., Parrillo, J. E., Bennett, J. E., & Masur, H. (1985). Cryptococcosis in the acquired immunodeficiency syndrome. *Annals of Internal Medicine, 103*, 533–538.

Kovacs, J. A., Ng, V. L., Masur, H., Leoung, G., Hadley, W. K., Evans, G., Lane, H. C., Ognibene, F. P., Shelhamer, J., Parrillo, J. E., & Gill, V. J. (1988). Diagnosis of *Pneumocystis carinii* pneumonia: Improved detection in sputum with use of monoclonal antibodies. *New England Journal of Medicine, 318*, 589–603.

Krech, U., (1973). Complement-fixing antibodies against cytomegalovirus in different parts of the world. *Bulletin of the World Health Organization, 49*, 103–106.

Luft, B. J., & Remington, J. S. (1988). Toxoplasmic encephalitis. *Journal of Infectious Diseases, 157*, 1.

279

Masur, H., Michelis, M. A., Greene J. B., Onarato, I., Stouwe, R. A. V., Holqman, R. S., Womser, G., Brettman, L., Lange, M., Murray, H. W., & Cunningham-Rundles, S. (1981). An outbreak of community-acquired *Pneumocystis carinii* pneumonia: Initial manifestations of cellular immune dysfunction. *New England Journal of Medicine, 305*, 1431–1438.

McArthur, J. C. (1987). Neurologic manifestations of AIDS. *Medicine* (Baltimore), *66*, 407–437.

Meuwissen, J. H. E., Tauber, I., Leewenberg, A. D. E. M., Beckers, P. J. A., & Sieben, M. (1977). Parasitologic and serologic observations of infection with *Pneumocystis* in humans. *Journal of Infectious Diseases, 136*, 43–49.

Richman, D. D., Fischl, M. A., Grieco, M. H., Gottlieb, M. S., Volberding, P. A., Laskin, O. L., Leedom, J. M., Groopman, J. E., Mildvan, D., Hirsch, M. S., Jackson, G. G., Durack, D. T., Nusinoff-Lehrman, S., & the AZT Collaborative Working Group. (1987). The toxicity of azidothymidine (AZT) in the treatment of patients with AIDS and AIDS related complex. A double-blind, placebo controlled trial. *New England Journal of Medicine, 317*, 192–197.

Rothenberg, R., Woelfel, M., Stoneburner, R., Milberb, J., Parker, R., & Trumen, B. (1987). Survival with the acquired immunodeficiency syndrome: Experience with 5833 cases in New York City. *New England Journal of Medicine, 317*, 1297–1302.

Selwyn, P. A., Hartel, D., Lewis, V. A., Schoenbaum, E. E., Vermund, S. H., Klein, R. S., Wlaker, A. T., & Friedland, G. H. (1989). A prospective study of the risk of tuberculosis among intravenous drug users with human immunodeficiency virus infection. *New England Journal of Medicine, 320*, 545–550.

Wharton, J. M., Coleman, D. L., Wofsy, C. B., Luce, J. M., Blumenfeld, W., Hadley, W. K., Ingram-Drake, L., Volberding, P. A., & Hopewell, P. C. (1986). Trimethoprim-sulfamethoxazole or pentamidine for *Pneumocystis carinii* pneumonia in the acquired immunodeficiency syndrome: A prospective randomized trial. *Annals of Internal Medicine, 195*, 37–44.

Young, L. S. (1988). *Mycobacterium avium* complex infections. *Journal of Infectious Diseases, 157*, 863–867.

19

BEHAVIORAL AND PSYCHOSOCIAL ISSUES AND DIRECTIONS IN HIV/AIDS RESEARCH

JOANNE E. MANTELL AND ANTHONY T. DIVITTIS

Due to society's efforts to control HIV infection and its consequences, increasing interest has been shown in the paradigms provided by the social and behavioral sciences. Behavioral and psychosocial research has played a pivotal role in the formulation of HIV-prevention strategies, reflecting society's need to do *something* in the absence of clearcut biomedical solutions to the disease.

Behavioral and psychosocial research serves a number of functions. First, it can help community-based organizations and governmental agencies deploy scarce resources effectively. With the prevalence of new HIV-related service and prevention programs, research is needed to evaluate the effectiveness of these programs, provide guidelines for improving programs, and identify programs that should be terminated and services that need to be provided.

The focus of behavioral and psychosocial research is to identify the determinants of sexual and drug-related high-risk behaviors and of adoption and maintenance of behavioral change; social perceptions of the disease, including perceived health beliefs; patients' and health care providers' reactions to the disease and its social, psychological, and behavioral consequences; individuals' reactions to knowledge of their HIV serostatus; and evaluation of HIV-prevention programs (Coxon & Carballo, 1989). Implementation of behavioral/psychosocial research findings has proven to be less than effective. This chapter discusses the environment in which HIV/AIDS behavioral and psychosocial research is flourishing; the need for integration of theory, research, and practice; bioethical issues associated with conducting AIDS research; selected data-collection methods; and directions for future research.[1]

RESEARCH CONTEXT

The environment in which HIV/AIDS research has emerged sets the tone for how research is conducted. Several factors have made it difficult to do research: (1)

stigmatization of persons with HIV/AIDS, (2) competition for scarce resources, (3) the allocation of funds for services with a limited or with no research component, (4) conservative sexual values and attitudes, (5) the negative experience of minority groups with respect to research, and (6) patient activism.

Stigmatization of HIV/AIDS. Because a large proportion of society associates HIV/AIDS with homosexual behavior and injection drug use, persons with HIV/AIDS have experienced stigmatization and discrimination. Such stigmatization has made it difficult to recruit subjects, who are afraid of being identified as disease carriers.

Competition for scarce resources. AIDS research has been plagued by fierce and sometimes bitter competitiveness over the allocation of resources (Lee, 1986; Krieger, 1988; Hay, 1989), and in the second decade of AIDS, the availability of both research and service funds is more limited (Navarro, 1992). This climate has resulted in a backlash toward HIV research (Murphy, 1991). Activists complain that federal research efforts have been insufficient, whereas others argue that social hysteria has inappropriately shifted research priorities (Grossman, 1990). However, it must be noted that more federal research monies have been spent on AIDS than on heart disease, even though the latter kills more Americans each year (Hatziandreu, Graham, & Stoto, 1988). Competition is also found within the field of AIDS research, where biological scientists, epidemiologists, and behavioral scientists compete for research funds (Pear, 1988).

Distribution of funds to research vs. service activities. Populations affected by HIV/AIDS usually perceive service provision as being more important than research programs (Mantell & DiVittis, 1992). Faced with the dilemma of spending money on direct services and therapy or on research and evaluation, providers and community-based organizations set patient needs as a priority and minimize or deny allocation of funds to research and evaluation.

Conservative sexual values and attitudes. The study of sexual behavior has been tainted by moral and puritanical notions ("Shouts and Whispers about Sex," 1988; Callero & Howard, 1989; Maddox, 1989). As a case in point, final approval of the Survey of AIDS Risk Prevalence has been delayed, despite its scientific merit, by the Office of Management and Budget and the Secretary of the Department of Health and Human Services because of controversy over the inclusion of sensitive questions about sexual practices, especially homosexual behaviors. Also, the government recently canceled its plans to conduct an $18 million survey on the sexual behavior of teenagers out of fear that the questions would be construed as offensive and that they might encourage casual sex ("Government Scraps Study," 1991). Unfortunately, such fears have impeded efforts to obtain systematic baseline measures of the prevalence of specific sexual practices that are a major factor in HIV transmission.

Sexual behavior data collected since the onset of the HIV epidemic have been geared primarily to information about viral transmission, to the exclusion of the social and psychological context within which transmission occurs (Gagnon, 1988;

Mantell, Tross, & Rapkin, 1989). A more recent example of governmental conservatism is the Bush Administration's proposed regulations limiting abortion counseling in federally funded family-planning clinics. Abortion counseling represents a viable option to HIV-positive women wishing to avoid perinatal transmission.

Sometimes, the political prejudices of a funding source can interfere with the integrity of a research project. For example, the conservative climate of the Reagan presidency led to the Helms Amendment to the 1988 Labor, Health and Human Services Appropriations Bill for AIDS education (Amendment 963), which prohibited the Centers for Disease Control (CDC) from funding programs that provided AIDS education, information, or prevention materials (Congressional Record, 1987; Koch, 1987; Rovner, 1987). A modified version of this legislation, which requires CDC-funded research and service initiatives to form local censorship panels to review these materials, is still in effect.[2]

Negative experience of minority groups. Blacks and Latinos frequently distrust research because they perceive such efforts as experimentation. AIDS is a highly sensitive topic, and many minority community members are suspicious that such research will result in exploitation similar to the Tuskegee syphilis experiments, in which the U.S. government deliberately withheld treatment from syphilitic black prisoners so as to observe the long-term effects of syphilis (Mantell & DiVittis, 1990a; Wilkerson, 1991). Although the belief that HIV is the product of a conspiracy of whites for the genocide of minorities has no basis, some minority persons believe this to be the case (Thomas, So'Brien van Putten, & Chen, 1991). Second, disillusionment with the health care system may be generalized to overall mistrust of service providers. Some people believe that behavioral and psychosocial research efforts are an example of outsiders "taking" information from a population or community without giving anything back in return.

Patient activism. The AIDS Coalition to Unleash Power (ACT UP) advocacy model has set the tone for patient activism (Gamson, 1989) and has challenged institutionalized ways of conducting research. It has provided a forum whereby people with HIV infection can mobilize and channel their anger toward the medical establishment for moving too slowly (Morgan, 1988; Crossen, 1989; Taylor, 1990; Astor, 1990; Hilts, 1991). Through AIDS activists' lobbying efforts, unprecedented changes in the rigid regulatory process of releasing experimental drugs on a compassionate-use basis have occurred (Byar et al., 1990; Edgar & Rothman, 1991; Chase, 1991). Some people with HIV-related diseases, primarily gay men, have become active in determining treatment decisions and advocated aggressively for research-based evaluation of alternative therapies.

Such efforts have created a climate of patient-driven research and an environment in which research bridges the gap between patients and providers. Given the emphasis on change and grass-roots activism, AIDS service providers are often forced to assume the role of researcher. The move toward client-centered research is also reflected in researchers' actively involving representatives from a population under study in the research process (Gagnon, 1988; Mantell & DiVittis, 1990a).

INTEGRATING THEORY, RESEARCH, AND PRACTICE

Theory-driven research, as opposed to trial-and-error programs, is essential for the development of effective clinical, psychosocial, and prevention programs for HIV-related disorders and their sequelae. A conceptual paradigm provides a unifying framework with which to understand behaviors such as sexual and drug-associated risk reduction, use of ambulatory care services, or compliance with an AZT or ddI regimen, and ultimately to attain program goals.

Research and practice are not well integrated in many human service settings. Service providers frequently do not want to be confined by the details and rigors of a research protocol. However, research can help broaden a practice base and improve its quality and effectiveness, and practice can generate hypotheses (O'Hare, 1991). Evaluation of client satisfaction with service delivery process and outcomes, that is, quality assurance, can assist clinicians in sharpening definitions of clients' problems and specification of treatment goals and intervention, thus increasing patients' use of services and achieving desired clinical outcomes.

Increased dialogue between clinicians and researchers assists in breaking down barriers between the two camps. The institutionalization of research in clinical service settings might demonstrate its relevance and generate more interest in or mitigate clinicians' ambivalence toward the need for research. Behavioral research findings can also be used to direct clinical interventions to individuals who engage in high-risk behaviors or to improve the quality of life of persons with AIDS. The integration of research findings into a knowledge base of clinical practice may lead to the development of new models of practice. For example, evaluation of a case-management system may highlight the need for different implementation strategies. Researchers can learn how clinicians use (or could use) research findings in their practice and help clinicians pose important unanswered questions.

THE NEED FOR CULTURAL SENSITIVITY IN DESIGN AND MEASUREMENT

Given the differential impact of HIV/AIDS on various communities and populations, the research process must be conducted dynamically, yet remain sensitive to the culture and acceptable to each group or community. Getting communities or populations involved in the research process is an important but often overlooked facet of research. Community leaders or "gatekeepers" should collaborate in the research process from the outset, including the design of studies, construction and translation of questionnaires, pretesting, data collection, interpretation of the data, and dissemination of results (Rogler, 1989; Mantell & DiVittis, 1990a).

An example of participatory research is the Galveston, Texas, Minority AIDS Education Project's use of community officials and "gatekeepers" to help ensure researchers' access to residents of a housing project for an AIDS survey, which generated a 75% response rate (Longoria, Turner, & Philips, 1991). When a new service with a research component is introduced into a community, both researchers and service providers must be cognizant of how to obtain community sanction and support. For example, when the New York City Department of Health's Perinatal HIV Prevention Project planned to open a prevention/research storefront, efforts were undertaken to assess and solidify community support. A comprehensive needs-assessment survey was conducted to determine where the storefront should be located; community-based organizations were recruited to assist in staffing; and meetings were held with representatives from community boards, churches, and other organizations (Ramos et al., 1991).

The need for cultural sensitivity is not limited to race or ethnicity, but applies as well to personal characteristics such as sexual orientation and behaviors. Because AIDS researchers are continuously exposed to sexual behavior and drug-use issues, they are sometimes insensitive to society's discomfort with these topics. This is especially true when vernacularisms are used to refer to sexual practices. For example, in our early HIV-related studies, to prepare a questionnaire for data entry, we assigned "street-term" mnemonics to code study variables.[3] When the data were sent to an outside organization for computer entry, their staff, largely composed of Moslem women, refused to do the work.

Cultural sensitivity is also required when dealing with research participants. Interviewers must treat all subjects with respect and be nonjudgmental in their interpersonal interactions. Subjects' attitudes about the cultural acceptability and compatibility of condoms and other contraceptive methods should be recognized. Failure to consider these factors may alienate participants.

BIOETHICAL CONCERNS

The HIV epidemic has raised a number of bioethical issues that researchers need to consider. The stigma attached to HIV/AIDS (Walkey, Taylor, & Green, 1990) requires special attention to the manner in which research is conducted. This section considers the special requirements associated with confidentiality and anonymity, notification, institutional review boards, service referrals, clinical trials, and affected communities.

CONFIDENTIALITY, ANONYMITY, IDENTIFICATION, AND DISCLOSURE

The stigmatization and discrimination that result when a person discloses his or her positive HIV serostatus make confidentiality and anonymity extremely sensitive issues (Melton & Gray, 1988). In confidential studies, knowledge of a participant's identifying information, such as name and address, is limited to staff. In anonymous studies, this information is not made available even to researchers.

Study designs must safeguard participants' confidentiality. Clinical research targeted to populations with high-risk behaviors (e.g., anal or vaginal intercourse without a condom, drug-injection, unprotected sex with an HIV-positive partner) must be set up in such a way that participants cannot automatically be identified as taking part in an AIDS study. Giving a research project a "neutral," nonstigmatizing name not associated with AIDS can help break down barriers to participation and protect

285

participants' confidentiality. For example, a project examining the social, psychological, and cultural barriers to HIV risk-reduction, testing, and notification was named the Cultural Network Project/Proyecto de Apoyo Cultural (Mantell, Tross, & Rapkin, 1989).

When the focus of research centers on a couple, the confidentiality of each partner can be difficult to protect. In one study that examined biological markers of heterosexual HIV transmission, HIV-discordant[4] couples were excluded or dropped from the study if the HIV-negative partner (1) used injectable drugs, (2) was not sexually monogamous with the positive partner, or (3) seroconverted. The only exception to this exclusion occurred if the HIV-negative partner did not want information disclosed about these three factors, as each partner had been guaranteed confidentiality. Disqualification from the study in midstream would result in tacit disclosure of information to the partner (Ramis et al., 1991).

Offering subjects anonymity may increase study participation rates, especially when the research assesses highly personal sexual behavior, illicit drug use, and HIV serostatus. Anonymity is no problem with cross-sectional designs because individuals are not followed over time. With longitudinal designs, creative approaches to data linkage are essential, because subjects' questionnaires are completed at different points in time and must be linked. Encrypted personal identifiers generated by subjects can be developed to match a subject's data from different assessment periods. These identifiers may be a numerical code based on the subject's date of birth, numerical position in the alphabet of the first initial of the first and last names (Mantell & DiVittis, 1990a, 1990b), or an algorithm of letters generated from factors such as birthplace, first primary grade school attended, number of siblings, and subject's mother's family name (Bharucha-Reid, Schork, & Schwartz, 1990). One problem with this method is that subjects who do not return for follow-up cannot be tracked. Linkage of the encrypted personal identifiers with a subject's demographic characteristics and geographical location has been suggested (Bharucha-Reid, Schork, & Schwartz, 1990). To link records from different sources, for example, hospital records with Medicaid records, Boruch (1988) suggested that all confidential information from one source be cryptographically encoded (hidden from the researcher), except for one individual identifier.

DUTY TO WARN

Duty to warn refers to the circumstances under which a health care provider is obligated to inform a sex partner or needle-sharing "buddy" of the serostatus of an HIV-infected person. This issue stems from the California court ruling—*Tarasoff v. the Regents of the University of California* (1976)—that when a patient threatens harm to a third party, the patient's therapist has the duty to warn the third party. Thus, researchers who learn the serostatus of a subject must consider whether they are obligated to reveal this information to the subject's partner, despite their obligation to protect medical confidentiality.

Given that most ELISA (enzyme-linked immunoabsorbent screening assay) screening includes a test for syphilis, the same issue of reporting is relevant. The difference is that in the event of a positive syphilis serology, the researcher/clinician may receive a call from the local department of health, because reporting of syphilis is mandatory. All staff who answer the phone must be trained to report that information about participants in a study cannot be released without the consent of the participant.

RECONCILIATION OF ANONYMITY AND/OR CONFIDENTIALITY VS. DUTY TO WARN

Although every effort must be made to ensure anonymity and/or confidentiality, the most important obligation of health workers is to be honest with their clients. Therefore, providers must notify potential research study participants of legal obligations, if any, to notify family, friends, or government authorities *before* an individual becomes a participant in a program. For example, does a health care worker have a moral or legal obligation to disclose to the wife of a male client with AIDS that he is infected if the wife says that she wants to become pregnant? What is the obligation of health authorities who conduct anonymous HIV screening of newborns to inform seropositive babies' mothers of their child's and, hence, their own serostatus? Obviously, health care providers must become cognizant of the laws of the jurisdictions in which they render services. Failure to disclose this critical information could lead to substantial attrition over the life of a study.

ACCESS TO CLINICAL TRIALS AND ADHERENCE TO THE TREATMENT REGIMEN

Until recently, injection drug users (IDUs) were rarely involved in clinical trials because of providers' perceptions that they would be noncompliant. Women have also been excluded because of concerns that the drugs provided to women of child-bearing age could have effects on future pregnancies. The clinical sequelae of most antiviral drugs have been assessed largely on populations of white homosexual and bisexual men.

A proposed solution to the problem of including IDUs and mothers in clinical trials (Craven et al., 1990) is for researchers to provide comprehensive, integrated primary care, drug treatment, psychosocial, and day-care services in the treatment setting as well as reimbursement for transportation costs.

Coercion is also an issue. Consent to participate in a clinical trial may be perceived as coerced if (1) no other treatment options are available, (2) the specific medication cannot be obtained through other means, or (3) subjects are unable to afford the medications (Arras, 1990). Community-based (parallel-track) trials[5] must be held to the same high standards as are those at university medical centers. A formal review by a qualified, independent institutional review board should be performed to protect the rights of subjects (Bayer, 1990). For example, requiring participants to waive their right to sue for damages could be construed as coercive and unethical.

OFFERING INCENTIVES TO STUDY PARTICIPANTS

Researchers need to come to grips with the ethical issues in providing incentives to study participants. Participation in HIV/AIDS research has become an important source of supplementary income to particular subgroups, for example, IDUs. The authors do not believe that it is appropriate to provide incentives to secure participants without full disclosure. Nor is it reasonable to offer some IDUs economic incentives that could be used to buy drugs, no matter how full and complete the disclosure is.

POLITICS OF INSTITUTIONAL REVIEW BOARDS

The fear and discrimination surrounding AIDS have resulted in greater scrutiny by institutional review boards (IRBs) of research involving HIV-infected subjects or those at high risk for HIV, especially when the protocol involves HIV testing. When dealing with an IRB, both researchers and clinicians are faced with conflicting issues. A researcher must be prepared to defend projects and convince the IRB that a project will be more beneficial than detrimental to the individual and community. Although an IRB's mission is to assess whether the protocol, questionnaires, and laboratory tests adequately protect the rights of human subjects, IRBs frequently go beyond their mandate and comment on study methods independent of subjects' concerns.

Institutional review boards are mandated by the federal government's Office of Protection of Research Risks to have a minimum of two community representatives. The members of the IRB and researchers have to negotiate language in the questionnaire and the study protocol. While responding to the IRB's needs, researchers must also ensure that research protocols are maintained. In presenting a research project to an IRB, the researcher should know if any parts of the project are expendable.

METHODOLOGIC ISSUES

In the following sections of this chapter, methodologic concerns that plague AIDS social science research are discussed: (1) gaps in specific types of research methods and topics, (2) sampling diversity, (3) recruitment and retention incentives, and (4) assessment. Various data-collection methods commonly used in AIDS behavioral and psychosocial research are reviewed and future research directions are suggested.

GAPS IN SPECIFIC TYPES OF RESEARCH METHODS AND TOPICS

AIDS treatment lacks systematic, well-planned, and controlled preventive interventions. Also, research is inadequate on the effectiveness of psychosocial interventions, such as support groups, stress-management training, and cognitive therapies; clinical service delivery (Kelly & St. Lawrence, 1988); the influence of social norms; the cultural and gender-role context of sexual risk-reduction behaviors (Mantell, Ramos, Majidi, Walton-Glover, & Leslie, 1992); and the social diffusion of HIV-prevention messages.

SAMPLING DIVERSITY

Rigorous sampling is often compromised in favor of convenience and "snowball"[6] samples because of the difficulty of identifying members of groups who practice high-risk and sometimes illegal behaviors. For example, men who have sex with men but who do not self-identify as gay because they are married bisexuals or have not publicly disclosed their sexual identity cannot be reached through an organization targeted to gay men. With street-based substance users who are not receiving drug treatment, random sampling is almost impossible to attain. This type of sampling selection bias has limited the diversity of populations under study and, thus, external validity of findings. Behavioral research to identify the determinants and barriers to AIDS prevention cannot rely solely on the findings from populations of gay and bisexual men. Ethnic differences in sexual behavior and political and economic needs particular to other groups must be considered. Surveys of people's knowledge, attitudes, practices, and needs are crucial to program development for specialized subsets of the population.

HIV testing notification procedures can affect the representativeness of a sample. Because some jurisdictions or agencies have laws that require tested patients to be notified of their test results (Windom, 1988; Faden & Kass, 1991), samples in such studies are limited to participants who are willing to be notified of their test results. This limits the generalizability of findings to this self-selected sample.

RECRUITMENT AND RETENTION INCENTIVES

The use of incentives to recruit and retain subjects is perceived by researchers as being a positive reinforcement strategy. Incentives can increase the appeal of a research project and motivate participation. Issues that need to be addressed include: (1) cost, (2) type, (3) timing (during recruitment, before or after an intervention, or during maintenance), (4) purpose (for participation in an interview or intervention), (5) relevance (HIV prevention related), and (6) noneconomic benefit (perceived value) for participants.

Various incentives that have been offered to participants in HIV/AIDS studies include money, carfare/tokens, condom key chains, personal hygiene kits, tote bags, fanny packs, and coffee mugs. Research with some populations, such as clients in methadone-maintenance programs, has employed monetary incentives. However, one study that conducted focus groups with both hospital staff and potential participants learned that participants felt that the success of the program should depend on the merits of the program (Mantell & Ramos, 1991).

Ultimately, the researcher must determine what is an appropriate incentive for participation. In cross-sectional, epidemiological research, in which the goal is to determine HIV seroprevalence without concomitant service provision, money may be an appropriate incentive. In community demonstration projects, in which the ultimate goal is to assess the cost effectiveness of a long-term behavioral intervention in a population, the use of an economic incentive may be contraindicated. With such research, it would be impossible to differentiate participation for monetary gain from the efficacy of an educational intervention.

The use of incentives can result in sampling bias in that incentives encourage self-selection; that is, participants in programs that provide incentives may differ from those who are willing to participate without an external reward. It would be naive for the clinician/researcher to believe that subjects are unaware of the economic incentives that the latter can accrue as a result of study participation. To circumvent the use of economic incentives, researchers should consider offering psychosocial services. For example, one New York City study offered individual and couples group counseling, a monthly support group, and child care to facilitate participation of HIV-discordant couples (Ramis et al., 1991). Psychosocial incentives should not only increase participation rates, but diminish participants' possible sense of being "guinea pigs."

Unfortunately, evaluation of the effects of incentives on response and retention has been inadequate. More controlled studies (e.g., Smith, Weinman, Johnson, & Wait, 1990) are needed to determine whether offering incentives increases subject enrollment and, in longitudinal studies, decreases subject attrition over time.

ASSESSMENT

Few researchers have addressed whether their data-collection instruments are reliable or valid. As a result, reported outcome variables may not be assessing that which they were intended to assess. Ideally, a separate psychometric study should be performed to assess the reliability of the instruments and, if possible, determine their validity. Given the economic and time constraints on most clinician/researchers, this may not be practical. A limited psychometric study, such as estimating reliability through internal-consistency item analysis, however, can be performed on the current research sample. Although this is not the preferred method, it is better than nothing.

In terms of what is actually assessed, outcome measures that tap appropriate variables need to be carefully defined. Behavioral variables, such as safer sex, have multiple meanings, depending on the operational definition used. In some research studies, success is defined as increased condom use. For others, success may be defined as 100% condom use. In reported findings, clear definition and interpretation of behavioral outcomes are necessary for comparison of results across projects. This caveat holds true for clinical and biological markers of HIV infection. Differences in laboratory methods may result in calibration errors across sites, especially in instances whereby a project changes labs in the middle of a study. The laboratory and testing method must always be reported with the findings.

DATA-COLLECTION METHODS

Research that incorporates both qualitative and quantitative techniques provides a more balanced, comprehensive view of the research problem than do studies based on only one of these techniques (Stange & Zyzanski, 1989). For example, qualitative research may be conducted concurrently with quantitative designs as a cross-validation technique (Webb, Campbell, Schwartz, & Sechrest, 1966). Or qualitative and quantitative techniques may be used sequentially.

QUANTITATIVE METHODS

The types of research designs and sampling techniques available to HIV clinician/researchers may be constrained by the difficulty of access to the target population and the type of preventive "treatment" intervention. Two major issues involve the use of randomized experiments.

Preexperimental and quasi experimental designs. Randomized, controlled interventions involve the comparison of one HIV-prevention strategy with the absence of that intervention, for example, type of care for persons with AIDS (home care vs. no home care or high-intensity case management vs. low-intensity case management). Classic randomization ensures that every participant has an equal chance of being in the treatment intervention and thus minimizes the chance of selection bias. Although this design is scientifically appropriate, it is often impossible to implement. Community concerns about the denial of care or substandard care to a group of people, even for a short period, can make this type of research protocol unacceptable. This perception may prevail even if the treatment has not been shown to be efficacious. The clinician/researcher is faced with the decision of limited generalization due to the lack of random sampling or not being able to study the target community at all. Further, given the demands faced by these communities, inconsistent attendance and high attrition are to be expected, which can make the statistical comparison of a treatment and control condition irrelevant.

Two approaches that help to mitigate these difficulties are to use study designs that compare two treatments, thus ensuring some kind of treatment to each group. If withholding treatment is essential, a reversal or wait-list[7] control group treatment design, which ultimately provides treatment to all participants, may be acceptable (Cook & Campbell, 1979). Clinicians might argue that because the "treatment" is untested, it is possible that it may help but also possible that it may hurt. Therefore, withholding treatment may not be perceived as denial of opportunity.

Single-subject designs. Single-subject, also known as single-case or idiographic, experimental designs used initially to evaluate behavior therapy and psychotherapy, assess AIDS-related behavioral change in the individual. This design is frequently used by providers (e.g., clinician, health educator, social worker) to evaluate the effectiveness of the practice (assess individual process and outcome) (Hersen & Barlow, 1977). In single-subject designs, individual outcomes are not obscured in group averages. Single-subject designs may use modified repeated-measures or time-series designs, whereby changes are observed from baseline until completion of the intervention. For example, in an equivalent time-series design, the impact of treatment on health outcomes (e.g., T4 cells or reduction in the number of lesions) is manipulated by withdrawing a treatment and introducing a second treatment, then returning to the first treatment.

Another example of a single-subject design might be a person with HIV infection who is taking AZT, for whom a clinician or researcher determines the effectiveness of treatment by monitoring CD4 (T4) count to determine whether the absolute number of T4 cells has increased as a result of the medication. In such research, the patient's body serves as a barometer of the effects of medication. By comparing data with a normal curve, the researcher can establish the presence of statistically significant changes in outcome (e.g., T4 cell count) over time. The provider and patient can use data to negotiate changes in treatment dosages. This type of evaluation is also useful in assessing alternative therapies such as high-dose vitamin-C injections.

Unlike a group-based design, cause–effect relationships in individual outcomes cannot be established and change cannot be attributed to an intervention. Further, the magnitude of change required to achieve statistical significance is greater for an individual than for a group. However, as with classic research methodology, consistency across individuals builds a body of evidence in support of the intervention under study.

Goal-attainment scaling is one method used in single-subject designs. In this type of idiographic assessment, the client helps establish the goals and outcomes of treatment. In many ways, the client serves as a barometer of treatment. In conjunction with the clinician, prior to intervention, the client sets his or her individual goals and criteria for improvements and behavioral changes over time. For example, if an HIV-infected participant is currently using condoms during 50% of his or her sexual encounters, improvement would be reflected by an increase to 75% condom use. Conversely, decrements over time might be reflected by a reduction in condom use to 25%. The set of goals and behavioral assessment over time serve as a measure to gauge the progress toward completion of goals. This technique has been used successfully in psychiatric research (Lewis, Spencer, Haas, & DiVittis, 1987).

Surveys. Surveys to assess levels of HIV-related knowledge, attitudes, and risk behaviors among the general population as well as specific groups believed to engage in high-risk practices are useful in determining baseline or preintervention information about a target population. These surveys are cross-sectional or longitudinal and entail either an interview or self-administered questionnaire. With questions about highly sensitive life-style practices, such as drug use, male-to-male sex, and heterosexual anal sex, respondents may answer the questions with socially desirable responses, thereby giving answers that the respondent believes the researcher wants to hear.

Questions are needed to determine the influence of social norms and perceptions, partners' attitudes, and acculturation issues in assessment tools for new populations. Such questions enable researchers and clinicians to view HIV-related diseases within the context of participants' lives.

Medical-record reviews. Analyses of medical records can yield valuable information about the service-utilization experiences of people with HIV. Acute-care hospitalizations and use of ambulatory-care services by persons with AIDS can be monitored over the course of the illness. These record reviews provide a quick method for culling important information, compared with expensive methods of enrolling a cohort of HIV-infected individuals and following them prospectively. For example, a study of hospitalized men with AIDS derived from a record analysis revealed that persons with a history of injecting drugs had longer hospital stays than did homosexual/bisexuals (Mantell, Shulman, Belmont, & Spivak, 1989).

Telephone screening. Due to their low cost, telephone interviews are a popular alternative to face-to-face interviews. Although some differences between the two interview methods exist, for example, greater response bias in telephone interview data (Jordan, Marcus, & Reeder, 1980), they are comparable (Aneshensel, Frerichs, Clark, & Yokopenic, 1982). A major question about the use of telephone surveys is their effectiveness in obtaining detailed information about a sensitive topic such as the sexual and drug-related risks for HIV infection. A recent telephone screening study for risk of HIV infection among 1,610 Los Angeles men resulted in a 50% completion rate; 96% of the respondents answered all of the sexually sensitive questions (Montgomery, Lewis, & Kirchgraber, 1991).

QUALITATIVE TECHNIQUES

Compared with survey interviews, qualitative techniques permit in-depth exploration of individuals' experiences from the respondents' perspectives. Popular qualitative approaches used in HIV/AIDS behavioral and psychosocial research include the focus group, ethnographic interview, diaries, and observation. Focus groups and ethnographic interviews are especially useful for rapid immersion in a culture.

Focus groups. Focus groups, a market-research technique, are now widely used by social scientists as an independent data-collection tool as well as an adjunct to individual surveys, qualitative interviews, and observation. Focus groups provide a quick way to gather data about a population or community with whom the researcher may be unfamiliar. The flexibility of this type of group interview enables the researcher to gather information on a broad range of topics and to initiate in-depth probing into the meaning of behaviors. Such groups serve a variety of purposes, including questionnaire development and piloting, program design and implementation, subject recruitment, materials development and evaluation, interpretation of study findings, and identification of cultural values of the target audience. Sensitive information may be discussed more openly in a group situation, in that people frequently feel more at ease in such settings and are encouraged to speak openly.

For example, the reactions of recovering substance users in a drug-free therapeutic community after having watched an AIDS video that followed the lives of two persons with AIDS until their deaths were discussed in a focus group (Mantell, DiVittis, & Ostfield, 1987). Although the intent of the video was to put a "face on the disease" by personalizing it, discussion revealed that the video precipitated feelings of hopelessness among group members. This evaluation of the video and its messages by the focus group led to its rejection for use in an HIV-prevention program.

Ethnographic interviews. Ethnographic research has achieved increased prominence (Weibel, 1988; Kenny, Mantell, Cortez, Gonzalez, & Brown, 1990; Sterk & Elifson, 1990; Mantell et al., 1990; Leonard, 1990) in HIV prevention and research programs, because traditional approaches, such as surveys, often fail to reach high-risk individuals who engage in behaviors that are illegal or viewed as

293

taboo or groups that are socially marginal or considered difficult to reach by traditional service providers (Schensul & Schensul, 1990). Information from ethnographic interviews can be used to generate questions for surveys, develop hypotheses, and modify the content of HIV-prevention programs (Williams et al., 1990).

For example, use of qualitative interviews to examine the social context of AIDS among a "hidden" high-risk group—lesbian IDUs—revealed that (1) lesbian drug users had distinct identification patterns (either lesbian, IDU, or neither); (2) these women were not greatly concerned about spreading HIV infection from woman to woman; and (3) sexual activity with men was not uncommon (Case, Downing, Fergussio, Lorvick, & Sanchez, 1988). Thus, these data were used to tailor HIV-prevention messages to the lesbian community.

Such qualitative interviews are especially useful in understanding the context and process of HIV, such as the "illness career" of a person with HIV. In-depth interviews, log documentation, or observational techniques illuminate the cultural and social context of health beliefs, attitudes, and behaviors; how women negotiate sexual encounters with their partners; attitudes about childbearing; interactions of male and female prostitutes with clients; barriers to condom use; and exchanges of sex for drugs. The conversational and process nature of the interviews allows respondents to present information grounded in *their* reality.

Qualitative methods can also be useful in understanding communities' and populations' values, including needle-sharing practices, crack use, condom use, contraceptive use, and social norms for HIV risk reduction. Conversations can be tape recorded or field notes taken. A coding system to uncover emergent themes is then constructed through a content analysis of the transcribed text by team consensus.

Interviews are open-ended and unstructured, with probe questions used to facilitate discussion. The flexibility of the interviewing process permits the interviewer to explore topics as they unravel during the course of the interview—topics that are grounded in the respondent's perspective and language rather than the researcher's. Single or multiple interviews may occur, depending upon the research objective (Conrad, 1990). For example, the study of behavioral change or the illness career of a person with AIDS would best be handled with multiple interviews.

Diaries. Personal diaries or logs have been used to document individuals' sexual and drug-using practices prospectively, rather than relying on their retrospective recall of these events. With the diary approach, respondents can record behavioral events contemporaneously and identify the social context in which having sex or using drugs occurred and the motivations for the behavior.

In an intervention with gay and bisexual men, a diary approach was used to identify the contingencies (e.g., when, where, why, and who) of sexual behaviors over a six-week period (Mantell et al., 1989). Like other qualitative methods, the diary approach can be used as an independent data-collection method or as a way to confirm and validate responses on a quantitative survey. The validity of the diary method, however, is dependent on highly motivated subjects who are willing to record their behaviors daily.

DIRECTIONS FOR FUTURE BEHAVIORAL/PSYCHOSOCIAL RESEARCH

Other areas of research that warrant future investigation include the following:
Social networks

◆ The impact of AIDS on the social networks of people with AIDS

◆ The impact of social-support systems on coping with HIV infection

◆ The effectiveness of dissemination of AIDS-prevention information through social networks

Psychological impact

◆ Bereavement and AIDS

◆ The impact of stress on the development of AIDS among asymptomatic HIV-seropositive individuals

◆ Psychosocial impact of AIDS on caregivers and families, including anticipatory grief and bereavement and their effects on social and psychological adjustment

◆ Short- and long-term mental health consequences among children who lose a parent and/or sibling to HIV/AIDS

◆ Impact of HIV on women's psychological well-being

◆ Effects of pregnancy on the self-esteem and psychological well-being of HIV-infected women

◆ Stress and burnout among health care providers

Service utilization

◆ Caregiver burden

◆ Quality of care

Behavioral impact

◆ Sexual behavior: Variations in sexual practices, rate of acquiring new sexual partners, frequency of sexual contacts, why some people continue to practice high-risk behaviors; determinants of behavioral change and sexual risk-reduction; normative beliefs and behaviors that govern communities

◆ The effect of partners' vulnerability to HIV infection, or actual risk status, on women's use of condoms

◆ Delay in seeking treatment

◆ Compliance with AIDS-treatment regimens

◆ Impact of partner's serostatus on HIV seroconversion rates

Case management

◆ Impact on service utilization and length of hospital stay

◆ Effectiveness of various case-management strategies with respect to clients' psychological, social, and physical functioning

◆ Effectiveness of case-manager functions (Sonsel, Paradise, & Stroup, 1988)

◆ The effects of early case-management intervention with HIV-infected individuals who have not yet had an episode of acute hospitalization on clients' access to services

◆ Effectiveness of an early-intervention model as a cost-containment mechanism

◆ Effects of case managers' qualifications and training on client and cost-containment outcomes (Conviser, Young, Grant, & Coye, 1991; Piette, Fleishman, Mor, & Thompson, 1992)

CONCLUSION

The urgency of the AIDS crisis demands aggressive, nationwide behavioral and psychosocial research efforts to guide the content and strategies of prevention programs to achieve effective HIV risk reduction. Research findings inform us about the development of appropriate population-specific interventions as well as the suitability of cross-cultural interventions.

Integration of research and practice is essential to improving the quality of clinical practice in the field of HIV/AIDS. Both quantitative and qualitative research methods serve to evaluate, and perhaps legitimate, practice wisdom frequently expressed by case illustrations (Scott, 1990). Practice-centered research is also responsive to the mounting demands for service and program accountability.

Our only hope for achieving HIV risk reduction is to integrate research with practice. Researchers must be sensitized to the practical problems faced by clinicians and realize that clinical colleagues can provide keen insights. Clinicians, in turn, must be convinced of the benefits of research and realize that without research, practitioners may continuously make the same mistakes and reinvent the same solutions.

NOTES

1. This work was supported in part by the U.S. Centers for Disease Control Cooperative Agreements #U62/CCU207163 and #U64/CCU203274, to Medical and Health Research Association of New York City, Inc., the New York City Department of Health, and the New York City Health and Hospitals Corporation (Woodhull Medical and Mental Health Center), respectively; and the National Institute on Drug Abuse, R-01-DA05995.

2. A 1992 federal court declared this activity censorship and the "offensiveness rule" to be unconstitutional (McFadden, 1992).

3. Examples of the variable mnemonic labels included "jerkoff," "masterba," "blow job," and "ass fuck."

4. HIV-discordant refers to the HIV status of a couple in which one partner is HIV-seropositive and the other HIV-seronegative.

5. Community-based trials refer to federally approved drug trials that are conducted in community rather than traditional university medical center settings. They are also referred to as a parallel-track system, because the same rigor and safeguards built in medical-center-sponsored trials are applied in community nonprofit settings. Parallel-track trials are frequently sponsored by a consortium of community-based physicians, and the protocols are reviewed by institutional review boards.

6. In snowball sampling, a person enrolled in the study nominates or suggests other people for the researcher to contact for recruitment purposes. This is sometimes referred to as chain-referral sampling.

7. In a reversal design, group A receives a treatment and group B serves as the control. After a period of study, group A becomes the control to group B. In a wait-list design, treatment to one or more groups is delayed. While waiting for treatment, the wait-list group(s) serves as the control.

REFERENCES

Aneshensel, C. S., Frerichs, R. R., Clark, V. A., & Yokopenic, P. A. (1982). Telephone versus in-person surveys of community health status. *American Journal of Public Health, 72,* 1017–1021.

Arras, J. D. (1990, September–October). Noncompliance in AIDS research. *Hastings Center Report, 20,* 24–32.

Astor, J. (1990, November 7). In Puerto Rico, grim AIDS stats yield activist fury. *OUTWEEK,* pp. 24–27.

Bharucha-Reid, R. P., Schork, A., & Schwartz, S. A. (1990). Data linkage and subject anonymity for HIV testing. *AIDS and Public Policy Journal, 5,* 189–190.

Bayer, R. (1990). The ethics of research on HIV/AIDS in community-based settings. *AIDS, 4,* 1287–1288.

Boruch, R. F. (1988, June 2–4). *Resolving privacy problems in AIDS research: A primer.* Paper presented at the National Center of Health Services Research and Health Care Technology Assessment's Health Services Conference (report No. A-453), University of Arizona, Tucson, AZ.

Byar, D. P., Schoenfeld, D. A., Green, S. B., Amato, D. A., Davis, R., De Gruttola, V., Finkelstein, D. M., Gatsonis, C., Gelber, R. D., Lagakos, S., Lefkopoulou, M., Tsiatis, A. A., Zelen, M., Peto, J., Freedman, L., Gail, M., Simon, R., Ellenberg, S. S., Anderson, J. R., Collins, R., Peto, R., & Peto, T. (1990). Design considerations for AIDS trials. *New England Journal of Medicine, 323,* 1343–1348.

Callero, P. L., & Howard, J. A. (1989). Biases of the scientific discourse on human sexuality: Toward a sociology of sexuality. In K. McKinney & M. Sprecher (Eds.), *Human sexuality: The societal and interpersonal contact* (pp. 425–437). Norwood, NJ: Ablex.

Case, P., Downing, M., Fergussio, B., Lorvick, J., & Sanchez, L. (1988, June). The social context of AIDS risk behavior among intravenous drug using lesbians in San Francisco, *Lesbian AIDS Project, San Francisco, CA.* Poster presented at the Fourth International Conference on AIDS, Stockholm, Sweden.

Chase, M. (1991, March 8). AIDS activists press boycotts of drug firms. *Wall Street Journal,* p. C-20.

Congressional Record. (S14216). (1987, October 14). Section (a) of Amendment 963, offered by Senator Helms.

Conrad, P. (1990). Qualitative research on chronic illness: A commentary on method and conceptual development. *Social Science and Medicine, 30,* 1257–1263.

Conviser, R., Young, S. R., Grant, C. M., & Coye, M. J. (1991, Winter). A hospital-based case management program for PWAs in New Jersey. *AIDS and Public Policy Journal, 4,* 148–158.

Cook, T. D., & Campbell, D. T. (1979). *Quasi-experimentation: Design and analysis issues for field settings.* Chicago, IL: Rand McNally.

Coxon, A. P. M., & Carballo, M. (1989). Research on AIDS: Behavioural perspectives. *AIDS, 3,* 191–197.

Craven, D. E., Liebman, H. A., Fuller, J., Hagerty, C., Cooley, T. P., Saunders, C. A., & Steger, K. A. (1990). AIDS in intravenous drug users: Issues related to enrollment in clinical trials. *Journal of Acquired Immune Deficiency Syndromes, 3*(suppl. 2), 545–550.

Crossen, C. (1989, December 7). AIDS activist group harasses and provokes to make its point. *Wall Street Journal,* pp. A1, A9.

Edgar, H., & Rothman, D. J. (1991). New rules for new drugs. The challenge of AIDS to the regulatory process. In D. Nelkin, D. P. Willis, & S. V. Parris (Eds.), *A disease of society: Cultural and institutional responses to AIDS* (pp. 84–115). Cambridge, England: Cambridge University Press.

Faden, R. R., & Kass, N. E. (1991). Bioethics and public health in the 1980s: Resource allocation and AIDS. *Annual Review of Public Health, 12,* 335–360.

Gagnon, J. H. (1988). Sex research and sexual conduct in the era of AIDS. *Journal of Acquired*

Immune Deficiency Syndromes, 1, 593–601.

Gamson, J. (1989, October). Silence, death, and the invisible enemy: AIDS activism and social movement "newness." *Social Problems, 36,* 351–367.

Government scraps study of teen-age sex. (1991, July 25). *New York Times,* p. B-8.

Grossman, H. (1990, August 19). Keep politics out of scientific research. *New York Times,* p. 13.

Hatziandreu, E., Graham, J. D., & Stoto, M. A. (1988, January–February). AIDS and biomedical research funding: Comparative analysis. *Review of Infectious Diseases, 10,* 159–167.

Hay, J. W. (1989, October 3). Is too much being spent on AIDS? *Wall Street Journal,* p. A22.

Hersen, M., & Barlow, D. H. (1977). *Single case experimental designs.* New York: Pergamon Press.

Hilts, P. (1991, August 4). Women with AIDS seize stage, asking Bush to help ease stigma. *New York Times,* pp. 1, 30.

Jordan, L. A., Marcus, A. C., & Reeder, L. G. (1980). Response styles in telephone and household interviewing: A field experiment. *Public Opinion Quarterly, 44,* 211–222.

Kelly, J. A., & St. Lawrence, J. S. (1988). AIDS prevention and treatment: psychology's role in the health crisis. *Clinical Psychology Review, 8,* 255–284.

Kenny, M., Mantell, J. E., Cortez, N., Gonzalez, V., & Brown, L. S., Jr. (1990, October). *HIV prevention among women at risk.* Paper presented at the 118th Annual Meeting of the American Public Health Association, New York.

Koch, E. L. (1987, November 7). Senator Helms's callousness toward AIDS victims. *New York Times,* p. 27.

Krieger, N. (1988). AIDS funding: Competing needs and the politics of priorities. *International Journal of Health Services, 18,* 521–541.

Lee, P. R. (1986). AIDS: Allocating resources for research and patient care. *Issues in Science and Technology, 2,* 66–73.

Leonard, T. L. (1990, March). Male clients of female street prostitutes: Unseen partners in sexual disease transmission. *Medical Anthropology Quarterly, 4,* 41–55.

Lewis, A., Spencer, J., Haas, G., & DiVittis, A. T. (1987) The reliability of goal attainment scaling with an inpatient population. *Journal of Nervous and Mental Diseases, 175,* 408–418.

Longoria, J. M., Turner, N. H., & Philips, B. U., Jr. (1991, May). Community leaders help increase response rates in AIDS survey. *American Journal of Public Health, 81,* 654–655.

Maddox, J. (1989, September 21). Sexual behavior unsurveyed. *Nature, 341,* 181.

Mantell, J. E., & DiVittis, A. T. (1990a, Summer). AIDS prevention programs: The need for evaluation in the context of community partnership. In L. C. Leviton, A. M. Hegedus, & A. Kubrin (Eds.), *Evaluating AIDS prevention: Contributions of multiple disciplines* (pp. 87–98). San Francisco: Jossey-Bass.

Mantell, J. E., & DiVittis, A. T. (1990b, August). *Prevention of HIV transmission: AIDS risk-reduction interventions with high-risk groups.* Final report to the Centers for Disease Control (#U62/CCU201065), Atlanta, GA.

Mantell, J. E., & DiVittis, A. T. (1992). *Evaluating AIDS prevention programs: A guidebook for the health educator.* New York: Gay Men's Health Crisis.

Mantell, J. E., DiVittis, A. T., & Ostfield, M. L. (1987, Spring). *Focus group with support group members of a drug-free therapeutic community.* Samaritan Village, New York.

Mantell, J. E., Kenny, M., Cortez, N., Shiflett, S., Ramos, S. E., Leonard, T., Tross, S., Gonzalez, V., Brown, L. S., Jr., Laqueur, P., Barton, E., Berman, S., & Sterk, C. (1990, October). *Using ethnography to understand reproductive and contraceptive practices among women at risk for HIV infection.* Paper presented at the 118th Annual Meeting of the American Public Health Association, New York.

Mantell, J. E., & Ramos, S. E. (1991, December). *Prevention of perinatal HIV infection demonstration project,* Cooperative agreement #U62/CCU207163, Final report submitted to the U.S. Centers for Disease Control, Atlanta, GA.

Mantell, J. E., Ramos, S. E., Majidi, K., Walton-Glover, C., & Leslie, S. (1992). *Gender and social power: Effects of inner-city women's HIV preventive, contraceptive and reproductive intentions and behaviors.* Bureau of Disease Intervention, New York City Department of Health, New York.

Mantell, J. E., Shulman, L., Belmont, M. F., & Spivak, H. B. (1989, February). Social work responses to the AIDS epidemic in an acute care hospital: Practice and system implications. *Health and Social Work, 14,* 41–51.

Mantell, J. E., Tross, S. E., & Rapkin, B. (1989, January). *Promoters and barriers to HIV testing and risk-reduction* (grant application R-01-DA05995). National Institute on Drug Abuse, Washington, DC.

McFadden, R. D. (1992, May 12). Judge overturns U.S. rule blocking "offensive" educational material on AIDS. *New York Times,* p. B-3.

Melton, G. B., & Gray, J. (1988, January). Ethical dilemmas in AIDS research. *American Psychologist, 43,* 60–64.

Montgomery, K., Lewis, C. E., & Kirchgraber, P. (1991, May). Telephone screening for risk of HIV infection. *Medical Care, 29,* 399–407.

Morgan, T. (1988, July 22). Mainstream strategy for AIDS group. *New York Times,* pp. B-1, B-4.

Murphy, T. M. (1991, March–April). No time for an AIDS backlash. *Hastings Center Report, 21,* 7–11.

Navarro, M. (1992, March 31). Fighting AIDS, and fighting one another. *New York Times,* pp. B-1, B-4.

O'Hare, T. M. (1991). Integrating research and practice: A framework for implementation. *Social Work, 36,* 220–222.

Pear, R. (1988, January 10). In AIDS research, money is just the start. *New York Times,* p. 36-E.

Piette, J., Fleishman, J. A., Mor, V., & Thompson, B. (1992, February). The structure and process of AIDS case management. *Health and Social Work, 17,* 47–56.

Ramis, C., DiVittis, A. T., Lee, G., Levitan, S., Hollingsworth, S., A-Wali, A., Cintron, V., Forte, S., & Morgan, A. (1991, July). *The Northern Brooklyn Partner Study: The study of the heterosexual transmission of HIV.* Brooklyn, NY: Woodhull Medical and Mental Health Center.

Ramos, S. E., Mantell, J. E., Pack, C., Ricardo, M., Cortez, N., Hernandez, A., & Laqueur, P. (1991, June). *A non-traditional approach to AIDS prevention service delivery.* Poster Session, Seventh International Conference on AIDS, Florence, Italy.

Rogler, L. H. (1989, March). The meaning of culturally sensitive research in mental health. *American Journal of Psychiatry, 146,* 296–303.

Rovner, J. (1987, December 5). Congress is stalemated over AIDS epidemic. *Congressional Quarterly,* pp. 2986–2988.

Schensul, J. J., & Schensul, S. L. (1990, Summer). Ethnographic evaluation of AIDS prevention programs: Better data for better programs. In L. C. Leviton. A. M. Hegedus, & A. Kubrin (Eds.), *Evaluating AIDS prevention: Contributions of multiple disciplines* (pp. 51–62). San Francisco: Jossey-Bass.

Scott, D. (1990, November). Practice wisdom: the neglected source of practice research. *Social Work, 35,* 564–568.

Shouts and whispers about sex. (1988, July 31). *New York Times,* p. 24-E.

Smith, P. B., Weinman, M. L., Johnson, T. C., & Wait, R. (1990). Incentives and their influence on appointment compliance in a teenage family-planning clinic. *Journal of Adolescent Health Care, 11,* 445–448

Sonsel, G. E., Paradise, F., & Stroup, S. (1988, June). Case-management practice in an AIDS service organization. *Social Casework, 69,* 388–392.

Stange, K. C., & Zyzanski, S. J. (1989, November–December). Integrating qualitative and quantitative research methods. *Family Medicine, 21,* 448–451.

Sterk, C. E., & Elifson, K. W. (1990). Drug-related violence and street prostitution. In M. De La Rosa, E. Y. Lambert, & B. Gropper (Eds.), *Drugs and violence: Causes, correlates, and consequences* (pp. 208–221). Research Monograph Series No. 103. Rockville, MD: National Institute on Drug Abuse.

Tarasoff v. Regents of the University of California. (1976). 17 Cal. 3d 425, 131 C.R. 14.

Taylor, P. (1990, November 12). AIDS guerrillas. *New York,* pp. 60–62; 67–73.

Thomas, S. B., So'Brien van Putten, J. M., & Chen, M. S. (1991). *A program planning and evaluation manual for HIV education programs: A primer for ethnic and racial minority community based organizations.* Columbus, OH: Ohio Department of Health.

Walkey, F. H., Taylor, A. J. W., & Green, D. E. (1990). Attitudes to AIDS: A comparative analysis of a new and negative stereotype. *Social Science and Medicine, 30,* 549–552.

Webb, E. J., Campbell, D. T., Schwartz, R. D., & Sechrest, L. (1966). *Unobtrusive measures: Nonreactive research in the social sciences.* Chicago, IL: Rand McNally.

Weibel, W. W. (1988). Combining ethnographic and epidemiologic methods in targeted AIDS interventions: The Chicago model. In R. J. Battjes & R. W. Pickens (Eds.), *Needle sharing among intravenous drug abusers: National and international perspectives* (pp. 137–150). (National Institute on Drug Abuse Research Monograph 80). Washington, DC: Department of Health and Human Services.

Wilkerson, I. (1991, June 1). Blacks assail ethics in medical testing. *New York Times,* p. A-12.

Williams, D. G., Best, J. A., Taylor, D. W., Gilbert, J. R., Wilson, D. M. C., Lindsay, E. A., & Singer, J. (1990, December). A systematic approach for using qualitative methods in primary prevention research. *Medical Anthropology Quarterly, 4,* 391–409.

Windom, R. E. (1988, May 9). *Policy on informing those tested about HIV serostatus.* Letter to PHS agency heads. Washington, DC.